MAGNETIC RESONANCE IMAGING OF THE SPINE

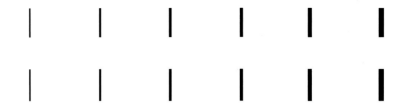

MAGNETIC RESONANCE IMAGING OF THE SPINE

Editors

Val M. Runge, MD
Rosenbaum Professor of Diagnostic Radiology
Director of the Magnetic Resonance Imaging
    and Spectroscopy Center
University of Kentucky
Lexington, Kentucky

Mark H. Awh, MD
Director of Magnetic Resonance Imaging
Associated Radiologists, P.C.
St. Thomas Hospital
Nashville, Tennessee

Donald F. Bittner, MD
Director of Magnetic Resonance Imaging
Northwest Center for Advanced Imaging
Franklin, Pennsylvania

John E. Kirsch, PhD
Assistant Professor of Diagnostic Radiology and Assistant Professor
    of Biomedical Engineering
Director of Research for the Magnetic Resonance Imaging
    and Spectroscopy Center
University of Kentucky
Lexington, Kentucky

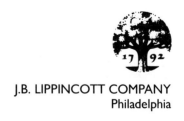

J.B. LIPPINCOTT COMPANY
Philadelphia

Acquisitions Editor: James D. Ryan
Developmental Editor: Kimberley Cox
Associate Managing Editor/Project Editor: Elizabeth A. Durand
Indexer: Alexandra Nickerson
Design Coordinator: Doug Smock
Cover Designer: Mark James
Production Manager: Caren Erlichman
Senior Production Coordinator: Kevin P. Johnson
Pre-press: Jay's Publishers Services, Inc.
Compositor: Compset, Inc.
Printer/Binder: Quebecor/Kingsport

6 5 4 3 2 1

Library of Congress Cataloging-in-Publication Data

Magnetic resonance imaging of the spine / Val M. Runge . . .
  [et al.].
    p.   cm.
   Includes bibliographical references and index.
   ISBN 0-397-51290-2
   1. Spine—Magnetic resonance imaging.   2. Spine—Magnetic
resonance imaging—Case studies.   I. Runge, Val M.
   [DNLM: 1. Spine—anatomy & histology.   2. Spinal Diseases—
diagnosis.   3. Magnetic Resonance Imaging.   WE 725 M196 1995]
RD768.M286   1995
617.3'7507548—dc20
DNLM/DLC
for Library of Congress   94-32067
                                       CIP

♾ This paper meets the requirements of ANSI/NISO Z39.48-1992 (Permanence of Paper).

The authors and publisher have exerted every effort to ensure that drug selection and dosage set forth in this text are in accord with current recommendations and practice at the time of publication. However, in view of ongoing research, changes in government regulations, and the constant flow of information relating to drug therapy and drug reactions, the reader is urged to check the package insert for each drug for any change in indications and dosage and for added warnings and precautions. This is particularly important when the recommended agent is a new or infrequently employed drug.

PREFACE

Magnetic resonance (MR) imaging has become firmly established as a major diagnostic modality for the spine, with current clinical use equal to that for the head. *Magnetic Resonance Imaging of the Spine* is designed to serve both as a primary text and as a reference source, covering in depth the diseases encountered in current clinical practice. Improvements in hardware and imaging technique have fueled the growth of MR, particularly in the spine. Recent advances, such as fast spin echo imaging, have had a major impact on clinical use, and are discussed in the context in which they are used today—as standard tools of the trade.

For ease of reference, *Magnetic Resonance Imaging of the Spine* is organized according to the pathology code of the *Index for Radiological Diagnoses,* 4th edition, as published by the American College of Radiology. The text is divided into four sections, beginning with a discussion of physics (code 30). This is followed by a discussion of normal anatomy and diseases specific to the cervical spine (code 31), thoracic spine (code 32), and lumbar spine (code 33). This division comes naturally, given the current use of local surface coils and limited anatomic coverage in any one scan. Within the cervical, thoracic, and lumbar sections, normal anatomy and congenital disease (code .1) are covered first, followed by inflammation (code .2), neoplasia (code .3), trauma (code .4), degenerative disease (code .7), and miscellaneous conditions, including specifically multiple sclerosis (code .8).

Each case begins with a short history, drawn from the patient's chart, that highlights clinical information important for scan interpretation. The film findings are then discussed in a succinct manner. MR images are correlated with conventional radiographs, CT, and gross pathology where applicable. The diagnosis is provided, followed by an in-depth discussion of the disease entity and its appearance on MR. Three special sections highlight important additional information regarding MR technique, pitfalls in image interpretation, and correlative pathology. Current references are provided to further guide the interested reader. In each case, the focus is on the MR images themselves, and their radiologic interpretation.

MR—with its use of nonionizing radiation, multiplanar imaging capability, high sensitivity to pathologic processes, and high intrinsic spatial resolution—has had a major impact on routine clinical care in spine disease over the past decade. Our knowledge base concerning normal and pathologic processes has also increased substantially. The future of MR continues to be bright, with current delivery of the next generation of scanners providing substantial further improvement in image quality and reduction in scan time.

Val M. Runge, MD

CONTENTS

Chapter One
Physics for Spine Magnetic Resonance *1*
John E. Kirsch

Chapter Two
Cervical Spine *53*
Val M. Runge
Mark H. Awh
Donald F. Bittner

Chapter Three
Thoracic Spine *171*
Mark H. Awh
Val M. Runge
Donald F. Bittner

Chapter Four
Lumbar Spine *231*
Val M. Runge
Mark H. Awh
Donald F. Bittner

Index *391*

MAGNETIC RESONANCE IMAGING OF THE SPINE

Magnetic Resonance Imaging of the Spine, by Val M. Runge,
Mark H. Awh, Donald F. Bittner, and John E. Kirsch.
J.B. Lippincott Company, Philadelphia © 1995.

CHAPTER
ONE

Physics for Spine Magnetic Resonance

John E. Kirsch

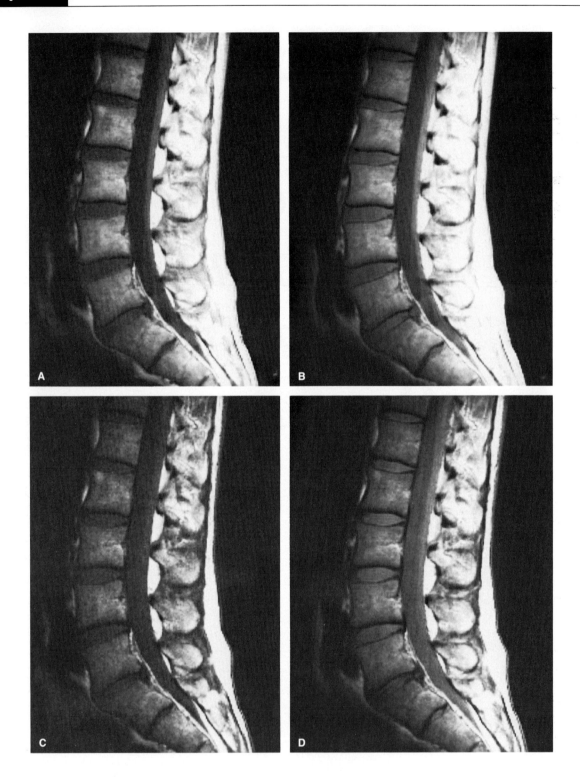

TOPIC

T1-weighted spin echo (SE) technique

FINDINGS

The effect of varying TR and TE on T1-weighted SE contrast is demonstrated on midline sagittal images through the lumbar spine that depict the thecal sac, nerve roots, and vertebral bodies (*A through D*). With short TR and short TE (TR/TE = 400/10), fat signal intensity is high and CSF is dark, while the cord and nerve roots possess intermediate signal (*A*). High intensity is seen in the bone marrow of the vertebral bodies, and the intervertebral disks are hypointense. Good contrast is observed in all structures of the spine. Lengthening TR (TR/TE = 1200/10) increases overall signal and improves the signal-to-

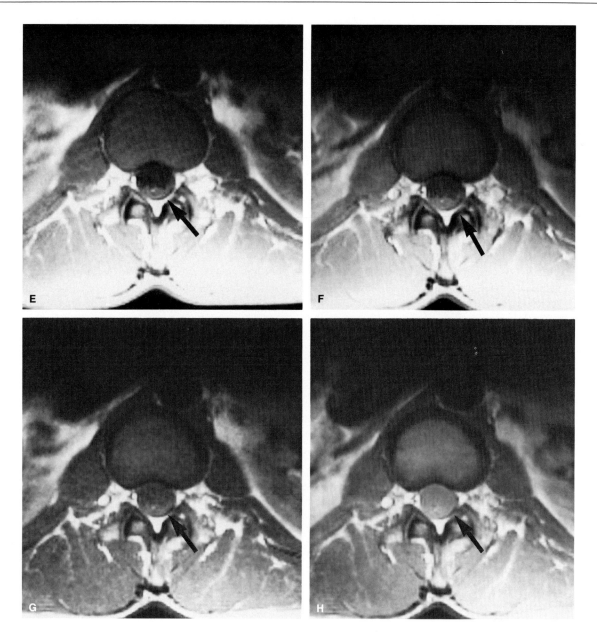

noise ratio (S/N) but reduces contrast, particularly between the vertebral bodies and disks (*B*). A slight increase in TE (TR/TE = 400/30) may substantially compromise S/N, with a loss in depiction of the cord and nerve roots (*C*). Use of a comparably long TR and TE (TR/TE = 1200/30) can increase vertebral disk and CSF signals relative to surrounding structures due to the introduction of T2 weighting, resulting in significant loss in overall contrast (*D*). Also shown are T1-weighted axial images through the L1–L2 intervertebral disk at a TR/TE of (*E*) 400/10, (*F*) 1200/10, (*G*) 400/30, and (*H*) 1200/30. Note the significant changes in contrast between the nerve roots, which are layered posteriorly, and CSF in the thecal sac (*arrows*).

CONCLUSION

Optimum T1-weighted SE contrast results when a short TR on the order of the T1 of the tissues is used and when TE is as short as possible.

DISCUSSION

Spin echo has historically been a primary technique in spine MRI because of its generally high signal and contrast compared with other techniques. SE is characterized by a 90° RF pulse followed by a 180° RF pulse, and generates a signal "echo" at the time TE. This pulsing is repeated at intervals of TR to obtain a two-dimensional image. Tissue signal is derived from the user-selectable parameters, TR and TE, and from the differences in the intrinsic NMR properties of hydrogen density, T1, and T2.[1-4] The tissue contrast is achieved by accentuating the differences in these properties with the proper manipulation of TR and TE.

Hydrogen (or spin) density, the number of hydrogen nuclei per unit volume of tissue, is linearly proportional to the MR signal. Although the amount of hydrogen present in the body is large (60% to 90% of the body is water by weight), the difference between tissues is small.

T1, also called longitudinal or spin-lattice relaxation time, is a characteristic property of tissues and refers to the amount of time it takes for the magnetization of a tissue to return to its original state of thermal equilibrium. The value of T1 for a given tissue depends on its molecular and thermal environment. In general, T1 will also increase with magnetic field strength. Tissues with short T1 values, such as fat, have a faster return to equilibrium and magnetization recovery than tissues with long T1, such as water.

The repetition time (TR) defines the time interval between successive 90° and 180° RF pulse pairs and determines the degree of T1 relaxation and the longitudinal magnetization recovery of the tissue. Signal increases with increasing TR. At short TR, few tissues possess fully recovered magnetization. Therefore, signal differences and the contrast will be "weighted" by T1 differences, and the overall signal will be relatively low due to partial recovery. At large TR, most of the magnetization reaches equilibrium recovery, resulting in high signal but reduced T1-weighted contrast.

T2 is another intrinsic property of tissues (see 30.121411-2). The echo time (TE) defines the time between the 90° pulse and the SE signal and determines the degree of T2 relaxation in a tissue. At short TE, large signal occurs due to little T2 dephasing, and tissue contrast associated with T2 differences is small.

In general, SE contrast is discussed in terms of the relative weighting of the intrinsic differences between hydrogen density, T1, and T2.[5] In most situations, it is advantageous to accentuate differences from only one property while minimizing the differences due to the others. T1-weighted contrast is achieved by maximizing signal variations due to different T1 values in the tissues using a short TR, while minimizing the signal differences due to T2 relaxation effects using a short TE. T1-weighted contrast tends to be used for obtaining good anatomic detail and contrast-enhanced information.[6,7] Fatty tissues that possess a short T1 will typically demonstrate large signals and bright pixel intensities due to fast longitudinal magnetization recovery, even with a short TR. On the other hand, water has a long T1 and will appear dark due to little recovery and small signal. Although TE should always be kept as short as possible, the TR may vary depending on the situation. Use of a longer TR results in greater slice coverage and improved overall signal but requires proportionately longer scan times and may reduce T1 weighting.

Technical References

1. Wehrli FW, MacFall JR, Glover GH, et al. The dependence of nuclear magnetic resonance (NMR) image contrast on intrinsic and pulse sequence timing parameters. Magn Reson Imaging 1984;2:3–16.
2. Wehrli FW, MacFall JR, Shutts D, et al. Mechanisms of contrast in NMR imaging. J Comput Assist Tomogr 1984;8:369–380.
3. Perman WH, Hilal SK, Simon HE, Maudsley AA. Contrast manipulation in NMR imaging. Magn Reson Imaging 1984;2:23–32.
4. Bradley WG. Effect of relaxation times on magnetic resonance image interpretation. Noninv Med Imaging 1984;1:193–204.
5. Hendrick RE, Raff U. Image contrast and noise. In: Stark DD, Bradley WG, eds. Magnetic resonance imaging, 2nd ed, vol 1. St. Louis: Mosby-Year Book, 1992.
6. Feinberg DA, Mills CM, Posin JP, et al. Multiple spin-echo magnetic resonance imaging. Radiology 1985;155:437–442.
7. Posin JP, Ortendahl DA, Hylton NM, et al. Variable magnetic resonance imaging parameters: effect on detection and characterization of lesions. Radiology 1985;155:719–725.

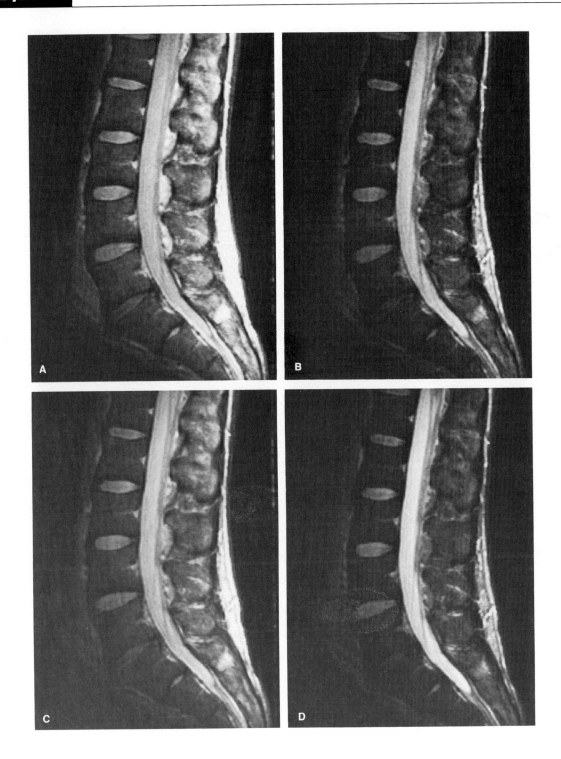

TOPIC

T2-weighted spin echo (SE) technique

FINDINGS

The effect of varying TR and TE on T2-weighted SE contrast is demonstrated with midline sagittal images through the lumbar spine that depict the thecal sac, nerve roots, and vertebral bodies (*A through D*). With long TR and intermediate TE (TR/TE = 2000/45), CSF signal intensity is high and fat is low, while the cord and nerve roots possess intermediate signal (*A*). Low intensity is seen in the bone marrow of the vertebral bodies, and the intervertebral disks are bright. Good contrast is observed in vertebral structures, but relatively poor depiction of the cord and nerve roots is demonstrated. Increased TE on the second echo (TR/TE = 2000/90) reduces overall signal and decreases the signal-to-noise ratio (S/N) but im-

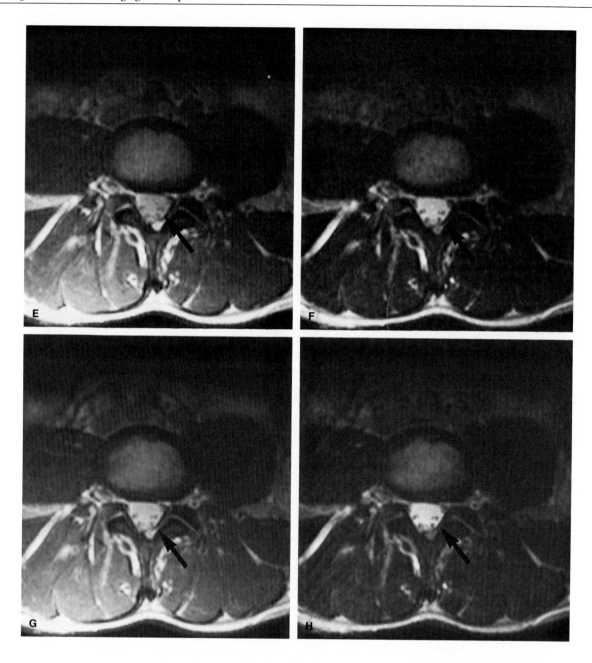

proves contrast (*B*). Lengthening TR (TR = 3500) increases S/N on the first echo (TE = 45) (*C*) and substantially improves T2-weighted contrast on the second echo (TE = 90) (*D*). The longest TR and TE demonstrate the highest degree of contrast between the cord, nerve roots, and CSF (*D*). Also shown are T2-weighted axial images through the L4–L5 intervertebral disk at a TR/TE of (*E*) 2000/45, (*F*) 2000/90, (*G*) 3500/45, and (*H*) 3500/90. Note the significant changes in contrast between the nerve roots and CSF in the thecal sac (*arrows*). The greatest delineation is observed with the strongest T2 weighting (*H*).

CONCLUSION

Optimum T2-weighted SE contrast results when a long TR and a long TE are used.

DISCUSSION

T2-weighted SE is a useful technique in spine MRI to characterize pathology and visualize CSF fluid. Spin echo is characterized by a 90° RF pulse followed by a 180° RF pulse that creates a signal "echo" at the time TE. This is repeated at intervals of TR to obtain a two-dimensional image. Tissue signal is derived from the selection of TR and TE and from the intrinsic differences in hydrogen density, T1, and T2.[1-3]

T1 is a characteristic property of tissues (see 30.121411-1). The repetition time (TR) that defines the time interval between successive 90° and 180° RF pulse pairs determines the degree of T1 relaxation and the longitudinal magnetization recovery of the tissue. Signal increases with increasing TR, and at large TR most of the magnetization reaches equilibrium recovery, resulting in high signal but minimal T1 weighting.

T2, also called transverse or spin–spin relaxation time, is another intrinsic property of tissues and refers to the amount of time it takes for magnetization lying in the transverse plane to dephase and lose its coherence. The value of T2 for a given tissue also depends on its molecular and thermal environment. Larger, more rigid molecules such as fat or solids tend to possess short T2 values, whereas smaller, freely mobile types such as water tend to have long T2 values. Tissues with shorter T2 values have faster dephasing of the magnetization. T2 is also generally considered to be relatively independent of field strength.

The echo time (TE) defines the time between the 90° pulse and the SE signal and determines the degree of T2 relaxation in a tissue. The MR signal, which is directly proportional to the magnitude of the transverse magnetization, decreases with increasing TE at a rate determined by the T2 of the tissue. At short TE, large signal occurs due to little T2 dephasing, and tissue contrast associated with T2 differences is small. At long TE, significant T2 relaxation results in T2-related contrast, and the overall signal is low due to substantial dephasing of the magnetization.

T2-weighted contrast is achieved by maximizing signal variations due to different T2 values in the tissues, using a long TE that allows sufficient dephasing of the transverse magnetization, while minimizing the signal differences due to T1 relaxation effects, using a long TR that will achieve near-complete longitudinal magnetization recovery. Fatty tissues that possess a short T2 will typically demonstrate low signals and dark pixel intensities due to rapid transverse magnetization decay at a comparably long TE. On the other hand, water has a long T2 and will appear bright due to little signal decay. Although TE should be kept relatively large for good T2 weighting, the overall signal in the image will be low. Use of a substantially large TE will result in poor image quality, decreased slice coverage, and contrast that will depict only structures that contain water, such as CSF. Scan times for T2-weighted studies tend to be quite long due to the need for a long TR to minimize T1 effects.

Technical References

1. Hendrick RE, Raff U. Image contrast and noise. In: Stark DD, Bradley WG, eds. Magnetic resonance imaging, 2nd ed, vol 1. St. Louis, Mosby-Year Book, 1992.
2. Feinberg DA, Mills CM, Posin JP, et al. Multiple spin-echo magnetic resonance imaging. Radiology 1985;155:437–442.
3. Posin JP, Ortendahl DA, Hylton NM, et al. Variable magnetic resonance imaging parameters: effect on detection and characterization of lesions. Radiology 1985;155:719–725.

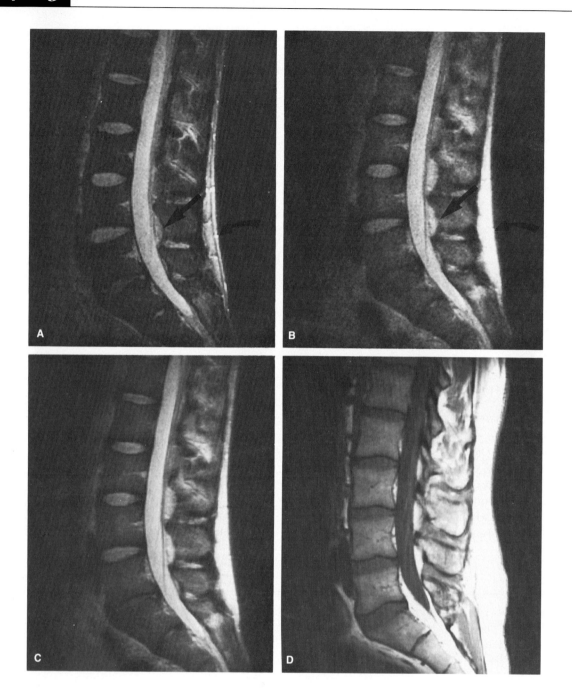

TOPIC

Fast spin echo (FSE) technique

FINDINGS

Comparison between (A) a conventional T2-weighted SE scan (TR/TE = 2500/90) and (B) a 12-echo FSE scan (TR/TE$_{eff}$ = 2500/90) reveals similar tissue contrast in midline sagittal images through the lumbar spine. Acquisition times were 10:04 minutes and 1:47 minutes respectively. The most noticeable characteristic of FSE is that fat is bright (*arrows*). Increase in nerve root delineation is also apparent due to the contribution of later echoes from the echo train used in FSE. Shorter acquisition times permit an increase in the number of acquisitions, which improves signal-to-noise ratio (S/N) and image quality, as shown in (C) using four acquisitions in a total scan time of 6:47 minutes. On a T1-weighted scan (TR/TE = 500/15) using conventional SE (D), nerve root structures in the thecal sac are well demonstrated. However, using a four-echo train FSE (TR/TE$_{eff}$ = 500/15), fine structure blurring due to T2 signal decay during data acquisition results in a near-complete loss in the depiction of the roots (E) in the phase-encoding direction (left to right). Switching the physical direction of frequency (left to right) and phase encoding (top to bottom) under otherwise identical ac-

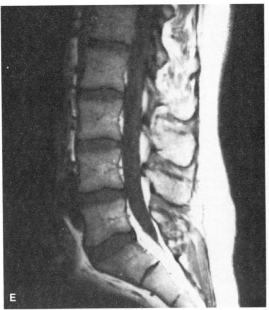
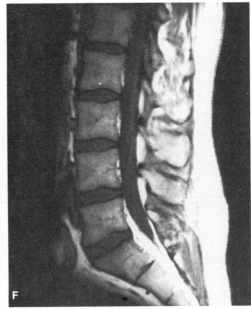

quisition conditions recovers the nerve root information (*F*).

CONCLUSION

Images are acquired in substantially reduced scan times with FSE, which has contrast characteristics similar to SE technique, although some blurring of structural detail may occur.

DISCUSSION

Fast spin echo (FSE) is a technique that uses the characteristics of SE while maximizing the efficiency of data collection. It was first introduced as RARE (rapid acquisition with relaxation enhancement).[1] In conventional two-dimensional spin echo, each phase-encoding step is acquired as a single 90° and 180° RF echo at an echo time (TE) by repeating the pulsing at a repetition rate of TR. In FSE, multiple spin echoes are generated by rapidly cycling the 180° pulse. Each successive RF echo is used to acquire additional phase-encoding steps within the same TR interval. For example, if 12 echoes are produced, one TR interval will yield 12 phase-encoding steps instead of one, as in a conventional SE technique. Therefore, the total scan time will be reduced in principle by a factor of 12.

FSE is typically used to reduce the scan time of a T2-weighted SE study. However, it can also be used to obtain T1-weighted images. With the substantial decrease in imaging time, protocols can be combined with multiple acquisitions to improve image quality of thin-section or high-spatial-resolution scans.

The contrast in FSE is similar to SE.[2,3] However, by producing an image based on multiple spin echoes that are used for acquiring the phase-encoding steps, the FSE image demonstrates several fundamental differences. Fat, which is normally dark on a T2-weighted SE image, will have high signal intensity in a comparable FSE image. Other tissue signal intensities may be slightly reduced with FSE; this is believed to be partially due to magnetization transfer effects.[4] Multi-echo techniques will generally have less signal loss associated with molecular diffusion and tissue susceptibility; this is also a characteristic of FSE.[5] Furthermore, since T2 signal decay occurs across different phase-encoding steps, preferential blurring of structures in the phase-encoding direction of the image may result.[6]

Technical References

1. Hennig J, Naureth A, Friedburg H. RARE imaging: a fast imaging method for clinical MR. Magn Reson Med 1986;3:823–833.
2. Melki PS, Mulkern RV, Panych LP, Jolesz FA. Comparing the FAISE method with conventional dual-echo sequences. J Magn Reson Imaging 1991;1:319–326
3. Jones KM, Mulkern RV, Schwartz RB, et al. Fast spin-echo MR imaging of the brain and spine: current concepts. Am J Roentgenol 1992;158:1313–1320.
4. Melki PS, Jolesz FA, Mulkern RV. Partial RF echo-planar imaging with the FAISE method. II. Contrast equivalence with spin-echo sequences. Magn Reson Med 1992;26:342–354.
5. Jones KM, Mulkern RV, Mantello MT, et al. Brain hemorrhage: evaluation with fast spin-echo and conventional dual spin-echo images. Radiology 1992;182:53–58.
6. Constable RT, Gore JC. The loss of small objects in variable TE imaging: implications for FSE, RARE, and EPI. Magn Reson Med 1992;28:9–24.

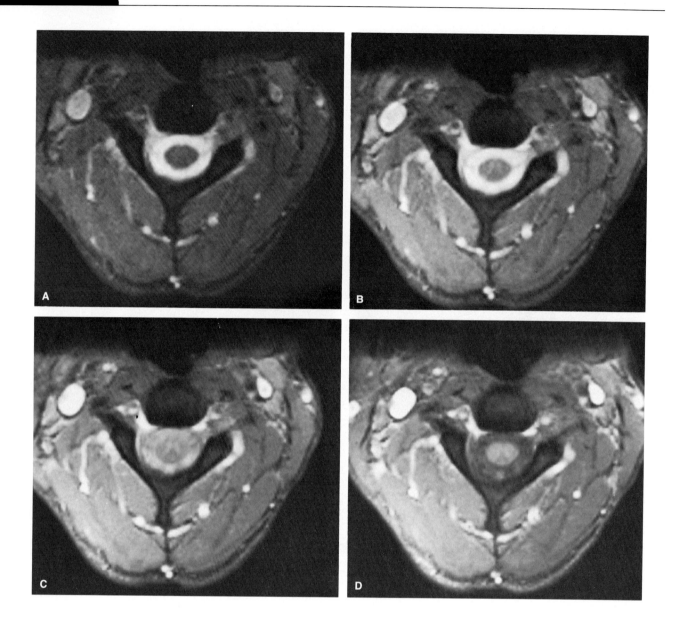

TOPIC

Spoiled gradient echo (GRE) technique

FINDINGS

Contrast changes are demonstrated by varying TR and RF flip angle (FA) in axial spoiled GRE scans through the cervical spine. At TR/TE = 400/10 (*A through D*), significant variation in tissue contrast is observed, particularly in the CSF and spinal cord. At a low FA of 10° (*A*), contrast is similar to a T2-weighted spin echo (SE) scan with high signal intensity in the CSF and dark surrounding tissue structures. As the FA is increased to (*B*) 20° and (*C*) 40°, the cord and muscle signal increases, whereas the CSF decreases. Tissue contrast approaches that of a T1-weighted SE scan when FA is 90° (*D*), with good depiction of internal structures of the cord. Subcutaneous fat, however, remains relatively dark due to the absence of a 180° RF pulse and rapid signal decay from a very short T2*. At a very short TR of 40 (*E through H*), the contrast changes observed with increasing FA are similar to a longer TR but approach a T1-related contrast at less of a flip angle. Signal from CSF is moderately hyperintense at 10° (*E*), decreases at 20° (*F*) and 40° (*G*), and is very low at 90° (*H*). Lower overall signal is observed at a very short TR. Note the substantial increase in vessel signal due to time-of-flight in-flow enhancement effects, similar to techniques used for two-dimensional MR angiography. Signal variations seen in the CSF are related to intravoxel phase dispersion and signal losses due to flow.

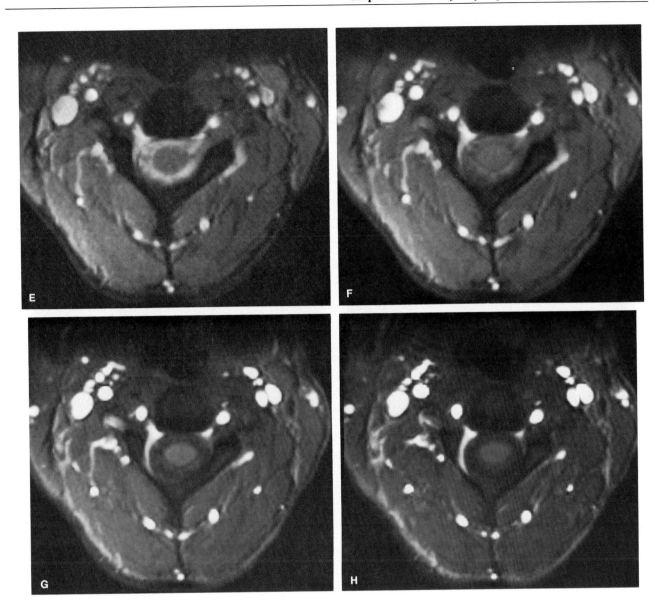

CONCLUSION

Spoiled GRE possesses similar contrast behavior to SE at a 90° FA or at a shorter TR with a reduced FA, and signal advantages at very short TR using low FA.

DISCUSSION

Gradient echo techniques, a valuable adjunct to SE in MRI (see 30.121411-1, 30.121411-2), are rapid imaging methods that primarily comprise two groups—spoiled and rephased (see 30.121412-2). The spoiled GRE technique, also called fast low angle shot (FLASH) or spoiled gradient recalled acquisition in the steady state (SP-GRASS), is based on T1 recovery and the free induction decay (FID) signal. It is characterized by the fact that only lon-

gitudinal magnetization is allowed to approach a steady state magnitude. Transverse magnetization is "spoiled" away before subsequent RF pulsing and therefore will not contribute to the FID signal and image.

Spoiled GRE is similar to SE with respect to signal generation and tissue contrast. Unlike SE, however, there is no 180° RF pulse that normally produces the RF echo, which must be created by the use of gradients. Because of the absence of the 180° pulse, the signal decays more rapidly with TE according to T2* instead of T2. In addition to TR and TE, the tissue contrast is further complicated by a dependence on the RF FA.[1]

At an RF FA of 90°, the contrast behavior is the same as in SE, except for the different TE dependencies between T2* and T2.[2,3] However, at a reduced FA, less time is required for full T1 recovery of the magnetization. Therefore, similar contrast can be achieved at a shorter

TR using a small FA. If the TR is short enough, the signal can even exceed what is attained with a 90° pulse at the same TR. Nevertheless, because only a portion of the magnetization becomes transverse after a small FA pulse, the maximum achievable signal at a sufficiently long TR will be less than for 90°. Thus, the only advantage of spoiled GRE is at short TR while using a reduced FA.

Because the origin of the FID signal is based on T1 recovery of the longitudinal magnetization, spoiled GRE can provide good T1-weighted contrast. At a reduced FA, T1 contrast can be maintained with a shorter TR, thereby reducing scan time, provided TE is kept shorter than for SE because of the faster $T2^*$ decay of the signal.[4,5] With a smaller FA, a very short TR can be used and still achieve T1-weighted contrast.[6] This enables rapid imaging for two-dimensional breathhold techniques and allows three-dimensional data to be acquired in reasonable scan times (see 30.12149-10).[7] With a very small FA, a TR normally used in SE for T1 weighting can provide proton density weighting. In conjunction with a moderately long TE, $T2^*$ weighting similar to T2 weighting can be obtained.[4,5,8]

Without a 180° pulse, the spoiled GRE signal is subject to dephasing based on all magnetic field inhomogeneities in addition to T2 and susceptibility that comprise $T2^*$. This includes chemical shift differences between fat and water that cause signal modulation with TE, bulk susceptibility artifacts, and accentuated artifacts from metal (see 30.121412-3). Normally, the 180° pulse in SE minimizes these effects, but in GRE techniques they can substantially reduce tissue signal, cause image distortions, and change contrast, particularly due to intrinsic tissue susceptibility differences.

Technical References

1. Buxton RB, Edelman RR, Rosen BR, et al. Contrast in rapid MR imaging: T1- and T2-weighted imaging. J Comput Assist Tomogr 1987;11:7–16.
2. Bydder GM, Young IR. Clinical use of the partial saturation and saturation recovery sequences in MR imaging. J Comput Assist Tomogr 1985;9:1020–1032.
3. Schorner W, Sander B, Henkes H, et al. Multiple slice FLASH imaging: an improved pulse sequence for contrast-enhanced MR brain studies. Neuroradiol 1990;32:474–480.
4. Stadnik TW, Luypaert RR, Neirynck EC, Osteaux M. Optimization of sequence parameters in fast MR imaging of the brain with FLASH. Am J Neuroradiol 1989;10:357–362.
5. Mills TC, Ortendahl DA, Hylton NM, et al. Partial flip angle MR imaging. Radiology 1987;162:531–539.
6. Van der Meulen P, Groen JP, Cuppen JJM. Very fast MR imaging by field echoes and small angle excitation. Magn Reson Imaging 1985;3:297–299.
7. Frahm J, Haase A, Matthaei D. Rapid 3D MR imaging using the FLASH technique. J Comput Assist Tomogr 1986;10:363–368.
8. Bydder GM, Payne JA, Collins AG, et al. Clinical use of rapid T2-weighted partial saturation sequences in MR imaging. J Comput Assist Tomogr 1987;11:17–23.

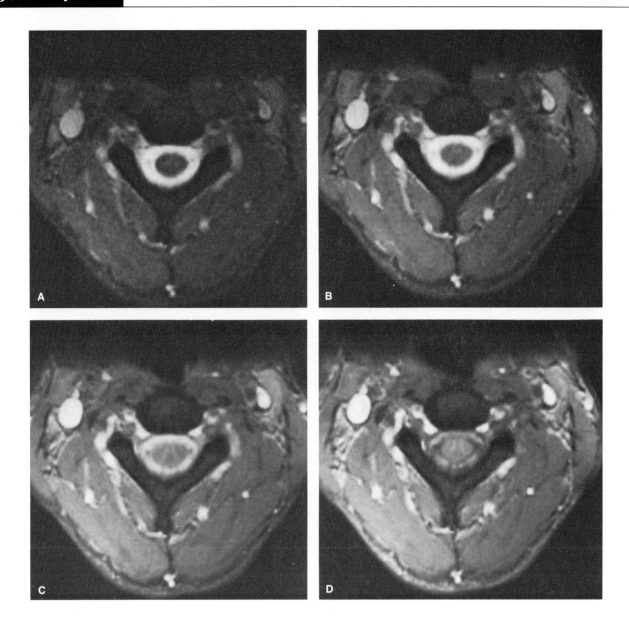

TOPIC

Rephased gradient echo (GRE) technique

FINDINGS

Contrast changes are demonstrated by varying TR and RF flip angle (FA) in axial rephased GRE scans through the cervical spine. At a TR/TE = 400/10 (*A through D*), significant variation in tissue contrast is observed, particularly in the CSF and spinal cord. At a low FA of 10° (*A*), contrast is similar to a T2-weighted spin echo (SE) scan with high signal intensity in the CSF and dark surrounding tissue structures. As the FA is increased to (*B*) 20° and (*C*) 40°, the cord and muscle signal increases, whereas the CSF decreases. Tissue contrast approaches that of a T1-weighted SE scan when the FA is 90° (*D*), with the exception of CSF, which remains moderately intense. TR and FA dependencies in contrast are similar to spoiled GRE, but also with the exception of CSF, especially at large FA. Subcutaneous fat remains relatively dark due to the absence of a 180° RF pulse and rapid signal decay from a very short T2*. At a very short TR of 40 (*E through H*), the primary contrast changes are observed in the CSF with increasing FA. Signal from CSF is moderately hyperintense at 10° (*E*) and progressively decreases at 20° (*F*), 40° (*G*), and 90° (*H*). Lower overall signal is also observed at a very short TR along with high vessel signal due to time-of-flight effects.

To eliminate artifacts from magnetic field inhomogeneities, only partial rephasing is normally imple-

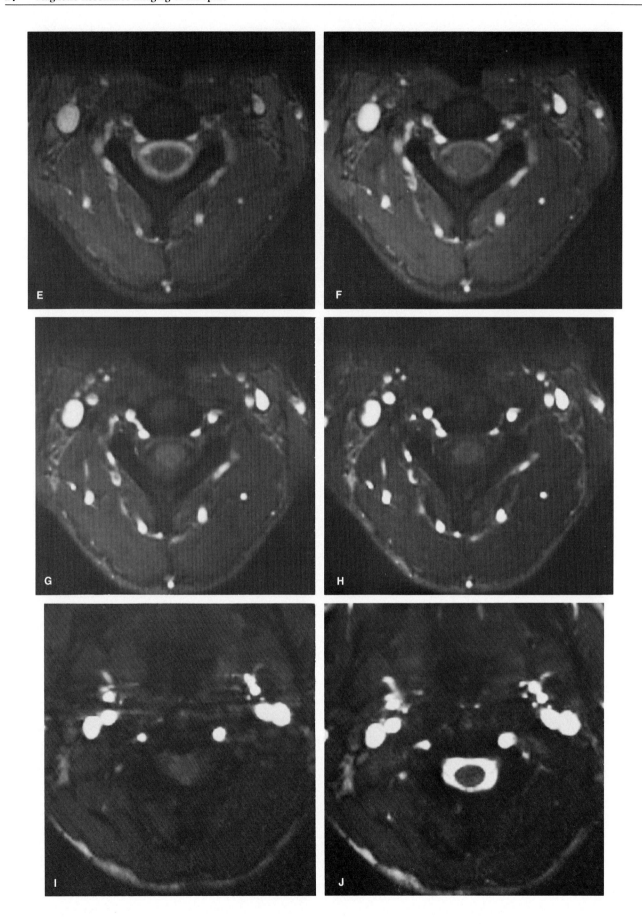

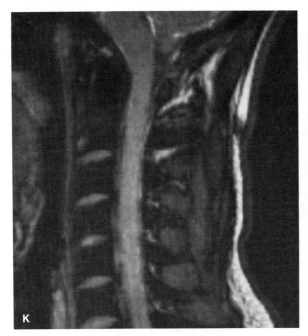

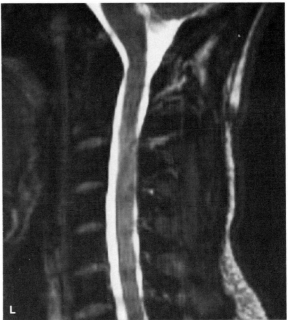

mented (*A through I*). As a result, significant signal loss then occurs in the CSF (*I*) related to intravoxel phase dispersion at very short TR (24) and high FA (90°). Some pulsation artifacts are also seen in major vessels. Complete rephasing recovers very high CSF signal (*J*), compared to partially rephased methods (*I*). This is well demonstrated on midline sagittal images of the cervical spine (TR/TE/FA = 24/12/90°), comparing partial rephasing (*K*) and complete rephasing (*L*). Note, however, the mottled appearance of the cord due to some phase dispersion signal losses that remain from magnetic field inhomogeneities.

CONCLUSION

Rephased GRE has similar contrast behavior to spoiled GRE at long TR with the exception of CSF, and very high water signal at very short TR when using large FA when a completely rephased GRE technique is used.

DISCUSSION

The rephased GRE technique, also called fast imaging with steady precession (FISP), Fourier acquired steady state (FAST), and gradient recalled acquisition in the steady state (GRASS), is a steady state free precession (SSFP) method based on T1 and T2 relaxation and the SSFP-free induction decay (FID) signal. It is characterized by the fact that both longitudinal and transverse magnetization approach a steady state. Contrary to spoiled GRE (see 30.121412-1), the transverse magnetization coher-

ency is maintained before subsequent RF pulsing and therefore contributes an additional T2-related signal component to the FID.[1]

When the transverse magnetization is preserved during pulsing, it can survive through multiple TR intervals. Every pair of adjacent RF pulses that constitutes a time of 2*TR will generate an RF SE based on the transverse magnetization called the SSFP-echo. Its strength will depend on T2 and the "echo time" of 2*TR. This signal adds to the FID signal created by each individual RF pulse which is based on the longitudinal magnetization and whose strength will depend on T1 and TR. Unlike the FID in spoiled GRE, the combined signal will therefore be additionally based on T2 and is called the SSFP-FID. Being a gradient echo technique, however, the signal decays faster with TE according to T2* instead of T2 due to the absence of the 180° pulse.

The difference in contrast between spoiled GRE and rephased GRE is the degree to which the SSFP-echo contributes to the FID signal. At long TR, little or no transverse magnetization survives through two TR intervals, even from tissues with long T2. In effect, T2 signal decay behaves like a "spoiling" mechanism. Therefore, the SSFP-echo becomes negligible and rephased GRE produces the same contrast as spoiled GRE with long TR. As TR is reduced, however, the contribution of the SSFP-echo increases, with highest signal coming from tissues with the longest T2. Furthermore, a higher RF FA—near 90°—will generate a greater SSFP-echo signal as well. Thus, the largest differences in tissue contrast between spoiled GRE and rephased GRE occur when a short TR and large FA are used. This is primarily seen as a combined T1 and T2 mixed weighting, and is more precisely a T2/T1 weighting.[1] Because free water such as CSF has the longest T2 and will generate the largest SSFP-echo signal, rephased GRE contrast is sometimes called water weighting.

When the transverse magnetization is completely rephased to generate as large an echo contribution as possible, constructive and destructive interference between the FID and the SSFP-echo occurs in the image as banding patterns due to signal modulations from external magnetic field inhomogeneities.[2] In standard rephased GRE techniques, this is circumvented by introducing partial spoiling with some compromise in the SSFP-echo portion of the signal. However, true rephased GRE images with maximal SSFP-echo signal are possible by combining two separate acquisitions that possess banding patterns that are the opposite of each other, but at the expense of doubling the imaging time.[2]

With its largest difference in tissue contrast being produced at very short TR, rephased GRE can be useful in rapid two-dimensional imaging for breathhold studies and in three-dimensional acquisitions.[3–5] However, with the absence of a 180° pulse, the rephased GRE technique is subject to the same magnetic field errors as is spoiled GRE (see 30.121412-1). This includes chemical shift differences between fat and water that cause signal modulation with TE, bulk susceptibility artifacts, and accentuated artifacts from metal (see 30.121412-3).

Technical References

1. Tkach JA, Haacke EM. A comparison of fast spin echo and gradient field echo sequences. Magn Reson Imaging 1988; 6:373–389.
2. Haacke EM, Wielopolski P, Tkach JA, Modic MT. Steady-state free precession imaging in the presence of motion: an application to cerebrospinal fluid. Radiology 1990;175:545–552.
3. Gyngell ML. The application of steady-state free precession in rapid 2DFT NMR imaging: FAST and CE-FAST sequences. Magn Reson Imaging 1988;6:415–419.
4. Steinberg PM, Ross JS, Modic MT, et al. The value of fast gradient-echo MR sequences in the evaluation of brain disease. Am J Neuroradiol 1990;11:59–67.
5. Hesselink JR, Martin JF, Edelman RR. Fast imaging. Neuroradiol 1990;32:348–355.

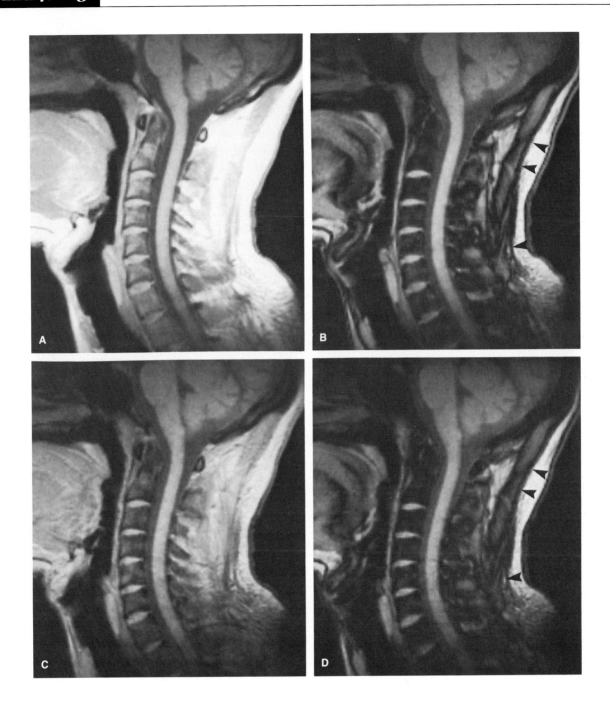

TOPIC

Image anomalies with GRE techniques

FINDINGS

Midline sagittal images of the cervical spine acquired with a spoiled GRE technique (TR/FA = 150/50°) exhibit significant signal intensity changes with a TE of (A) 4.5, (B) 7.0, (C) 9.0, and (D) 11.5. Tissue contrast appears the same in the cervical cord, CSF, and vertebral disks. However, large variations are observed in regions of tissues that contain both fat and water, such as the vertebral bodies and surrounding muscle, due to phase cycling from chemical shift between the two species. At specific echo times, the fat signal adds to the water signal when they are in phase (A and C), but they subtract from each other when they are out of phase (B and D). At specific boundaries between fat and water, large cancellation of signal can be seen (arrowheads). This artifact is not seen when signals are in phase (A and C). General T2* signal decay in all tissues occurs with increased TE. Lower overall signal intensity in the vertebral body bone marrow compared to conventional spin echo is also demonstrated with GRE techniques regardless of the TE based on localized magnetic susceptibility effects. Intravoxel phase dispersion and T2* shortening lead to the reduction in signal intensity, which becomes significant with increased TE (*D*).

CONCLUSION

Signal varies with TE in a gradient echo technique due to chemical shift when both fat and water are present. Localized tissue magnetic susceptibility also shortens T2* and results in decreased signal.

DISCUSSION

In all gradient echo techniques (see 30.121412-1 and 30.121412-2), the signal evolves as a free induction decay (FID). The characteristic time related to the decay for a given tissue is T2*. Owing to the absence of a 180° RF pulse used in spin echo techniques (see 30.121411-1 through 30.121411-3), T2* dephasing of the transverse magnetization is comprised of all magnetic field inhomogeneities, macroscopic and microscopic, and the FID signal is subject to these factors. Image artifacts can be observed as regional distortions or voids due to external magnetic field inhomogeneities and the presence of metal. Image signal intensity and contrast anomalies may occur due to magnetic susceptibility field variations and chemical shift.

Magnetic susceptibility (χ) is a property of tissues that defines the degree to which a material becomes magnetized. Not all tissues or substances experience the same magnetic field internally, even though they exist in the presence of the same external field. Differences in χ result in field gradients across boundaries, no matter how slight or small. These localized regions of field inhomogeneity can lead to T2* shortening, spin dephasing, and potential losses in MR signal.[1] The degree of signal loss will depend on the degree of difference in susceptibility between two regions. Air, for example, has a value of χ significantly different from most tissues. Thus, air/tissue interfaces show large susceptibility effects.[2,3]

Macroscopic susceptibility signal voids and image distortion artifacts are influenced in several ways. If TE is increased, signal errors will accumulate and artifacts become more prominent. Also, if the sampling bandwidth (see 30.12149-2) is lowered, thereby increasing the overall magnetic field sensitivity, regions with errors induced by susceptibility will be observed to a larger degree. These artifacts can be minimized by using a short TE or higher bandwidth.[4]

Microscopic susceptibility differences can lead to image intensity and contrast anomalies rather than regional artifacts. Most tissues have similar intrinsic χ values. However, in areas of complicated molecular structures such as trabecular bone, the overall signal may become re-

duced due to T2* shortening. Tissues may also be introduced with substances that change their susceptibility. The presence of ferromagnetic or paramagnetic material, either biochemically (e.g., hemosiderin) or artificially (e.g., contrast agents), can generate microscopic susceptibility-induced field inhomogeneities on a molecular level that can lead to enhanced contrast.[5]

If both fat and water components are present, the FID may possess an oscillatory behavior as a function of TE. When the gradient echo is collected at a TE when the signal is a peak, fat and water signals are combined and the image will be hyperintense. On the other hand, if the echo is generated when the signal is a minimum, the fat and water signals will cancel and the image will have a certain degree of suppression.[6–8] All gradient echo techniques have this anomaly.

It is well known that a distinct chemical shift of the Larmor frequencies of fat (primarily the $-CH_2$ moiety) and water ($-OH$) exists that may cause a pixel misregistration in the frequency encoding direction of the image (see 30.12149-2). In addition, a cycling of the relative phase difference between the two signals will occur based on their relative frequency difference. Following an RF pulse, the fat and water signal will begin in phase. As one signal precesses at a faster rate than the other, the signals will progress out of phase and the FID will oscillate in amplitude as it decays. Peaks will occur when they are in phase, and minimums will occur when they are 180° out of phase.

The chemical shift of fat and water is about 3.5 to 3.7 ppm, which corresponds to a 230-Hz frequency difference at 1.5T. Thus, the FID will oscillate about every 4.3 msec. Choosing the appropriate TE will determine the intensity of the fat/water region, being relatively bright at TE = 4.3, 8.7, 13.0, ... msec and suppressed at TE = 6.5, 10.9, 15.2,... msec. The degree of signal oscillation will depend on the fat and water present. None will occur if one of the two is absent from the region, and complete suppression will occur if the signal is composed of 50% fat and 50% water. This is most prevalent in trabecular structures that possess tissues of both chemical species.[9,10]

Technical References

1. Ludeke KM, Roschmann P, Tischler R. Susceptibility artifacts in NMR imaging. Mag Reson Imaging 1985;3:329–343.
2. Schick RM, Wismer GL, Davis KR. Magnetic susceptibility effects secondary to out-of-plane air in fast MR scanning. Am J Neuroradiol 1988;9:439–442.
3. Czervionke LF, Daniels DL, Wehrli FW, et al. Magnetic susceptibility artifacts in gradient-recalled echo MR imaging. Am J Neuroradiol 1988;9:1149–1155.
4. Haacke EM, Tkach JA, Parrish TB. Reduction of T2* dephasing in gradient field-echo imaging. Radiology 1989;170:457–462.
5. Young IR, Bydder GM, Khenia S, Collins AG. Assessment

of phase and amplitude effects due to susceptibility variations in MR imaging of the brain. J Comput Assist Tomogr 1989;13:490–494.

6. Wehrli FW, Perkins TG, Shimakawa A, Roberts F. Chemical shift-induced amplitude modulations in images obtained with gradient refocusing. Magn Reson Imaging 1987;5: 157–158.

7. Wehrli FW. Fast-scan magnetic resonance: principles and applications. Magn Reson Q 1990;6:165–236.

8. Szumowski J, Simon JH. Proton chemical shift imaging. In: Stark DD, Bradley WG, eds. Magnetic resonance imaging, 2nd ed, vol 1. St. Louis, Mosby-Year Book, 1992.

9. Wehrli FW, Ford JC, Attie M, et al. Trabecular structure: preliminary application of MR interferometry. Radiology 1991;179:615–621.

10. Sebag GH, Moore SG. Effect of trabecular bone on the appearance of marrow in gradient-echo imaging of the appendicular skeleton. Radiology 1990;174:855–859.

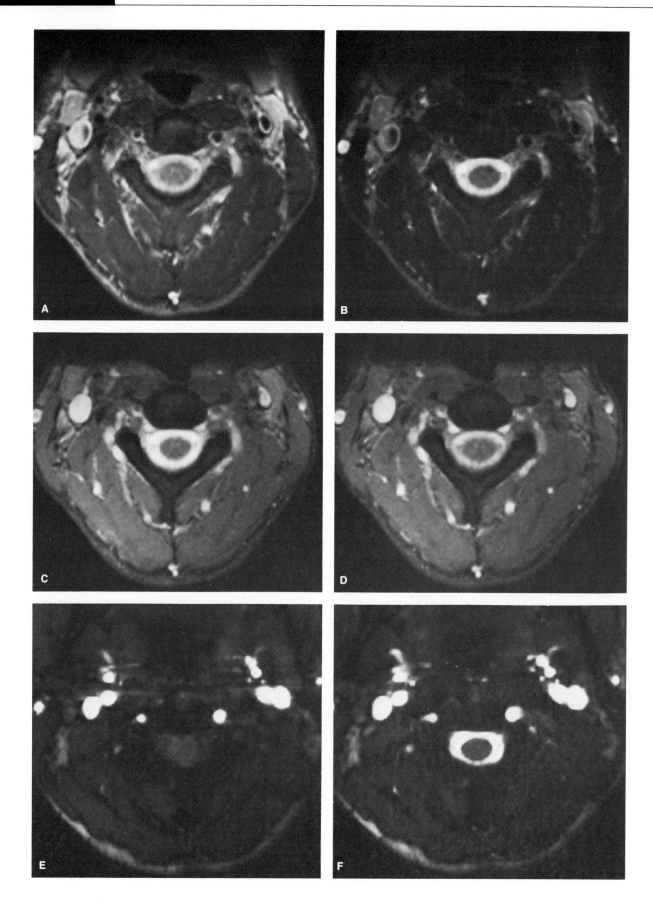

TOPIC

Cerebrospinal fluid (CSF) visualization with GRE and SE techniques

FINDINGS

Comparison among techniques in visualizing CSF is demonstrated in axial sections through the cervical spine. Using a conventional T2-weighted double echo SE acquisition, high CSF signal is observed with moderate signal intensity from surrounding tissues on the first echo (TR/TE = 2500/45), with intermediate T2-weighted cord and CSF contrast (*A*). On the second echo (TR/TE = 2500/90), contrast between CSF and the spinal cord is high due to stronger T2 weighting where neighboring tissue intensity is low (*B*). Using low RF flip angles (FA) with spoiled GRE techniques (TR/TE/FA = 400/10/20°), T2-like contrast with high CSF signal is observed with a reduced TR (*C*). Rapid scan GRE (TR/TE/FA = 40/10/10°) still enables CSF and cord contrast to be well visualized, although it is reduced (*D*). Use of a very short TR and large FA with rephased GRE techniques (TR/TE/FA = 24/12/90°) yields extremely high CSF signal relative to other tissues, but with partial rephasing flow-related phase dispersion can eliminate the signal altogether (*E*). With complete rephasing (*F*), CSF demonstrates maximum intensity while the spinal cord and other tissues remain dark.

CONCLUSION

CSF is visualized with a long TR/long TE spin echo (SE) technique, and a low FA GRE technique at a reduced TR. Reduced scan times are possible with GRE. Very high CSF contrast is obtained using completely rephased GRE at a very short TR and a high FA.

DISCUSSION

CSF is composed primarily of water; therefore, it has a characteristically long T1 and long T2. To delineate CSF from surrounding tissues, it is necessary to reduce their signal while maintaining the signal from CSF. With conventional SE, this requires the use of a large TR due to the long T1 of CSF to ensure sufficient growth of its longitudinal magnetization, and a large TE to reduce the sig-

nal from surrounding tissues.[1] Because of its long T2, CSF signal remains high and will then be well visualized on a T2-weighted SE image (see 30.121411-2). A major disadvantage of SE is the necessarily large TR, which leads to long scan times. This can be substantially improved by using fast SE methodology (see 30.121411-3), but still requires imaging times on the order of several minutes and can be subject to subtle blurring artifacts.[2]

In GRE imaging, with either spoiled (see 30.121412-1) or rephased (see 30.121412-2) techniques, CSF can be visualized by using a reduced FA.[3] Small angle excitations require less time for full longitudinal magnetization recovery, thereby allowing a shorter TR to be used. This reduces scan time significantly. At very short TR with scan times on the order of less than a minute, CSF can still be observed, but with an overall loss in signal and slice coverage. This can be improved by using a rephased GRE technique at high FA that retains a signal contribution from the SSFP-echo, largely from the CSF due to its long T2 (see 30.121412-2). By maintaining complete transverse coherency in rephased GRE, extremely large CSF signal can be observed.[4] Although this requires two independent scans that must be combined to eliminate phase-related banding artifacts due to magnetic field inhomogeneities, its scan time can still remain well under a minute.

The primary disadvantage of GRE techniques in visualization of CSF is the fact that they do not possess a 180° RF pulse that generates an echo in SE to eliminate signal dephasing due to field inhomogeneities. The FID decay is dictated by T2* instead of T2 and is subject to modulation from chemical shift, bulk magnetic susceptibility, external field variations, and metal-related field distortions (see 30.121412-3).

Technical References

1. Wehrli FW, MacFall JR, Shutts D, et al. Mechanisms of contrast in NMR imaging. J Comput Assist Tomogr 1984;8:369–380.
2. Jones KM, Mulkern RV, Schwartz RB, et al. Fast spin-echo MR imaging of the brain and spine: current concepts. Am J Roentgenol 1992;158:1313–1320.
3. Buxton RB, Edelman RR, Rosen BR, et al. Contrast in rapid MR imaging: T1- and T2-weighted imaging. J Comput Assist Tomogr 1987;11:7–16.
4. Haacke EM, Wielopolski P, Tkach JA, Modic MT. Steady state free precession imaging in the presence of motion: an application to CSF. Radiology 1990;175:545–552.

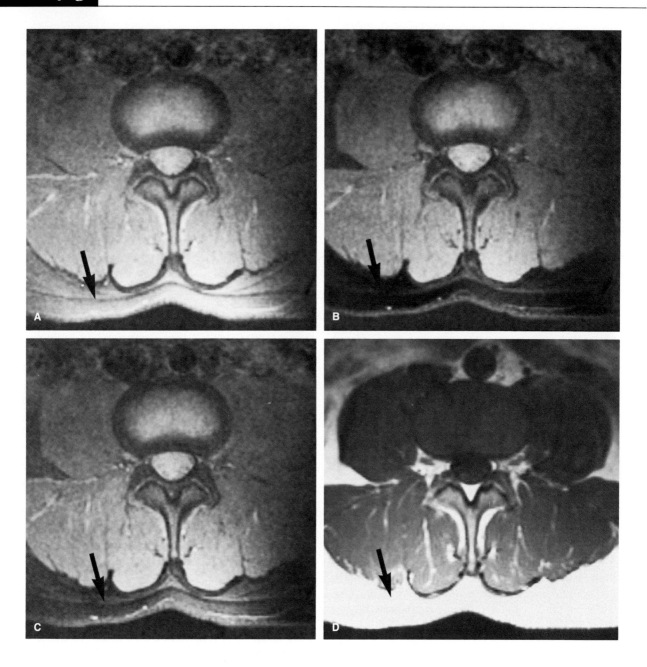

TOPIC

Short tau inversion recovery (STIR) for fat suppression

FINDINGS

Axial lumbar spine images through the L4–L5 intervertebral disk demonstrate fat suppression using the STIR technique (*A through C*), as compared to a conventional T1-weighted spin echo (SE) technique (*D*). With magnitude reconstruction, a short inversion time (TI) yields a tissue contrast inversion anomaly that depicts negative signals as positive. CSF intensity is bright because its signal is most negative, even though the contrast is actually strongly T1-weighted. If TI is too short (TR/TE/TI = 2000/20/130), fat signal does not reach the null point (*arrow*), resulting in poor suppression (*A*). If TI is too long (TR/TE/TI = 2000/20/170), fat signal goes beyond the null point (*arrow*) and is not well suppressed (*C*). However, at precisely the correct TI (TR/TE/TI = 2000/20/150), fat becomes uniformly suppressed (*arrow*), allowing surrounding structures to be well depicted (*B*). Note that contrast in the intervertebral disk and most tissues remains relatively similar because the TI differences are slight. On a T1-weighted SE acquisition (TR/TE = 400/10), the fat is very bright (*arrow*) and can obscure structures of interest (*D*).

CONCLUSION

Good suppression of fat signal is obtained with STIR using the correct inversion time, TI.

DISCUSSION

Certain MR techniques are designed to be well suited for enhancing contrast related specifically to either T1 or T2 differences in tissues. Inversion recovery (IR) is inherently a technique that offers exceptional T1 weighting and superb anatomic detail.[1] In general spine imaging, IR has received less attention than SE because in many cases pathology is better visualized on T2-weighted studies (see 30.121411-2). Also, T1 contrast, which is favored for anatomic depiction, can be achieved with SE in substantially less scan time (see 30.121411-1). Nevertheless, IR may offer an advantage in certain clinical situations.

The IR pulse sequence is characterized by a 180°-90° RF pulsing. The initial 180° pulse inverts the longitudinal magnetization. Because no signal can be detected in MRI until magnetization lies in the transverse plane, this is followed by a 90° RF pulse at the inversion time (TI). The signal is then collected as an SE or GRE. By initially inverting the magnetization, the time it takes for full T1 recovery is longer than in SE, thereby allowing a much greater degree of T1 contrast to be obtained. However, this also necessitates the use of a long TR, leading to increased scan times. The echo time (TE) is typically kept as short as possible to minimize introduction of T2-related contrast.

A unique aspect of IR is that the inverted magnetization will recover longitudinally according to T1 relaxation, and must cross through a null point or "bounce point" as it grows. This will occur when there is the same amount of magnetization in the negative direction as in the positive direction, with a net effective longitudinal magnetization of zero. If the TI is chosen so that signal is acquired precisely when a specific tissue of a given T1 value possesses zero net longitudinal magnetization, the result is a minimal signal output and selective suppression of that tissue in the image. This phenomenon has been used to specifically suppress fat signal and is called STIR (short tau inversion recovery).[1] It has been primarily used for better visualization of the optic nerves[2] and hepatic lesions.[3–5]

Fat characteristically has the shortest T1 value and therefore is the first magnetization to pass through the null point during the TI interval. As a result, all neighboring tissues will still possess negative magnetization and generate negative signals. An absolute or magnitude reconstruction of the STIR image will invert all the tissue signals that are negative to positive values. This will produce reversed tissue contrast that may lead to difficult interpretation. Phase-sensitive reconstruction allows the sign of the tissue signals to be preserved, thereby producing true T1 weighting.[6] When suppressing fat with the STIR technique, all tissues other than fat will exhibit negative pixel intensity, and background noise will have the highest pixel intensity. This, too, can prove difficult to interpret. In most uses, magnitude reconstruction is employed. Nevertheless, provided the correct TI is used, fat will be suppressed in both methods of reconstruction.

A very precise TI is necessary to effectively null a given tissue signal, and it depends on both TR and T1. It is roughly equal to 70% of the T1 if a long TR is used. Because T1 depends on field strength, the correct TI for good fat suppression also depends on field strength. If a larger TI is used, the fat signal will become positive while all the other tissues will still be negative. An absolute reconstruction and display of the STIR image will then produce boundary artifacts at interfaces.[7,8] Even small deviations from the proper TI will substantially compromise the suppression of the tissue.[5,9] On the other hand, this precise relationship between T1 and TI makes it possible to selectively suppress not only fat but certain types of lesions as well, potentially increasing specificity.[5]

Technical References

1. Bydder GM, Young IR. MR imaging: clinical use of the inversion recovery sequence. J Comput Assist Tomogr 1985; 9:659–675.
2. Atlas SW, Grossman RI, Hackney DB, et al. STIR MR imaging of the orbit. Am J Roentgenol 1988;151:1025–1030.
3. Dwyer AJ, Frank JA, Sank VJ, et al. Short-TI inversion-recovery pulse sequence: analysis and initial experience in cancer imaging. Radiology 1988;168:827–836.
4. Dousset M, Weissleder R, Hendrick RE, et al. Short TI inversion-recovery imaging of the liver: pulse-sequence optimization and comparison with spin-echo imaging. Radiology 1989;171:327–333.
5. Patrizio G, Pavone P, Testa A, et al. MR characterization of hepatic lesions by t-null inversion recovery sequence. J Comput Assist Tomogr 1990;14:96–101.
6. Park HW, Cho MH, Cho ZH. Real-value representation in inversion-recovery NMR imaging by use of a phase-correction method. Magn Reson Med 1986;3:15–23.
7. Hearshen DO, Ellis JH, Carson PL, et al. Boundary effects from opposed magnetization artifact in IR images. Radiology 1986;160:543–547.
8. Droege RT, Adamczak SM. Boundary artifact in inversion-recovery images. Magn Reson Med 1986;3:126–131.
9. Shuman WP, Lambert DT, Patten RM, et al. Improved fat suppression in STIR MR imaging: selecting inversion time through spectral display. Radiology 1991;178:885–887.

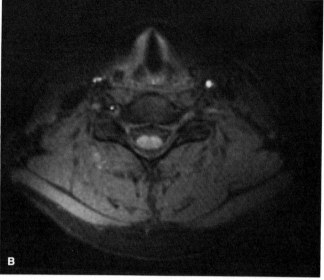

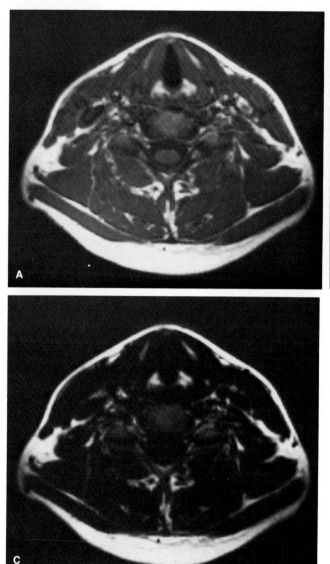

TOPIC

Chemical shift imaging of fat and water by spectral saturation

FINDINGS

Use of chemical shift spectral saturation to produce fat-only and water-only images is demonstrated in axial spin echo (SE) scans (TR/TE = 400/15) of the cervical spine (*A through C*) and midline sagittal scans (TR/TE = 600/15) of the lumbar spine (*D through F*). Without saturation (*A and D*), tissues containing both fat and water are observed. With T1 weighting, fat is high intensity whereas CSF is dark and the spinal cord and nerve roots are moderately bright. With saturation of the fat signal (*B and E*), tissues containing water are unaffected and the images yield better delineation of central structures. The intensity of the cord is the same but appears increased due to different windowing. Some variations in the efficiency of fat suppression are seen left to right on the axial scan (*B*) and near the surface coil (*arrow*) on the sagittal scan (*E*) due to magnetic field inhomogeneities. On fat-only images that have water suppression (*C and F*), the cord, CSF, and vertebral disks are devoid of signal, indicating that these tissues are mostly composed of water.

CONCLUSION

Effective fat or water suppression by spectral saturation in chemical shift imaging can be achieved, but with varying degrees of regional suppression due to sensitivity to external field inhomogeneities.

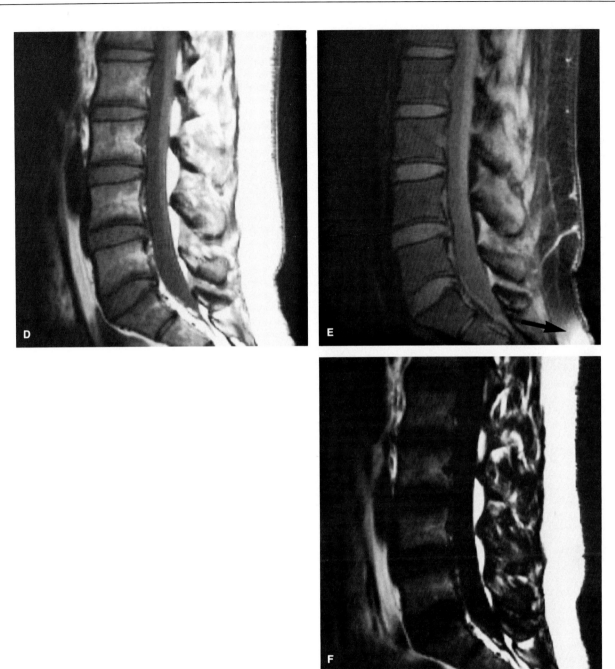

DISCUSSION

MRI can selectively isolate and image fatty tissues or water because of the fundamental differences between their NMR properties. Not only are their T1 and T2 values substantially different, but their inherent Larmor precessional frequencies are also different because of their chemical (spectral) shifts. Fat or water suppression techniques can offer enhanced diagnostic capabilities and ease of interpretation. Aside from providing fundamental information about the chemical nature of the tissue, they can allow increased conspicuity of structures otherwise obscured by fat or water.

Numerous techniques for suppressing fat or water have been developed.[1] All have met with varying degrees of success. Chemical shift selective (CHESS), frequency selective, or spectral saturation exploits the slight differences in the Larmor frequencies of fat and water and directly saturates the signal of either by applying a presaturation pulse before the imaging pulsing.[2-4] This can be incorporated into any conventional technique and is similar to spatial presaturation (see 30.12149-7), differing only in the fact that one is a spatial technique and the other is spectral.

If a 90° RF pulse is applied immediately preceding a standard imaging technique (such as SE), it will initially saturate the magnetization, leading to an effectively reduced signal. If this pulse is applied only to the fat spins, the fat signal will then be suppressed. Conversely, if it is applied to the water magnetization, then that will be reduced. Without spatial excitation of the presaturation pulse, this can be performed on a given chemical species throughout the imaging volume.

This method of selective saturation, however, is difficult to achieve uniformly throughout the image. It is well known that free water ($-$OH) and lipids ($-$CH$_2$, for example) have sufficient differences in their chemical environments that the hydrogen protons associated with each complex have resonant frequencies that differ by about 3.5 ppm. At 1.5T, this corresponds to a spectral frequency difference of only about 220 to 240 Hz. For spectral saturation to be effective, the presaturation pulse must be applied only to one chemical species and not the other. Therefore, it requires a very narrow bandwidth RF saturation pulse. If the magnetic field changes slightly, the pulse will not be on resonance with the species and the desired suppression will not occur and could potentially simulate pathology.[5,6] This requires a high degree of field homogeneity throughout the imaging volume.

Localized inhomogeneities such as those caused by susceptibility (see 30.121412-3) and metal will compromise this technique further.

Technical References

1. Szumowski J, Simon JH. Proton chemical shift imaging. In: Stark DD, Bradley WG, eds. Magnetic resonance imaging, 2nd ed. Vol 1. St. Louis, Mosby-Year Book, 1992.
2. Rosen BR, Wedeen VJ, Brady TJ. Selective saturation NMR imaging. J Comput Assist Tomogr 1984;8:813–818.
3. Frahm J, Haase A, Hanicke W, et al. Chemical shift selective MR imaging using a whole-body magnet. Radiology 1985;156:441–444.
4. Keller PJ, Hunter WW, Schmalbrock. Multisection fat/water imaging with chemical shift selective presaturation. Radiology 1987;164:539–541.
5. Joseph PM, Shetty A. A comparison of selective saturation and selective echo chemical shift imaging techniques. Magn Reson Imag 1988;6:421–430.
6. Anzai Y, Lufkin RB, Jabour BA, Hanafee WN. Fat-suppression failure artifacts simulating pathology on frequency-selective fat-suppression MR images of the head and neck. Am J Neuroradiol 1992;13:879–884.

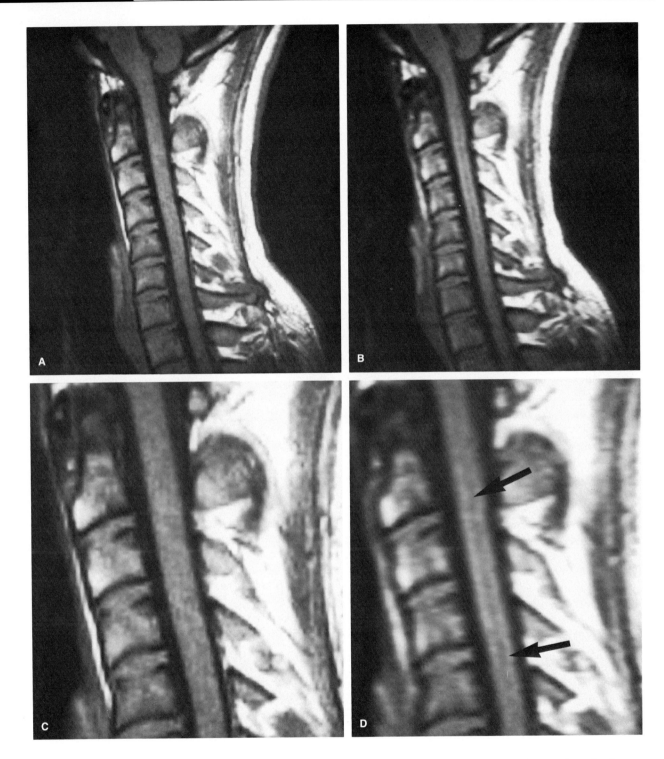

TOPIC

Matrix size, spatial resolution, truncation artifact, and scan time

FINDINGS

Midline sagittal T1-weighted spin echo images in the cervical spine (TR/TE = 450/12) demonstrate differences between using a 256 × 256 (*A and C*) and a 128 × 256 (*B and D*) acquisition matrix. Obtained with the same square field of view (250 mm), the pixel dimensions and spatial resolution are 0.96 × 0.96 mm and 1.92 × 0.96 mm respectively. Loss of edge definition, particularly in the spinal cord, and poor delineation of small structures are clearly apparent with the larger pixel dimensions shown left to right in images *B* and *D*. However, scan time is roughly halved, from 7:42 minutes to 3:52 minutes, because the matrix reduction of a factor of two is in the phase-encoding direction. Signal-to-noise ratio (S/N) is also higher by a factor of 1.41. Nevertheless, in addition to poorer spatial resolution, truncation artifacts in the reduced matrix direction can be observed (*B and D*). When the coarser resolution is left to right, this may lead to an artifact that runs longitudinally through the cord (*D*), simulating a syrinx (*arrows*).

CONCLUSION

Higher spatial resolution is achieved with a larger matrix at the expense of reduced S/N and longer scan times. Smaller matrices may demonstrate truncation artifact.

DISCUSSION

The effect of matrix size on S/N, spatial resolution, and imaging time is straightforward. However, determining the appropriate matrix size for a specific clinical study is not as easy. The detectability of a lesion is mainly associated with the contrast resolution, which is dependent on S/N, and the true spatial resolving power, which is not necessarily equal to the size of a pixel or voxel (see 30.12149-5). The influence of matrix size on these diagnostically relevant parameters is not intuitive and ultimately depends on the individual case being investigated.[1,2] A further complication is the general fact that a reduced matrix in digital imaging may lead to a phenomenon known as truncation artifact.[3]

The pixel dimensions of an MR image are determined by the field of view (FOV) divided by the matrix size in each direction (see 30.12149-3). If the FOV, along with other user-selectable parameters, is held constant, then the S/N increases with reduced matrix size.[1,4,5] Higher S/N may improve detection because of better contrast resolution, but a larger pixel size may counter this because of the loss in spatial resolution, particularly with small structures.

The total scan time also depends on the matrix size. A two-dimensional MR image is acquired by encoding one dimension in frequency and the other in phase. Three-dimensional MR incorporates a third dimension of phase encoding (see 30.12149-10). The number of phase-encoding steps equals the number of pixels in the phase-encoding directions of the image, provided partial data methods are not used. The total imaging time is directly proportional to the total number of phase-encoded signals that are acquired. Therefore, although some advantages can be gained by using large matrix sizes, the drawback of increased imaging time limits their routine use.

Truncation artifacts may become evident when using a smaller matrix; this is a frequently observed phenomenon in MRI.[3,6–8] It is also referred to as "ringing" or Gibbs artifact and can be recognized by a characteristic rippling of signal intensity in the vicinity of and parallel to high-contrast tissue boundaries, such as in the region of the spinal cord, particularly on T1-weighted scans.[8]

Signals in MRI are digitally sampled during the acquisition. Starting and stopping the sampling necessarily truncates some of the signal, which does not become processed in the image. This lost information may lead to a truncation artifact, and its severity depends on the pixel size and the spatial geometry of the tissue. The truncated signal is usually associated with the fine detail of edges and small structures throughout the image. Without this information, there is a potential loss or blurring of edge definition. In addition, the truncation results in a digital approximation error of edges during image reconstruction. This is seen as a rippling effect that emanates away from the edge and eventually dies away at a certain distance.

The ringing or rippling of edges will be larger if the truncation of the sampled data is greater. It occurs to a larger degree if high tissue contrast exists at sharp boundaries. The artifact is less severe if only smooth boundaries exist. Ringing can also exist in either the frequency or phase-encoding direction of an MR image. Although conspicuous, it may mimic pathology such as a syrinx in the spinal cord on sagittal T1-weighted scans.[8]

In terms of imaging parameters, truncation artifact is associated with the pixel size. Little artifact occurs if the pixel dimension is small relative to the tissue structures. Acquiring the data with a smaller FOV or larger matrix can minimize truncation artifact. However, reducing the FOV may cause image aliasing (see 30.12149-3), larger matrices will result in longer imaging times, and the inherent loss in S/N may compromise the image quality at the expense of removing the ringing.

Technical References

1. Bradley WG, Kortman KE, Crues JV. CNS high-resolution MRI: effect of increasing spatial resolution on resolving power. Radiology 1985;156:93–98.
2. Owen RS, Wehrli FW. Predictability of SNR and reader preference in clinical MR imaging. Magn Reson Imag 1990; 8:737–745.
3. Wood ML, Henkelman RM. Truncation artifacts in MRI. Magn Reson Med 1985;2:517–526.
4. Crooks LE, Hoenninger J, Arakawa M, et al. High-resolution MRI: technical concepts and their implementation. Radiology 1984;150:163–171.
5. Constable RT, Henkelman RM. Contrast, resolution, and detectability in MR imaging. J Comput Assist Tomogr 1991; 15:297–303.
6. Lufkin RB, Pusey E, Stark DD, et al. Boundary artifact due to truncation errors in MR imaging. Am J Roentgenol 1986;147:1283–1287.
7. Czervionke LF, Czervionke JM, Daniels DL, Haughton VM. Characteristic features of MR truncation artifacts. Am J Neuroradiol 1988;9:815–824.
8. Levy LM, DiChiro G, Brooks RA, et al. Spinal cord artifacts from truncation errors during MR imaging. Radiology 1988;166:479–483.

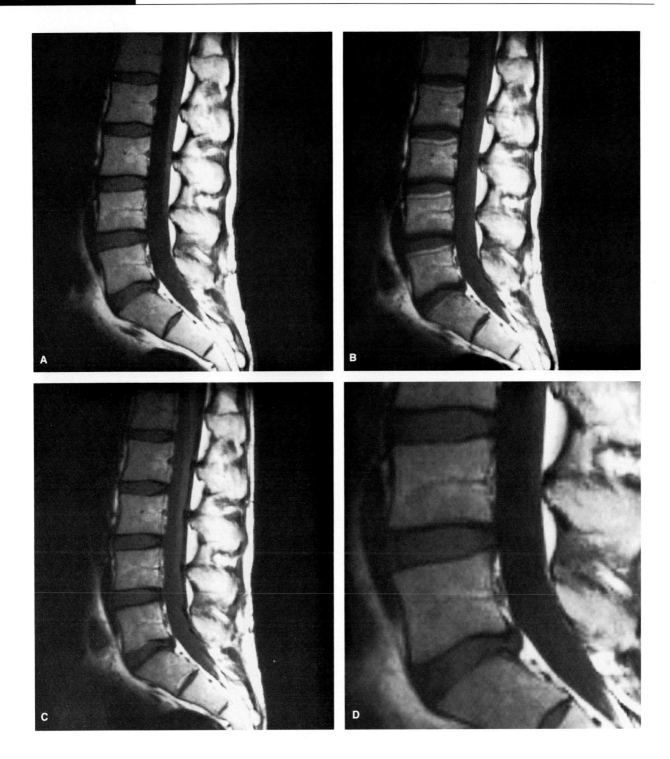

TOPIC

Sampling bandwidth and chemical shift artifact

FINDINGS

The effect of sampling bandwidth is demonstrated in midline sagittal T1-weighted spin echo images (TR/TE = 420/24) through the lumbar spine. At high sampling bandwidth (390 Hz/pixel), high contrast between the in-

tervertebral disks and vertebral bodies is observed with good delineation of the spinal cord (*A and D*). Note the symmetry of the vertebral end plates. Frequency encoding was top to bottom. With low sampling bandwidth (56 Hz/pixel), severe chemical shift misregistration artifact in fatty tissues is seen (*B, C, E, and F*). When frequency encoding is top to bottom (*B and E*), asymmetry in the vertebral end plates is particularly apparent (*arrow in E*), along with a decrease in the detail of the basivertebral veins (*E*). When frequency encoding is left to right (*C*

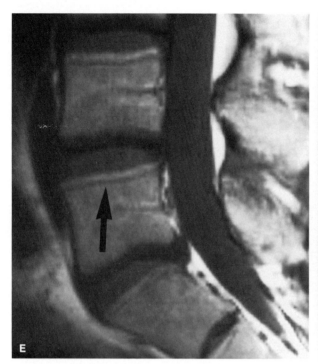

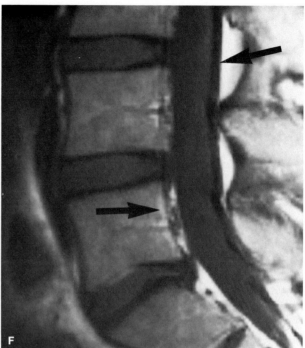

and F), no asymmetry in the end plates is observed, but a significant left-to-right shift in the position of the disk itself is apparent. Posterior and anterior epidural fat is severely shifted (*arrows*), leading to artifactual changes in neighboring structures (*F*). Similar image quality was obtained at both low and high sampling bandwidth in this example due to signal averaging. The substantially higher noise content in the images associated with high bandwidth was reduced by increasing the number of acquisitions and scan time by a factor of 6.

CONCLUSION

Reduced sampling bandwidths lead to improved signal-to-noise ratios (S/N) but may produce pixel misregistration between tissues containing fat and water.

DISCUSSION

The MRI signal must be digitally sampled to ultimately process it into an image. The sampling frequency bandwidth of the image, usually discussed in terms of Hz/pixel, is defined by the total amount of time that is allowed to acquire the signal. The primary advantage of using a small sampling bandwidth is that it substantially reduces the statistical noise of the image. This increases the S/N and contrast-to-noise ratio (C/N) and may improve overall image quality.[1,2] However, all magnetic field errors that result in signal frequency shifts will become accentuated. Extrinsic factors such as field inhomogeneity and metal objects warp the magnetic field, causing large distortions and signal loss in the image when low bandwidth sampling is used. Intrinsic field differences such as chemical shift between fat and water can lead to image pixel misregistrations and chemical shift artifact.

Reduced bandwidth imaging is frequently implemented on the later echoes of a T2-weighted study, where S/N is inherently low (see 30.121411-2).[2,3] At short TE and long TR in spin density weighting, overall S/N is large enough so that low sampling bandwidths tend not to be used. Although the S/N is relatively low on T1-weighted studies (see 30.121411-1), they have a substantial amount of fat signal that may cause large chemical shift artifacts and are thus typically acquired at high bandwidths. A further consideration is that lower bandwidths require proportionately longer sampling times, thereby limiting the minimum TE that can be used and reducing the number of slices that can be obtained.

A common artifact in MRI is chemical shift pixel misregistration. Early investigations showed wholesale shifts in regions of images between tissues containing fat and water.[4–6] This pixel misregistration is caused by a spectroscopic chemical shift magnetic field phenomenon, and its severity will depend on the sampling frequency bandwidth.

All MR signals carry spectroscopic information about the chemical nature of the tissue. At imaging field strengths, tissue lipids and water make up the majority of the hydrogen MRI signal. The spectral, or frequency, difference between the two species is about 3.5 ppm, or roughly 230 Hz at 1.5T (see 30.121414). Because one of the two directions of an MR image is spatially mapped according to signal frequency, this difference causes the fat and the water signals to be mismapped into two different pixel positions of the frequency-encoded direction in the image (see 30.12149-9). No pixel misregistration occurs in the phase-encoding direction of the image. In an imaging technique that uses a low sampling bandwidth, the 230-Hz chemical shift will lead to a large pixel shift. Conversely, if the sampling bandwidth is larger than 230 Hz, both species will be correctly mapped to the same pixel in the image.

Depending on the chemical makeup and anatomic structure of the tissues, chemical shift artifacts can have varying appearances, producing edge artifacts[7] or misleading subdural enhancement.[3] Errors are most prominent in regions containing fat and water, such as the pituitary,[8] the optic nerve,[9] and vertebral disks. The artifact is usually exhibited to a lesser degree on T2-weighted scans because most of the signal from fat has decayed.

Technical References

1. Hendrick RE. Sampling time effects on signal-to-noise and contrast-to-noise ratios in spin-echo MRI. Magn Reson Imag 1987;5:31–37.
2. Simon JH, Foster TH, Ketonen L, et al. Reduced-bandwidth MR imaging of the head at 1.5T. Radiology 1989;172:771–775.
3. Smith AS, Weinstein MA, Hurst GC, et al. Intracranial chemical-shift artifacts on MR images of the brain: observations and relation to sampling bandwidth. Am J Roentgenol 1990;154:1275–1283.
4. Soila KP, Viamonte M, Starewicz PM. Chemical misregistration effects in MRI. Radiology 1984;153:819–820.
5. Dwyer AJ, Knop RH, Hoult DI. Frequency shift artifacts in MR imaging. J Comput Assist Tomogr 1985;9:16–18.
6. Weinreb JC, Brateman L, Babcock EE, et al. Chemical shift artifact in clinical magnetic resonance images at 0.35T. Am J Roentgenol 1985;145:183–185.
7. Babcock EE, Brateman L, Weinreb JC, et al. Edge artifacts in MR images: chemical shift effect. J Comput Assist Tomogr 1985;9:252–257.
8. Haughton VM, Prost R. Pituitary fossa: chemical shift effect in MR imaging. Radiology 1986;158:461–462.
9. Daniels DL, Kneeland JB, Shimakawa A, et al. MR imaging of the optic nerve and sheath: correcting the chemical shift misregistration effect. Am J Neuroradiol 1986;7:249–253.

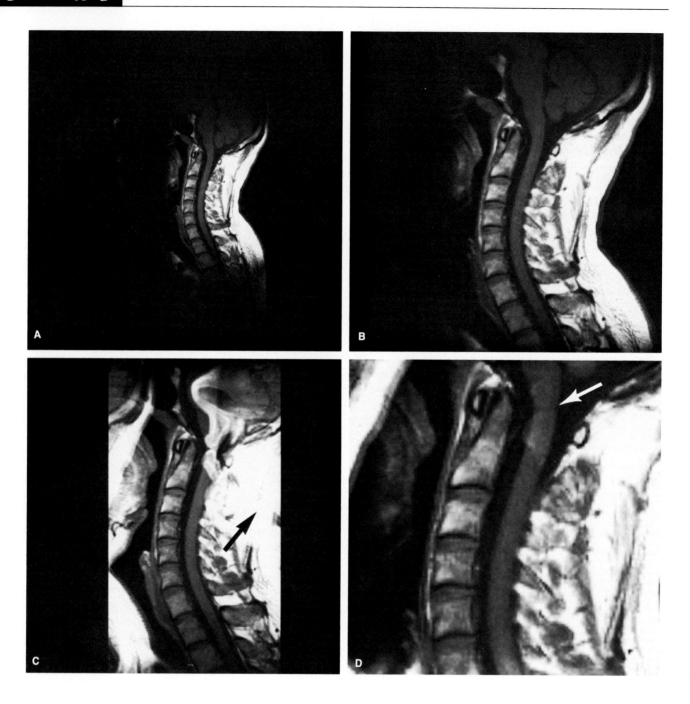

TOPIC

Field of view (FOV), spatial resolution, and image aliasing

FINDINGS

Midline sagittal T1-weighted spin echo scans through the cervical spine show the effects of changing the field of view (FOV). At large FOV (512 mm), the imaging volume lies well within the boundaries of spatial encoding (*A*), but requires a larger acquisition matrix to maintain spa-tial resolution (512 × 512, 2 acquisitions). With a more appropriate FOV (256 mm), the tissues remain within the boundaries (*B*), but this choice of FOV requires addi-tional acquisitions and signal averaging to maintain sig-nal-to-noise ratio (S/N) and image quality (256 × 256, 4 acquisitions). Further reduction of the FOV in the phase-encoding direction (128 × 256 mm) may cause tissue signal to extend beyond the boundaries of encoding (*C*), leading to aliasing or "wraparound" (*arrow*). If a re-duced FOV is used in both directions (128 mm), aliasing can occur at all four boundaries of the image (*D*) and may even simulate abnormalities (*arrow*).

CONCLUSION

Higher spatial resolution can be achieved with a smaller FOV, but at the expense of reduced S/N. Aliasing artifact may occur in tissues that extend beyond the FOV.

DISCUSSION

In MRI, the FOV can be easily prescribed to achieve any degree of spatial resolution within the constraints of the system hardware. The pixel dimensions in the image are determined by the FOV divided by the acquisition matrix in each direction (see 30.12149-1). If the matrix size is held constant, the spatial resolution is increased with a smaller FOV, allowing better visualization of small structures. However, determining the appropriate FOV for a clinical study is not easy. With all other measurement parameters held constant, the S/N reduces dramatically with FOV. The detectability of a lesion is associated not only with the spatial resolution, but also with the contrast resolution, which depends on the S/N (see 30.12149-5). The influence of FOV on the diagnostically relevant resolving power is complex and ultimately depends on the individual case being investigated.[1-3]

The most severe compromise with a reduced FOV is in the S/N.[1,3,4] If the FOV is halved, the S/N is reduced by a factor of four. As the pixel size decreases, the amount of signal representing the pixel reduces in two dimensions. Simple geometry dictates that the area of a square reduces as the product of its sides. Therefore, the total signal representing the pixel drops accordingly. Background noise, however, remains the same because the amount of noise in a pixel is associated with the characteristics of the data sampling. As a result, S/N reduces as the square of the FOV for a given matrix size. This large compromise may outweigh the benefits of increased spatial resolution.

High-resolution MRI is difficult to accomplish without necessarily lengthening scan times. Because of the substantial loss in S/N with a reduced FOV, good image quality may be attainable only by increasing the number of acquisitions to gain back the S/N. This inevitably increases the imaging time (see 30.12149-5). At a short TR, T1-weighted scans with multiple acquisitions may still be obtained in a reasonable amount of time. On the other hand, T2-weighted studies that have inherently long scan times may not benefit from higher resolution at the expense of prohibitively long exams. Therefore, T1-weighted protocols tend to be used to yield high spatial resolution images, unless increased signal sensitivity can be gained by the use of specialized coils (see 30.12149-11 and 30.12149-12).

If the FOV is reduced to the extent that tissue signal lies beyond the boundaries of spatial encoding, aliasing artifacts will occur. Aliasing, sometimes referred to as foldover or wraparound, is a digital phenomenon well known in MRI.[5,6] Signal is typically encoded with frequency and phase information associated with its spatial origin within the body. The digital sampling of the signal is at times not fast enough to uniquely represent the highest frequencies and largest phases of signals that come from regions far from the center of the image. As a result, signal from outside one boundary of the FOV becomes wrapped to the opposite boundary, overlaying itself on the image and obscuring details.

The use of a small FOV runs the highest risk of an aliasing artifact, but several methods exist that can minimize it. The most direct way is to increase the amount of sampling, or to "oversample" the signal. Aliasing will then be reduced in the frequency-encoding direction of the image. This can be achieved with no compromise in S/N or imaging time. Oversampling in the phase-encoding direction may also be done, but at the expense of imaging time, because more phase-encoding steps in the acquisition would be required to accomplish the task.

Another strategy is to ensure that signals from beyond the boundaries are suppressed and do not obscure the underlying structures when they become aliased. This can be accomplished by using spatial presaturation to reduce the signal outside of the boundaries (see 30.12149-7).[7] Use of surface coils may offer an effective way of minimizing aliasing by receiving signal only from a small region near the coil (see 30.12149-11). Filters can also be used to reduce the signals that lie beyond the FOV, although only in the frequency-encoding direction.

Technical References

1. Bradley WG, Kortman KE, Crues JV. CNS high-resolution MRI: effect of increasing spatial resolution on resolving power. Radiology 1985;156:93–98.
2. Runge VM, Wood ML, Kaufman DM, et al. The straight and narrow path to good head and spine MRI. Radiographics 1988;8:507–531.
3. Owen RS, Wehrli FW. Predictability of SNR and reader preference in clinical MR imaging. Magn Reson Imag 1990; 8:737–745.
4. Constable RT, Henkelman RM. Contrast, resolution, and detectability in MR imaging. J Comput Assist Tomogr 1991; 15:297–303.
5. Henkelman RM, Bronskill MJ. Artifacts in MRI. Rev Magn Reson Med 1987;2:1–126.
6. Bellon EM, Haacke EM, Coleman PE, et al. MR artifacts: a review. Am J Roentgenol 1986;147:1271–1281.
7. Edelman RR, Atkinson DJ, Silver MS, et al. FRODO pulse sequences: a new means of eliminating motion, flow, and wraparound artifacts. Radiology 1988;166:231–236.

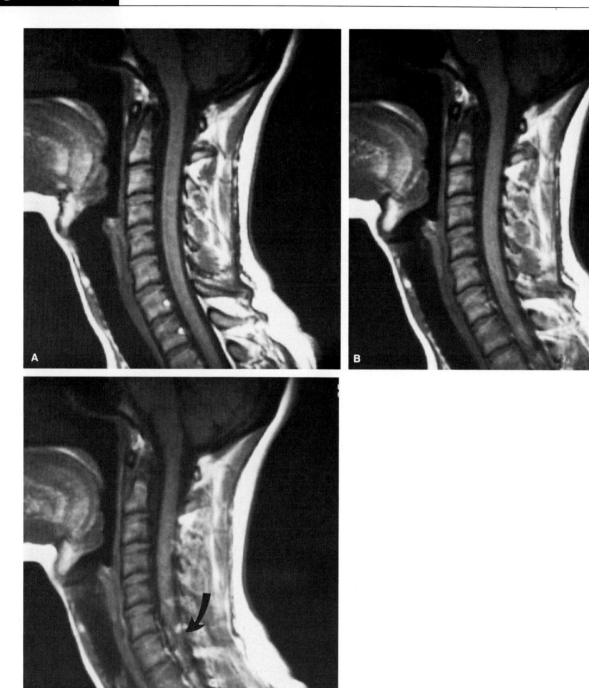

TOPIC

Slice thickness, volume averaging, and signal-to-noise ratio (S/N)

FINDINGS

The effect of slice thickness is demonstrated on T1-weighted sagittal spin echo scans (TR/TE = 200/12) through the cervical spine. In a 3-mm–thick midline section (A), the spinal cord is sharply defined throughout the image. Small structures are easily observed. With a 6-mm slice (B), slight curvature of the spine leads to volume averaging and loss of some structural definition of the cord inferiorly and of small structures. At 12 mm (C), a large degree of volume averaging is observed through most of the spine (*curved arrow*). Reduced S/N is associated with reduced slice thickness, and similar image quality in these examples was maintained by signal averaging. Images were acquired with (A) 16 acquisitions (13:41 minutes), (B) 4 acquisitions (3:26 minutes), and (C) 1 acquisition (53 seconds).

CONCLUSION

S/N increases with slice thickness. Volume averaging using thick sections results in loss of detail and contrast.

DISCUSSION

Selective excitation of larger sections of tissue leads to a linear increase in signal. Therefore, the S/N of the image is generally proportional to the slice thickness.[1] If the slice thickness is doubled, the S/N is doubled. This can lead to improved overall image quality and greater coverage. However, contrast, lesion detectability, and even image quality may actually decrease with an increase in slice thickness due to volume averaging, or partial voluming. This is particularly true when the region of interest contains anatomic structures that are small with respect to the slice thickness.[1–4]

Each pixel displayed in an image is a representation of the average signal produced by all the structures within the slice. The image, therefore, depicts a projection of all the anatomic detail contained within the section thickness. If structures are much smaller than the slice thickness, their conspicuity is compromised by averaging it with all the neighboring tissues.[3,4] Furthermore, edges that traverse through the slice in a curved fashion—such as at the boundary between CSF and the spinal cord—will tend to be blurred with large slice thicknesses. This results in a loss of boundary definition due to partial voluming.

Reduction in the slice thickness may aid in differentiating small structures, enhancing tissue boundaries, and increasing contrast, but the resulting loss in S/N may negate these advantages. Increasing the number of acquisitions to regain the S/N may be sufficient (see 30.12149-5), but the longer imaging time may not always be an option, as in the case of lengthy T2-weighted studies. Protocols are properly designed with thicknesses that will minimize volume averaging effects while still maintaining S/N so that imaging time is not unreasonable. Small structures such as the spinal cord and its respective nerve roots require thin sections in order to be well visualized, and this inevitably leads to long scan times. However, thicker slices may be necessary for obtaining sufficient coverage.

Technical References

1. Crooks LE, Watts J, Hoenninger J, et al. Thin-section definition in MRI. Radiology 1985;154:463–467.
2. Feinberg DA, Crooks LE, Hoenninger JC, et al. Contiguous thin multisection MR imaging by two-dimensional Fourier transform techniques. Radiology 1986;158:811–817.
3. Bradley WG, Glenn BJ. The effect of variation in slice thickness and interslice gap on MR lesion detection. Am J Neuroradiol 1987;8:1057–1062.
4. Webb WR, Moore EH. Differentiation of volume averaging and mass on MRI of the mediastinum. Radiology 1985;155:413–416.

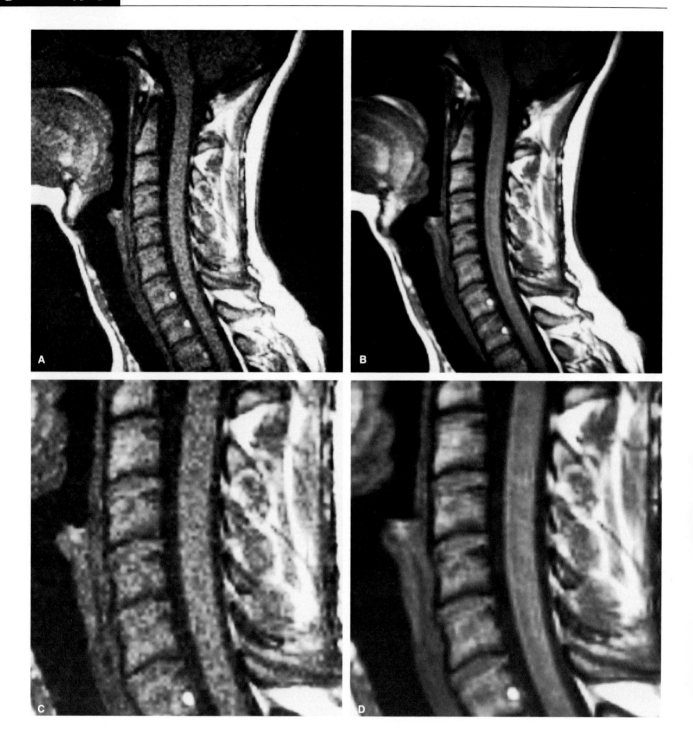

TOPIC

Acquisitions, imaging time, and signal-to-noise ratio (S/N)

FINDINGS

T1-weighted sagittal images (TR/TE = 200/12) were acquired with one acquisition (*A and C*) and 16 acquisitions (*B and D*) through the cervical spine. Scan times were 53 seconds and 13:41 minutes respectively. The difference in the S/N is a factor of four. Similar intrinsic contrast is observed, but the lower S/N associated with fewer acquisitions leads to an overall mottled appearance of nearly all tissues due to signal variations from pixel to pixel in the image. With low S/N, loss of subtle contrast differences can be seen, particularly in the vertebral bodies, and detail is degraded in the vertebral end plates (*C*).

CONCLUSION

Multiple acquisitions and signal averaging lead to higher S/N at the expense of imaging time.

DISCUSSION

S/N is an important consideration in maximizing the contrast-to-noise ratio (C/N) and lesion detectability and improving overall tissue delineation and image quality. Aside from the intrinsic signal and contrast of an image, the noise plays an equally important role. Even if there is high signal, a large noise component can negate its effect on image quality. Uncorrelated or random statistical noise results in pixel-to-pixel signal variability that occurs uniformly throughout the image. This is primarily introduced by the imaging system hardware. Correlated or systematic noise—such as from moving tissue structures, blood flow, or CSF—can obscure regional anatomic detail (see 30.12149-8). Averaging of the signals by using multiple acquisitions, or number of excitations, reduces the uncorrelated noise component in the image and increases the S/N and C/N.[1,2] Signal averaging may also minimize correlated noise but will not eliminate it.[3-5]

The main drawback of using multiple acquisitions is that it compromises the scan time. Imaging time is linearly proportional to the number of acquisitions. A factor of 4 increase in the number of acquisitions will double the S/N, but the total scan time will also lengthen by a factor of four. In many cases, increasing acquisitions can lead to prohibitively long scans. This is particularly true in T2-weighted studies, where TR tends to be large. It is used more frequently in T1-weighted scans with short TR, where an increase still allows reasonable imaging times.

Using multiple acquisitions can also have diminishing returns. If the tissue signal is intrinsically large compared to the image noise, or if the correlated noise is sufficiently large, then signal averaging by increasing the number of acquisitions may not necessarily enhance S/N, C/N, or image quality.[5,6] Thus, it would result in lengthened scan time with little added benefit.

Technical References

1. Edelstein WA, Bottomley PA, Hart HR, Smith LS. Signal, noise, and contrast in NMR imaging. J Comput Assist Tomogr 1983;7:391–401.
2. Hendrick RE, Raff U. Image contrast and noise. In: Stark DD, Bradley WG, eds. Magnetic resonance imaging, 2nd ed, vol 1. St. Louis, Mosby-Year Book, 1992.
3. Wood ML, Henkelman RM. Suppression of respiratory motion artifacts in MRI. Med Phys 1986;13:794–805.
4. Stark DD, Hendrick RE, Hahn PF, Ferrucci JT. Motion artifact reduction with fast spin-echo imaging. Radiology 1987;164:183–191.
5. Wood ML. Ineffectiveness of averaging for reducing motion artifacts in half-Fourier MR imaging. J Magn Reson Imag 1991;1:593–600.
6. Nalcioglu O, Cho ZH. Limits to signal-to-noise improvement by FID averaging in NMR imaging. Phys Med Biol 1984;29:969–978.

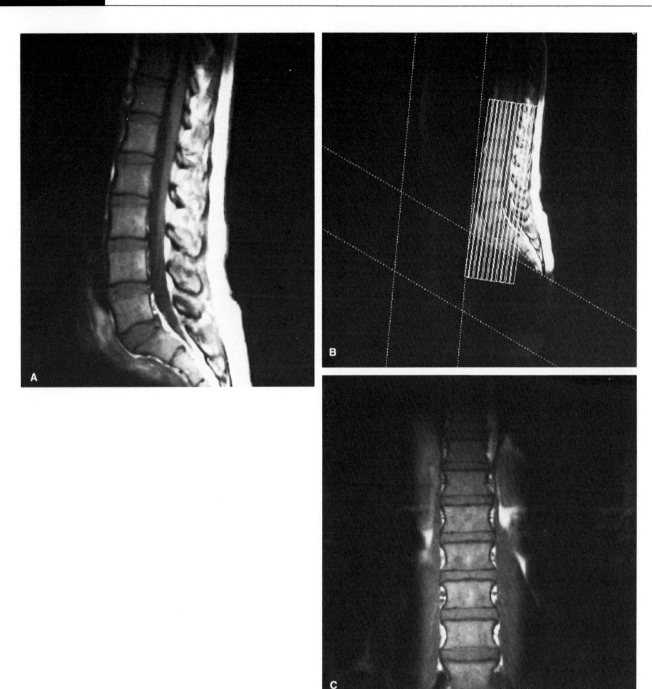

TOPIC

Multiple acquisition planes

FINDINGS

Two-dimensional T1-weighted spin echo scans (TR/TE = 400/10) were acquired in various planes through the lumbar spine. Sagittal scans (*A*) well depict the length of the spinal cord, intervertebral disks, and vertebral bodies and are useful to identify subsequent planes of acquisition (*B and D*). In oblique coronal sections through the vertebrae (*C*), complete cross sections of the disks are observed. Multi-angled scans, shown graphically in *D*, allow axial sections through multiple disks to be acquired simultaneously in a single acquisition. Accurate positioning enables full depiction of the disk and its relation to the cord and CSF (*E*).

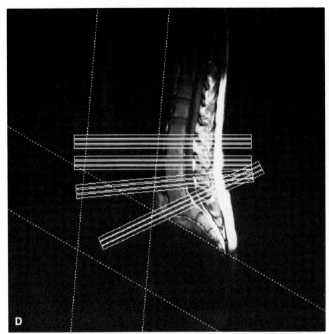

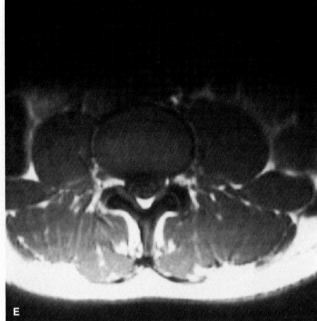

CONCLUSION

MRI has the unique ability to acquire sections in any planar orientation.

DISCUSSION

In addition to the use of nonionizing radiation, MRI has an intrinsic advantage over x-ray or CT because of its capability of obtaining images in any orientation or position of three-dimensional space without moving the patient.[1,2] Multiple planes can also be acquired simultaneously. In spine imaging, this can be particularly useful to image sections directly through the vertebral disks—for example, in the lumbar region, where they are positioned at different angles.

In MR, the magnetization is affected by the application of an RF field (excitation) only when the RF frequency matches the characteristic Larmor frequency of the magnetization. This is known as the resonance condition. Selective excitation in a specific region of tissue is accomplished by applying a gradient magnetic field that varies linearly in space during the RF transmission. Superimposed on the main external magnetic field, the gradient field causes each position along the gradient to experience a different net magnetic field. The magnetization from the tissues at each location will therefore have different Larmor frequencies, being directly proportional to the magnetic field strength according to the gyromagnetic ratio.

A spatially selective RF transmission pulse possesses a finite frequency bandwidth centered around a specific frequency.[1] During the application of a gradient field,

only one position in space will be excited that matches the center RF frequency. The width of the excited region that defines the thickness of the slice is determined by the RF frequency bandwidth. Changing the center frequency excites different spatial positions, whereas changing the bandwidth excites different thicknesses. Because this requires only the application of a gradient field during RF transmission, the patient is never required to move.

All MRI scanners contain gradient hardware that allows spatial variation of the external magnetic field in all three directions (X, Y, and Z). Therefore, to excite a sagittal section, the X gradient is applied during RF. Alternatively, the Y gradient is applied for a coronal section, the Z gradient for a transverse section. If an oblique orientation is required at any angle in three-dimensional space, two or three gradients are turned on simultaneously during RF transmission to achieve a gradient field that varies the magnetic field linearly along the respective oblique direction.[3] Furthermore, because the RF for each slice is transmitted in succession with a multislice technique, multiple planes can be acquired in the same acquisition by applying different gradients for each RF pulse.

Technical References

1. Wehrli FW. Principles of magnetic resonance. In: Stark DD, Bradley WG, eds. Magnetic resonance imaging, 2nd ed, vol 1. St. Louis, Mosby-Year Book, 1992.
2. Wood ML. Fourier imaging. In: Stark DD, Bradley WG, eds. Magnetic resonance imaging, 2nd ed, vol 1. St. Louis, Mosby-Year Book, 1992.
3. Edelman RR, Stark DD, Saini S, et al. Oblique planes of section in MR imaging. Radiology 1986;159:807–810.

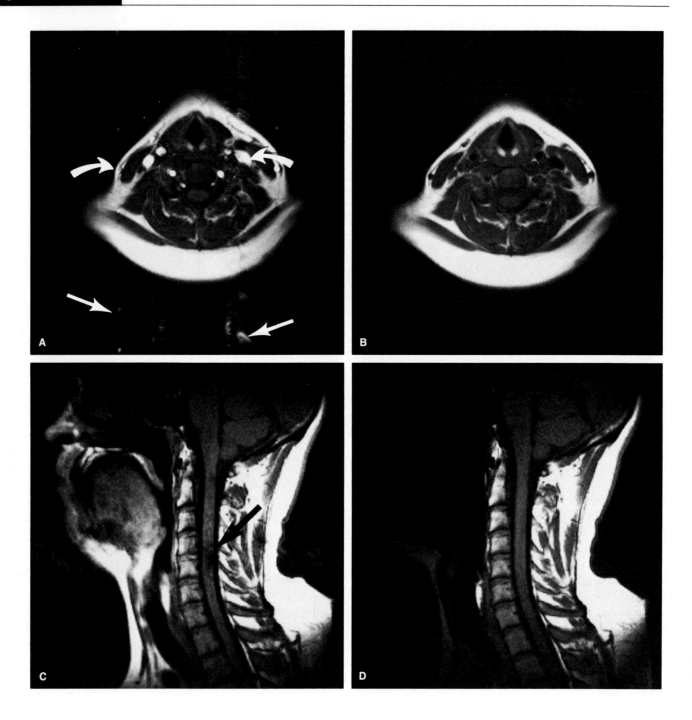

TOPIC

Spatial presaturation (SAT) for suppression of undesirable signal

FINDINGS

Use of SAT pulsing is demonstrated for the purposes of reducing flow artifacts (A and B) and bulk motion artifacts (C through F). In axial T1-weighted scans through the cervical spine (A), flow-related artifacts are observed (*straight arrows*) from arterial and venous pulsation (*curved arrows*) without SAT pulsing. Application of SAT pulses parallel to the plane of acquisition significantly reduces the artifacts without altering the image quality of the scan otherwise (B). In a midline sagittal image through the cervical spine (C), motion artifacts from high signal regions such as the chin also obscure relevant anatomic structures and may even simulate abnormalities (*arrow*). SAT pulses strategically placed perpendicularly in regions to void such signals substantially improve image quality (D). Respiratory motion of large body regions can lead to near-complete loss of detail in the spine on a coronal acquisition (E), but can be recovered with the use of SAT pulses placed over both kidneys (F).

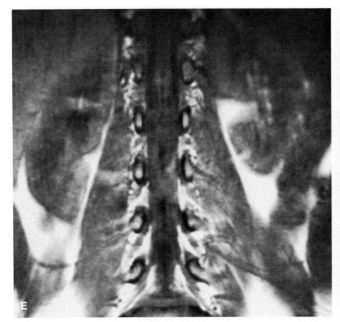

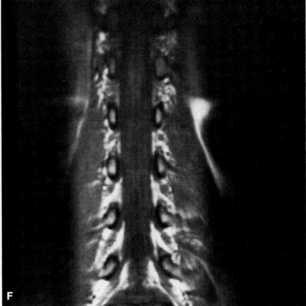

CONCLUSION

SAT pulsing that is either parallel or perpendicular to the imaging plane can substantially reduce flow- or motion-related artifacts.

DISCUSSION

Spatial presaturation[1-3] is an effective way to minimize certain types of artifacts that would otherwise obscure image details and make interpretation difficult. The concept of presaturation is to reduce the magnitude of the unwanted signal that produces the artifact. This is accomplished by preceding the RF pulsing used for imaging with a spatially selective RF pulse that is applied only in the region that produces the artifact. This is performed during each TR interval. The additional pulse prevents the growth of longitudinal magnetization by presaturating the spins in the region just before executing the imaging technique, thereby reducing the signal contribution.[4] SAT can be introduced into any MRI technique and can be applied to multiple regions within the same scan.

Flow-related artifacts are a result of blood flowing through vessels that traverse the slice.[1-3] If the signal originating from inflowing blood is suppressed, then the motion artifact associated with it will be suppressed in the image. This can be accomplished by applying presaturation pulses parallel to the plane of imaging and is sometimes referred to as flow voiding. The degree of signal and thus the flow artifact suppression achieved depends in a complex manner on the imaging technique parameters (e.g., TR and TE), the T1, velocity, and direction of the blood being saturated, the distance between the saturation plane and the imaging plane, and the delay time between the presaturation and the imaging pulses.[4] In a multislice technique, it is usually most effective in voiding flow that traverses perpendicular to the slices that are physically closest to the presaturation pulses.

SAT is also an effective method for minimizing motion (see 30.12149-8) or aliasing (see 30.12149-3) artifacts coming from signal within the imaging plane.[2] If this is suppressed by the application of SAT pulses perpendicular to the imaging plane, then the artifact associated with it will also become minimized. Although no flow may be involved, the effectiveness of the presaturation still depends in a complicated manner on the imaging technique parameters, the T1 relaxation time of the tissue being saturated, and the delay time between the presaturation and the imaging pulses.

Several disadvantages exist with the introduction of a presaturation pulse into an MR technique. Each pulse that is applied to suppress a region requires additional time. The use of many pulses will reduce the total slice capability of the technique. Presaturation pulsing will also increase the specific absorption rate and may significantly increase the RF exposure to the patient. Nevertheless, SAT can effectively reduce artifacts from unwanted tissues by suppressing their signal and may greatly enhance the diagnostic image quality.

Technical References

1. Felmlee JP, Ehman RL. Spatial presaturation: a method for suppressing flow artifacts and improving depiction of vascular anatomy in MR imaging. Radiology 1987;164:559–564.
2. Edelman RR, Atkinson DJ, Silver MS, et al. FRODO pulse sequences: a new means of eliminating motion, flow, and wraparound artifacts. Radiology 1988;166:231–236.
3. Ehman RL, Felmlee JP. Flow artifact reduction in MRI: a review of the roles of gradient moment nulling and spatial presaturation. Magn Reson Med 1990;14:293–307.
4. Mugler JP, Brookeman JR. The design of pulse sequences employing spatial presaturation for the suppression of flow artifacts. Magn Reson Med 1992;23:201–214.

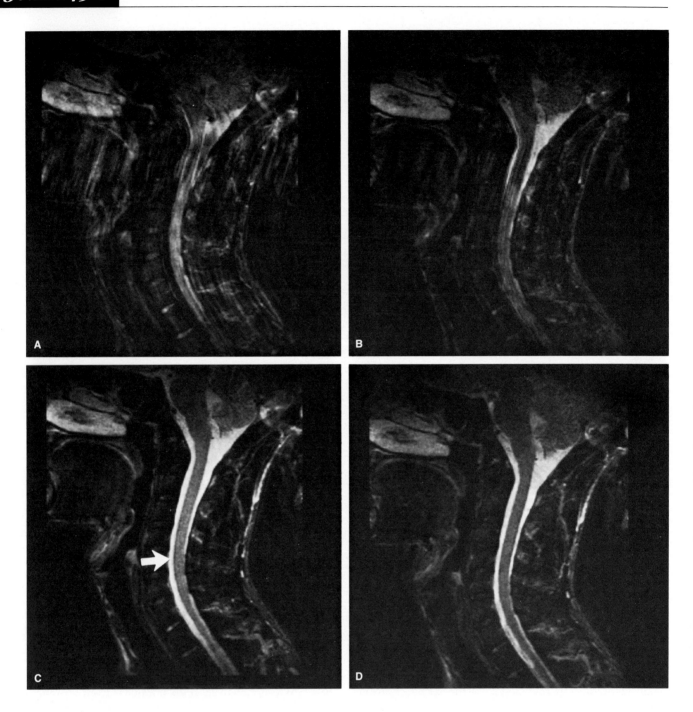

TOPIC

CSF-related artifacts, gradient moment nulling, and ECG triggering

FINDINGS

Midline sagittal T2-weighted spin echo scans through the cervical spine demonstrate CSF-related flow artifacts. Without any compensation or correction (A), severe artifacts are observed left to right in the phase-encoding direction throughout the image. Total loss of detail in the spinal cord is seen. With ECG triggering (B), improvement is seen, particularly in regions of high pulsation. Using first-order gradient moment nulling in both the frequency-encoding and slice-excitation directions (C), much of the CSF-related artifact is reduced throughout the spine, although some subtle false signal intensity variations are still observed from pulsation (arrow). With the combination of ECG triggering and gradient moment nulling (D), marked improvement in overall image quality is obtained, leading to optimal depiction of the spinal cord, CSF, and vertebral structures.

CONCLUSION

Motion artifacts such as from CSF flow and pulsation on T2-weighted studies are reduced with gradient moment nulling compensation and ECG triggering, improving overall image quality and CSF visualization.

DISCUSSION

The MRI signal from any moving tissue, such as blood, CSF, or the body, will deviate from stationary tissues and become mismapped as ghost artifacts in an image. Motion generated in any direction will always manifest itself as an artifact in the phase-encoding direction of the image in a conventional two-dimensional acquisition if it remains uncorrected (see 30.12149-9). These signal errors may constructively add to the static tissues to yield higher image intensity, or destructively cancel to create regions of signal void. In both cases, motion-related artifacts will give the image an overall splotchy appearance, obscure structures, and make interpretation difficult.

In most situations, bulk motion can be substantially minimized by proper patient set-up. However, in imaging of the spine, physiologic motion from CSF flow and pulsation is unavoidable. This particularly becomes a factor in T2-weighted studies (see 30.121411-2), where, of all tissues, CSF possesses the highest signal intensity. Because the CSF and surrounding structures such as nerve roots, cord, and vertebral bodies are of primary interest, it is crucial to implement methods to minimize the flow-related artifacts from CSF in spine MRI.

A commonly employed method to compensate for motion error in MRI is gradient moment nulling, also described as flow compensation, gradient motion rephasing, motion artifact suppression technique (MAST), and gradient motion refocusing.[1,2] By incorporating additional gradient pulses into an MRI technique, the phase error induced in moving spins can be eliminated, or nulled, without compromising the spatial encoding of static spins. As a result, signal caused by motion will be mapped in the correct position of the image along with the signal from stationary tissue, improving overall image quality.[3–5] Most MRI techniques can be implemented with gradient moment nulling.

Motion has numerous components associated with it. First-order motion pertains to velocity. Second-order motion refers to acceleration. Higher orders of motion also exist, particularly in areas of random, pulsatile, or turbulent flow. In most imaging techniques, only the first order, or moment, is nulled. Motion also tends to be multidirectional. To compensate for the error, gradient pulses must be added in each direction to gain the full advantage of artifact removal.[6] Difficulty arises in accomplishing motion reduction in T1-weighted studies, where TE is kept as short as possible, but lends itself well to T2-weighted studies, where TE tends to be long. Neverthe-less, T1-weighted scans that generate large signal from fat or regions of contrast agent uptake may benefit from gradient moment nulling if a small compromise in TE is tolerable.[7]

Pulsatile flow from either blood or CSF typically possesses higher-order components of motion. Gradient moment nulling by itself may have only limited success in correcting for pulsatility, either because of gradient hardware limitations or because the flow characteristics are too complex. If the pulsatile motion follows the cardiac cycle, the data collection can be synchronized so that each time the signal is collected, the motion error will be approximately the same. By monitoring an ECG trace, the acquisition can be triggered off the cyclic QRS complex for each phase-encoding step.[8,9] This can effectively minimize the largest contributions of motion artifact from blood or CSF that occur from one TR interval to another, but by itself cannot eliminate the phase errors that occur in a given TE interval.[3] However, by combining ECG triggering with gradient moment nulling, maximum reduction in CSF or blood flow-related artifacts can be achieved. Because triggering necessarily is synchronized to the cardiac cycle, the minimum TR that is possible using this technique is defined by the cardiac rate. Thus, triggering is used primarily in either T2-weighted studies or situations that do not require a very short TR.

Technical References

1. Pattany PM, Phillips JJ, Chiu LC, et al. Motion artifact suppression technique (MAST) for MR imaging. J Comput Assist Tomogr 1987;11:369–377.
2. Haacke EM, Lenz GW. Improving MR image quality in the presence of motion by using rephasing gradients. Am J Roentgenol 1987;148:1251–1258.
3. Elster AD. Motion artifact suppression technique (MAST) for cranial MR imaging: superiority over cardiac gating for reducing phase-shift artifacts. Am J Neuroradiol 1988; 9:671–674.
4. Colletti PM, Raval JK, Benson RC, et al. The motion artifact suppression technique (MAST) in MRI: clinical results. Magn Reson Imag 1988;6:293–299.
5. Quencer RM, Hinks RS, Pattany PH, et al. Improved MR imaging of the brain by using compensating gradients to suppress motion-induced artifacts. Am J Neuroradiol 1988; 9:431–438.
6. Duerk JL, Pattany PM. Analysis of imaging axes significance in motion artifact suppression technique (MAST): MRI of turbulent flow and motion. Magn Reson Imag 1989;7:251–263.
7. Richardson DN, Elster AD, Williams DW. Gd-DTPA-enhanced MR images: accentuation of vascular pulsation artifacts and correction by using gradient-moment nulling (MAST). Am J Neuroradiol 1990;11:209–210.
8. Lanzer P, Barta C, Botvinik EH, et al. ECG-synchronized cardiac MR imaging: method and evaluation. Radiology 1985; 155:681–686.
9. Njemanze PC, Beck OJ. MR-gated intracranial CSF dynamics: evaluation of CSF pulsatile flow. Am J Neuroradiol 1989; 10:77–80.

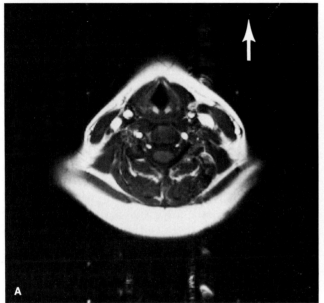

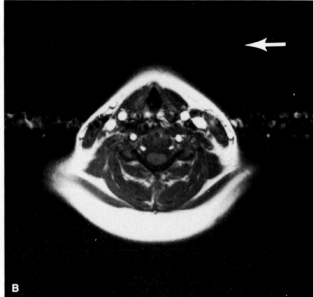

TOPIC

Phase- and frequency-encoding direction

FINDINGS

Phase- and frequency-encoding direction as it relates to flow and motion artifacts is shown in axial T1-weighted spin echo images of the cervical spine (*A and B*). Without any correction, significant pulsation artifacts are observed in the phase-encoding direction (*arrows*) across the entire image. Phase encoding can be acquired from top to bottom (*A*) or from left to right (*B*). The orientation of encoding is selected to reduce motion-related artifacts in regions of interest.

CONCLUSION

Motion and flow artifacts occur in the phase-encoding direction of the image. Swapping the phase- and frequency-encoding direction changes the direction of the artifact accordingly.

DISCUSSION

The MRI signal possesses three types of information: magnitude, frequency, and phase. In most conventional MR imaging techniques, the MR image is normally acquired in such a manner that the signal magnitude becomes mapped as pixel intensity, and the phase and frequency information determines where the pixel is

located in the image. In other words, one direction defines a phase axis, the other a frequency axis.

To generate a two-dimensional image, the signal must be encoded with a defined range of frequencies and phases. In conventional techniques, encoding of all the frequencies can be accomplished in a single pass each time a signal is collected, but only one piece of phase information is possible. Therefore, to collect enough information to spatially encode the full range of phases, the acquisition must be repeated (at a rate of TR, the repetition time), each time encoded with the full range of frequency information but with a different piece of phase information until all the phase information is obtained to map the full image. The vast majority of MRI techniques acquire data in this manner, called spin-warp imaging.

Motion induces changes in the MR signal if it is not compensated for or corrected in some way (see 30.12149-8).[1] Because frequency encoding occurs over a very short period of time, typically milliseconds, little change due to motion is detected. However, phase encoding is repeated at every TR interval and is collected over the entire scan time, which may span minutes. Because of this, each data acquisition of phase encoding from TR to TR will possess an error due to unpredictable motion. When the image is reconstructed, the signal associated with the motion will spread across the entire direction of phase encoding in the image. In other words, signal errors due to motion will cause the image to be mismapped in the phase-encoding direction, thereby obscuring anatomic structures in that respective direction. Motion occurs in all directions and will inevitably induce an error in the signal. Therefore, motion-related signal will be mismapped in the phase-encoding direction of the image regardless of its direction.[2]

Phase and frequency encoding of the spatial signal information is accomplished with linearly varying magnetic field gradients in the respective physical directions. Similar to slice excitation (see 30.12149-6), they can be applied in any direction and in any combination. Therefore, the physical direction that is defined as phase encoding that may contain artifacts due to motion can be swapped with the physical direction that is frequency encoding so that the artifacts become rotated by 90° in the image. Anticipating motion or flow in the acquisition enables the strategic decision as to which direction is to be phase-encoded with the associated artifacts. Doing so will not reduce the artifacts, but it may lead to their being rotated away from regions of interest, thereby improving the diagnostic utility of the image.

Knowledge of which direction is the phase and which is the frequency axis may be important in interpreting the results.[3] Motion- and flow-related artifacts are depicted in the phase-encoding direction, but the frequency-encoding direction also possesses a unique artifact. Chemical shift pixel misregistration (see 30.12149-2) is caused by a difference between the Larmor frequencies of lipids and water. This artifact will occur only in the frequency-encoding direction of the image. If the encoding is swapped, chemical shift pixel errors will rotate accordingly.

Technical References

1. Wood ML, Ehman RL. Effects of motion in MR imaging. In: Stark DD, Bradley WG, eds. Magnetic resonance imaging, 2nd ed, vol 1. St. Louis, Mosby-Year Book, 1992.
2. Wood ML, Henkelman RM. MR image artifacts from periodic motion. Med Phys 1985;12:143–151.
3. Thickman D, Rubinstein R, Askenase A, et al. Effect of phase-encoding direction upon MRI quality of the heart. Magn Reson Med 1988;6:390–396.

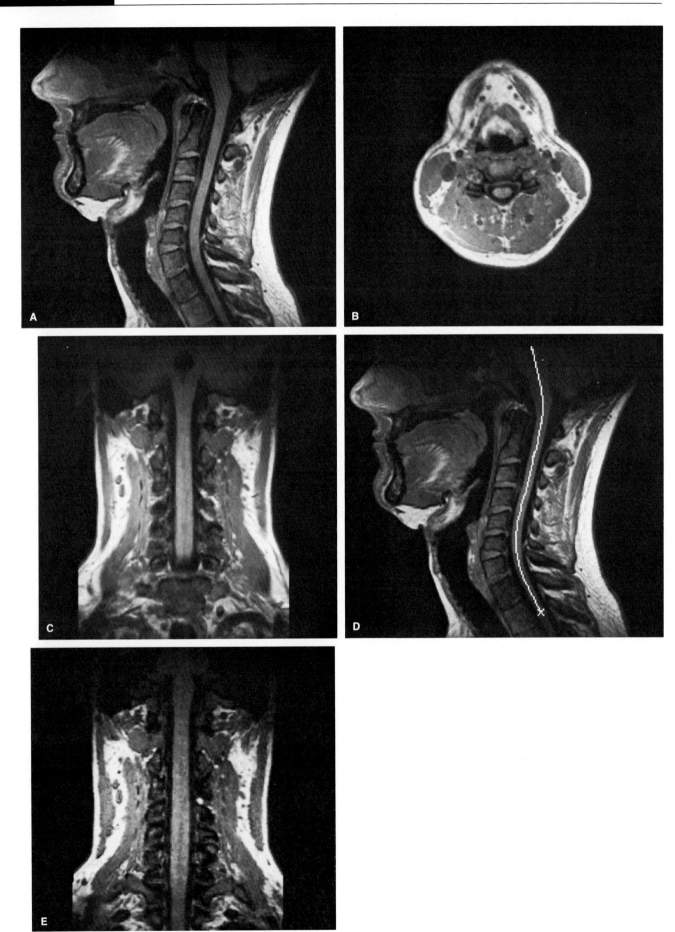

TOPIC

Three-dimensional imaging and multiplanar reformatting (MPR)

FINDINGS

Three-dimensional T1-weighted images of the cervical spine were acquired in the sagittal orientation with 1-mm isotropic resolution (*A*). MPR allows the display of axial (*B*), coronal (*C*), or oblique sections (*images not shown*) for better symmetry or visualization of structures. Isotropic acquisition maintains spatial resolution in all directions. Free curvilinear MPR is also demonstrated along the curve drawn along the axis of the spinal cord (*D*) and displayed in (*E*). This allows projection of the complete spinal cord, which is otherwise not possible to display on planar coronal reformatting (*C*).

CONCLUSION

Three-dimensional imaging allows MPR in any plane, including nonrectilinear formats for complete depiction of curved structures.

DISCUSSION

The primary advantage of three-dimensional MRI is its capability of attaining high spatial resolution in the slice direction without slice gaps or information loss. In conventional multislice two-dimensional MRI, each slice is a separate and independent excitation volume, with the image pixels representing the projected sum of the signals through the entire section thickness. This leads to slice-to-slice interference that prevents contiguous cuts from being obtained and limits the ability to acquire thin sections, resulting in partial voluming effects of small structures (see 30.12149-4).

The main constraint on three-dimensional MRI is the need for very rapid data acquisition. With the introduction of gradient echo techniques that allow rapid acquisition with a very short TR, large-volume three-dimensional image data sets can be acquired in reasonable scan times in a variety of ways with both T1- and T2-related contrast.[1-3]

In three-dimensional MRI, the third dimension becomes spatially phase-encoded. When reconstructed, the sections or partitions uniquely represent true contiguity. Partition thicknesses can routinely be as thin as the in-plane dimensions of the pixels. Isotropic encoding yields voxels of equal dimensions on all three sides and is primarily limited by signal-to-noise ratio (S/N) issues. To achieve reasonable imaging times, however, three-dimensional MRI requires a very short TR technique that generates good contrast and sufficient S/N. This currently restricts it to gradient echo methods using small RF flip angles (see 30.121412-1 and 30.121412-2) and therefore suffers the same potential artifacts as its two-dimensional counterpart (see 30.121412-3).

Because of its true contiguity and high resolution in the third dimension, three-dimensional imaging allows MPR without a loss in spatial resolution from thick slices or poor image quality from information voids between sections. With the appropriate post-processing capabilities, any plane through space can be visualized.[4-7] Free formatting of nonlinear planes can also be routinely achieved, which allows, for example, the complete visualization of the spinal cord. Partition averaging also allows multiple sections to be combined, which yields slightly thicker slice representations for higher S/N and superior image quality. Furthermore, volume and surface rendering of structures can be processed for three-dimensional visualization.[5-7] These image processing capabilities may further aid in diagnosis as well as treatment and surgical planning.

Technical References

1. Frahm J, Haase A, Matthaei D. Rapid 3D MR imaging using the FLASH technique. J Comput Assist Tomogr 1986; 10:363–368.
2. Runge VM, Kirsch JE, Thomas GS, Mugler JP. Clinical comparison of 3D MP-RAGE and FLASH techniques for MR imaging of the head. J Magn Reson Imag 1991;1:493–500.
3. Menick BJ, Bobman SA, Listerud J, Atlas SW. Thin-section, 3D Fourier transform, steady-state free precession MR imaging of the brain. Radiology 1992;183:369–377.
4. Sherry CS, Harms SE, McCroskey WK. Spinal MR imaging: multiplanar representation from a single high-resolution 3D acquisition. J Comput Assist Tomogr 1987;11:859–862.
5. Runge VM, Wood ML, Kaufman DM, et al. FLASH: clinical 3D MRI. Radiographics 1988;8:947–965.
6. Runge VM, Gelblum DY, Wood ML. 3D imaging of the CNS. Neuroradiol 1990;32:356–366.
7. Bomans M, Hohne K-H, Laub G, et al. Improvement of 3D acquisition and visualization in MRI. Magn Reson Imag 1991;9:597–609.

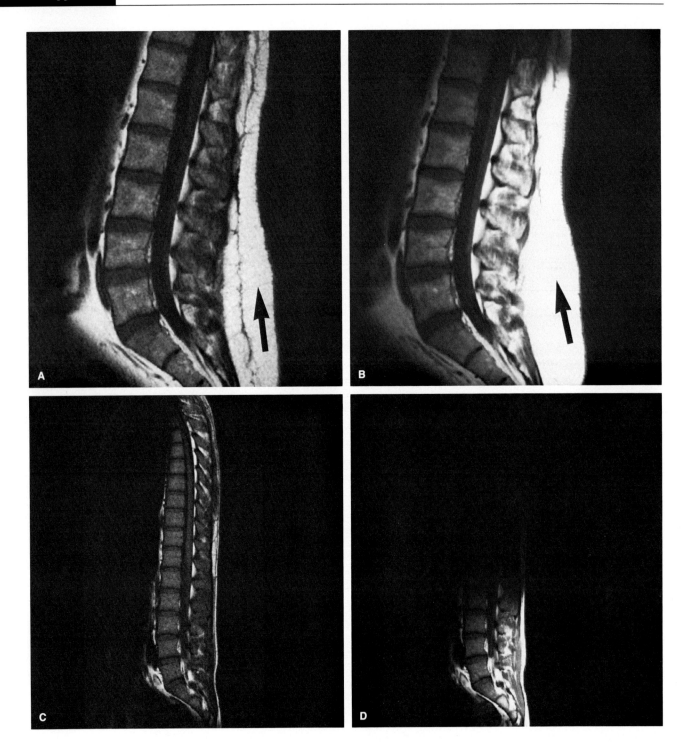

TOPIC

Coils and sensitivity

FINDINGS

Midline sagittal T1-weighted spin echo images through the spine are compared using a whole-body RF coil (transmitting and receiving) and a localized surface RF coil (receive only). Image uniformity is observed with the whole-body coil (*A*) at the expense of signal-to-noise ratio (S/N) due to reduced sensitivity. The surface coil image of the same anatomic region (*B*) shows significantly improved image quality, but with nonuniform signal intensity from regions in close proximity to the coil (*arrow*). A large whole-body coil can image the entire length of the spine in a single acquisition (*C*), whereas a surface coil can acquire information only in localized regions, typically covering only the lumbar (*D*), thoracic (*E*), or cervicothoracic (*F*) spine in any given acquisition.

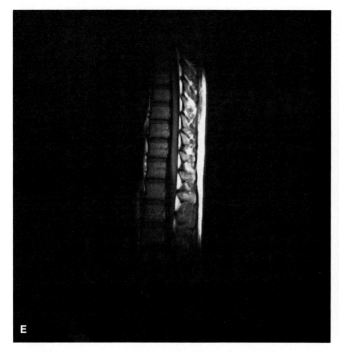

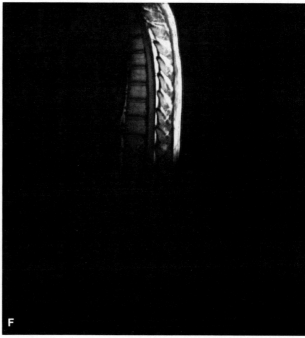

CONCLUSION

A whole-body RF coil provides uniformity and coverage at the expense of sensitivity; a surface coil is nonuniform and highly localized but provides much greater sensitivity.

DISCUSSION

When the body is placed in a static external magnetic field, it becomes magnetized. More specifically, bulk magnetization that points in the direction of the external field, known by convention as the B_0 field, is created in the tissues for all nuclei that possess a dipole moment, such as hydrogen. In this state of thermal equilibrium, nothing happens. Therefore, no information about the body and its hydrogen content can be detected.

Affecting the position of the bulk magnetization is possible only by creating a second magnetic field, known as the B_1 field, perpendicular to the main external field. Maximum efficiency in tilting the bulk magnetization away from the direction of B_0 by B_1 occurs when the frequency of the B_1 field equals the Larmor frequency of the magnetization. For hydrogen at a B_0 field strength of 1.5 Tesla, this is about 63 MHz, which lies in the RF range of the electromagnetic spectrum. Therefore, B_1 is sometimes referred to as the RF field, and the pulsing of such a field constitutes RF pulsing. The amount that the magnetization tilts is known as the RF flip angle.

When the bulk magnetization tilts away from B_0, it becomes possible to observe it. The magnitude of the detected signal will be proportional to the amount of bulk magnetization that exists perpendicular to the direction of B_0. This is known as the transverse component of the bulk magnetization. The remaining longitudinal component that points in the direction of B_0 is undetectable, just as it was during thermal equilibrium, when all the magnetization pointed in the direction of B_0.

RF antenna coils are used both to generate a B_1 field and to detect the transverse magnetization. A conducting wire that has electrical current running through it creates a magnetic field around it. Similarly, the same wire will create an electrical current through it when it experiences a magnetic field around it. RF coils are simply wire configurations that generate magnetic fields by transmitting current (the B_1 field) and sense magnetic fields by receiving current (the transverse magnetization coming from the body). The ability, or sensitivity, of a coil to create a B_1 field or detect the magnetization and generate a current from it is primarily based on its geometry and size. Large coils characteristically sense magnetization far from the coil, but with poor sensitivity. On the other hand, small coils can only pick up signal near the coil, but with high sensitivity. The MR signal that ultimately makes up the pixel intensities in a reconstructed image is based on the intensity of the voltage coming from the current picked up by the coil.

Several coils with a variety of geometric configurations are available for different clinical applications with most whole-body MR imaging systems. In most situations in imaging, a spatially uniform RF excitation is necessary to produce spatially consistent tissue contrast. This requires a transmitting coil that generates a uniform B_1

field. Large body coils have been designed to produce homogeneous B_1 fields that blanket large regions of the body but with relatively poor sensitivity, whereas smaller head coils that can be positioned closer to the tissues for greater sensitivity are usually used to create uniform B_1 fields over smaller regions.

S/N is a crucial factor in producing good image quality and diagnostically useful information, and is greatly influenced by coil sensitivity. Therefore, the type of coil used for a given application can at times be the most important factor in optimizing an MRI protocol. Imaging the spine requires thin slices with high spatial resolution for good diagnosis, both of which lead to very low inherent S/N. A uniform B_1 field is required for RF excitation, so a large body coil must be used for transmission. If the same coil is used for receiving the signal, very poor image quality would result due to the intrinsically low sensitivity of the large body coil.

Surface coils, which are much smaller than a body coil, have been specially designed to increase coil sensitivity if the regions of interest are near the surface of the coil.[1–3] In the case of the spine, surface coils are ideal for receiving the signal. With such a coil, the S/N can be substantially increased in the region of the spine, thereby resulting in good image quality even when thin slices and high resolution are demanded. Surface coils are characteristically one-sided and produce a very nonuniform area of sensitivity. As a result, they are rarely used as transmission coils, and as receivers produce images with a large degree of pixel intensity fall-off away from the location of the coil.[3]

Technical References

1. Axel L. Surface coil MRI. J Comput Assist Tomogr 1984; 8:381–384.
2. Schenck JF, Foster TH, Henkes JL, et al. High-field surface coil MR imaging of localized anatomy. Am J Neuroradiol 1985;6:181–186.
3. Fisher MR, Barker B, Amparo EG, et al. MR imaging using specialized coils. Radiology 1985;157:443–447.

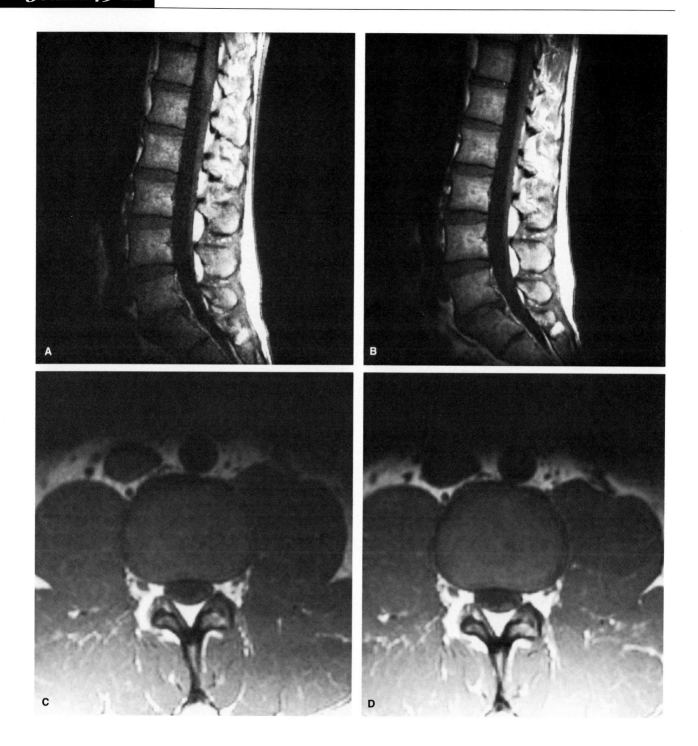

TOPIC

Linearly and circularly polarized coils

FINDINGS

Sagittal (*A and B*) and axial (*C and D*) T1-weighted images through the lumbar spine demonstrate image quality differences between scans obtained with linearly polarized (LP) and circularly polarized (CP) surface coils.

Although the extent of the volume of sensitivity is very similar, images acquired with an LP coil (*A and C*) are inferior to those acquired with a CP coil (*B and D*). Intrinsic contrast is identical, but LP coils have reduced sensitivity compared with CP coils, yielding images with less signal-to-noise ratio (S/N) and poorer image quality.

CONCLUSION

CP surface coils have superior sensitivity and S/N compared with LP coils of similar configuration.

DISCUSSION

In MRI of the spine, the acquisition of thin sections at high spatial resolution is necessary for accurate diagnosis. Such constraints result in poor overall S/N. Image quality can be improved by increasing the number of acquisitions (see 30.12149-5), but at the expense of scan time. Surface coils provide significant increases in S/N due to their enhanced sensitivity (see 30.12149-11). Because the areas of interest in the spine are close to the surface of the body, surface coils can greatly improve the image quality in spine applications. These specially designed coils are characteristically one-sided and produce a very nonuniform area of sensitivity. As a result, they are rarely used as transmission coils, and as receivers produce images with a large degree of pixel intensity fall-off away from the location of the coil. However, if the region of interest is in the vicinity of the coil, extremely high S/N can be achieved.

The signals detected by the coil and ultimately converted into pixel intensities in the image are based on the transverse component of the magnetization. The coil senses this transverse magnetization as a magnetic field that induces a current in the coil, the voltage of which makes up the MR signal. As with any electromagnetic field, the magnetization is composed of two more fundamental fields oriented 90° from each other in the transverse plane, and the total field is considered to be circularly polarized.

In its simplest form, the surface coil is a linearly polarized antenna.[1] In other words, it can sense only one of the two components of the circularly polarized transverse magnetization. Although the surface coil itself improves S/N due to its geometric configuration, having a linearly polarized sensitivity means that it does not take advantage of sensing the total transverse magnetization available to it. Improvements in design are possible that enable surface coils to be circularly polarized in their sensitivity, capable of detecting both components of the transverse magnetization simultaneously. Therefore, a circularly polarized surface coil has not only the S/N enhancement based on its geometry, but also has an additional 40% improvement over a linearly polarized surface coil of similar configuration.[1,2] In general, such coils are more difficult to design and construct and are substantially more expensive to build than linearly polarized coils. As a result, they are not as readily available commercially.

Technical References

1. Glover GH, Hayes CE, Pelc N, et al. Comparison of linear and circular polarization for MRI. J Magn Res 1985;64:255.
2. Chen CN, Hoult DI, Sank VJ. Quadrature detection coils: a further $\sqrt{2}$ improvement in sensitivity. J Magn Res 1983;54:324.

Magnetic Resonance Imaging of the Spine, by Val M. Runge,
Mark H. Awh, Donald F. Bittner, and John E. Kirsch.
J.B. Lippincott Company, Philadelphia © 1995.

CHAPTER
TWO

Cervical Spine

Val M. Runge
Mark H. Awh
Donald F. Bittner

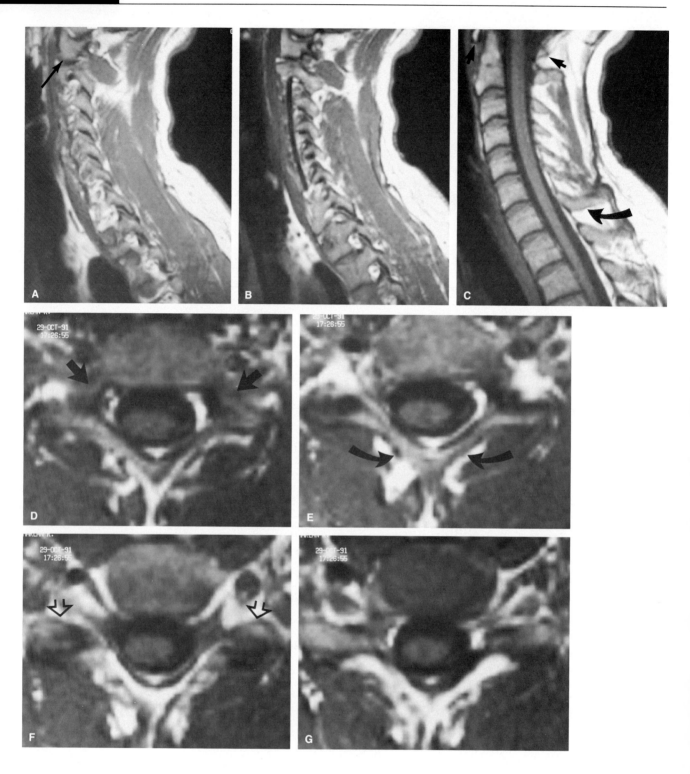

HISTORY

Noncontributory

FINDINGS

Sagittal T1-weighted images are presented from lateral to medial, depicting (A) the facet joints, (B) the neural for-amina, and (C) the central spinal canal. On A, the lateral mass of C1 (*arrow*) is seen at the top of the image, with the superior and inferior articular processes of C2–7 well depicted in sequence below. On B, the vertebral artery is seen passing through the foramen transversarium of the cervical vertebrae. The neural foramina are poorly visualized due to their oblique orientation. On C, the an-terior and posterior arches of C1 (*arrows*) are seen at the top of the image, with the scan encompassing C1 to T2. The spinal cord is of intermediate signal intensity, sur-

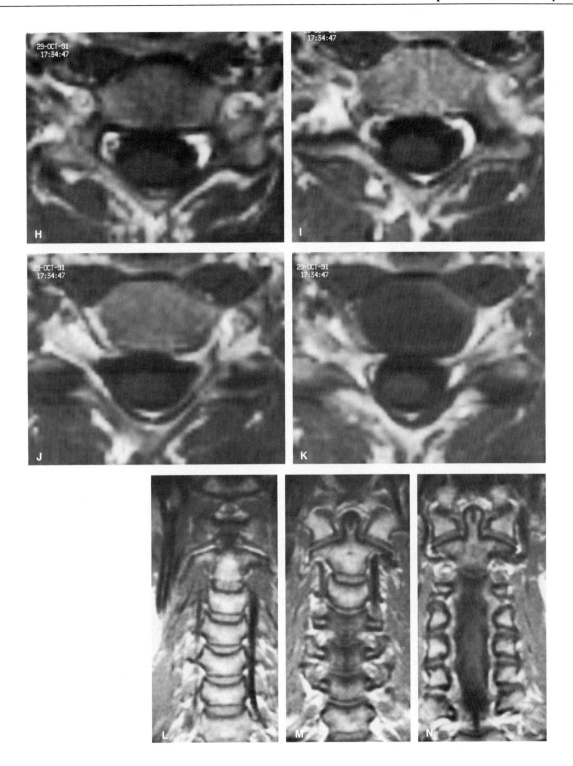

rounded by low-signal-intensity cerebrospinal fluid (CSF). The intervertebral disks are also of intermediate signal intensity. Marrow is of slightly higher signal intensity than the cord and intervertebral disks, with the spinous processes (*curved arrow,* spinous process of C7) well differentiated from surrounding fat within the posterior soft tissues.

Four adjacent axial sections (3-mm slice thickness) are presented from the T1-weighted scans both before (*D through G*) and after (*H through K*) IV contrast administration. *D* is through the superior C5 vertebral body, *E* is through the middle of the vertebral body, *F* is through the inferior body, and *G* is through the C5–6 disk. *H* through *K* correspond in position to *D* through *G*. The pedicles (*arrows*) are seen in *D*, the lamina (*curved arrows*) in *E*, and the facets (*open arrows*) in *F*. The level

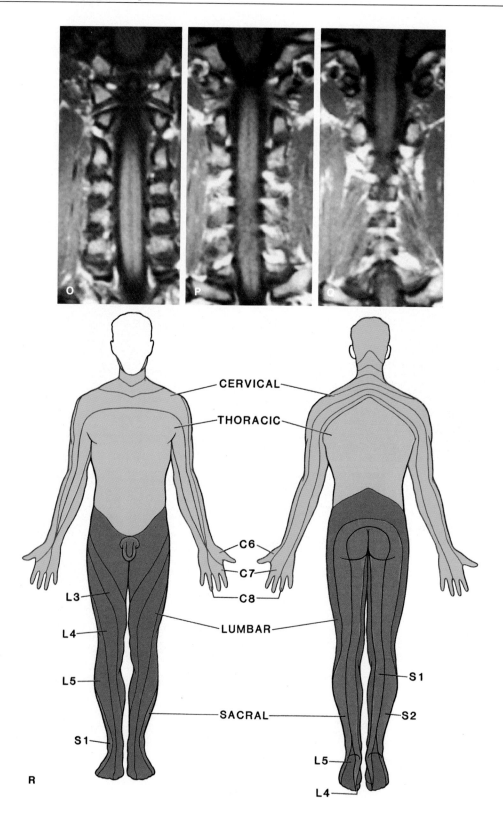

of the intervertebral disk (*G*) can be identified due to the lower signal intensity of disk material as compared to vertebral body marrow. Segments of the dorsal and ventral nerve roots can be seen within the subarachnoid space in *D* and *E*. After contrast, the most prominent change is noted at the level of the neural foramen (*J and*

K). Enhancement of the epidural venous plexus markedly improves visualization of the bony margins of the foramina. There is also slight improvement of the disk–thecal sac interface after contrast.

Six adjacent coronal sections (3-mm slice thickness) are presented in an anterior to posterior sequence from an unenhanced T1-weighted scan (*L through Q*). In *L*, the most anterior section (obtained through the midsection of the C4–6 vertebral bodies), the left vertebral artery is well seen within the foramen transversarium. In *M* and *N*, the tip of the odontoid is identified. In *N* and *O*, the articulation between the inferior facets of C1 (atlas) and the superior facets of C2 (axis) is best depicted. The cord in *O* and *P* has low signal intensity centrally, due to partial volume imaging of central gray matter. The cerebellar tonsils are seen lying in a normal relationship relative to the skull base in *Q*.

DIAGNOSIS

Normal cervical spine—T1-weighted spin echo imaging

DISCUSSION

T1-weighted spin echo images of the cervical spine can be obtained in a relatively short scan time with both high signal-to-noise ratio and high spatial resolution. The intrinsic contrast between fat, soft tissues, and fluid is high, with these three entities encompassing the range of signal intensity from high (white) to low (black). T1-weighted spin echo images are thus of great clinical utility for the detection of structural abnormalities, marrow infiltration (with normal marrow of high signal intensity due to its fat content), and degenerative disease, the latter including both disk herniation and cervical spondylosis. Gadolinium chelates, used intravenously as contrast agents, affect principally the spin-lattice relaxation time (T1). Contrast enhancement is thus best evaluated on T1-weighted spin echo scans.

There is excellent depiction of the vertebral elements and the intervertebral disks on T1-weighted scans. The spinal cord is also well evaluated on T1-weighted scans, in particular with regard to size, compression or deformity, and intrinsic structural abnormalities. In the cervical region, a single number cannot be used as the reference for normal in the evaluation of the spinal cord size.[1] Measurements should be compared to the normal range established for each anatomic level. Mean values for anteroposterior and transverse dimensions at C2 are 9 mm × 12 mm, at C4 are 9 mm × 14 mm, and at C7 are 7 mm × 11 mm. There is a slight increase in the cervical cord size normally from C4 to C6.

Dorsal and ventral nerve roots can be consistently identified on high-quality axial T1-weighted images traversing the subarachnoid space.[2] The epidural venous plexus is prominent in the cervical spinal canal, with intravenous administration of a gadolinium chelate providing enhancement. Contrast injection can thus improve both the depiction of the neural foramina and visualization of the disk–thecal sac interface.[3] Oblique plane imaging has also been suggested for improved depiction of nerve roots within their respective foramina in the cervical spine.

Anatomic Correlate

A dermatome is that anatomic area supplied by a single spinal nerve. A schematic of dermal segmentation (adapted from F. H. Netter) is presented in *R*. Although there is substantial variability and overlap of dermatomes, knowledge of their distribution aids in localization of lesions affecting the spinal cord and nerves. The dermatomes of the hand and foot deserve special attention, with the hand innervated by C6 (thumb), C7 (middle finger), and C8 (little finger) and the foot innervated by L4 (medial big toe), L5 (midfoot), and S1 (little toe).

Clinical References

1. Sherman JL, Nassaux PY, Citrin CM. Measurements of the normal cervical spinal cord on MR imaging. AJNR 1990; 11:369–372.
2. Flannigan BD, Lufkin RB, McGlade C, et al. MR imaging of the cervical spine: neurovascular anatomy. AJR 1987;148: 785–790.
3. Czervionke LF, Daniels DL, Ho PSP, et al. Cervical neural foramina: correlative anatomic and MR imaging study. Radiology 1988;169:753–759.

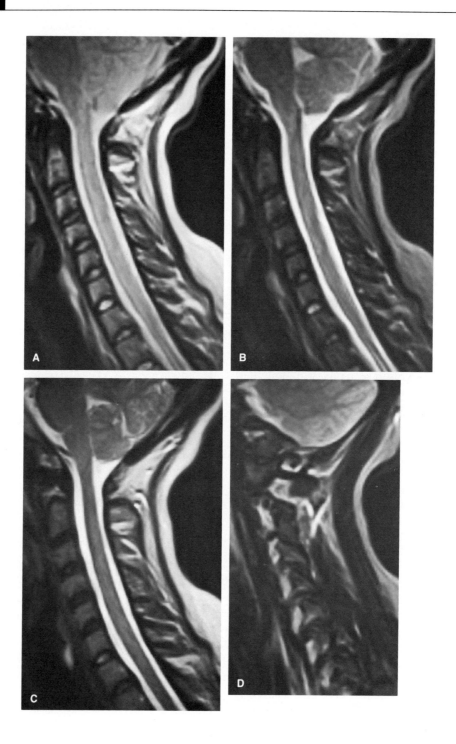

HISTORY

Normal volunteer

FINDINGS

On T2-weighted spin echo images, whether acquired with conventional or newer "fast" techniques, cerebrospinal fluid (CSF) and hydrated disks are high signal in-tensity, the spinal cord and most soft tissue structures are intermediate signal intensity, and vertebral body marrow is intermediate to low signal intensity. Since the clinical introduction of cervical spine imaging (*A and B*), dual spin echo ECG or pulse-triggered techniques have been the mainstay for T2-weighted imaging. This approach is slowly being replaced by (*C*) fast or turbo-spin echo techniques, which can be acquired in a shorter scan time and are less susceptible to motion artifacts, especially from CSF pulsation. For example, the (*A*) 45 and (*B*) 90 msec

TE conventional scan required about three times as long to acquire as the (*C*) 90 msec fast scan (9 versus 3 minutes), yet the fast scan demonstrates superior image quality. CSF pulsation artifacts are present on the second echo of the conventional spin echo exam, despite excellent triggering, and are conspicuously absent on the fast spin echo exam. Close inspection of midline T2-weighted sagittal images continues to be crucial for clinical diagnosis, with attention to cord/CSF and spinal canal/CSF interfaces. However, scrutiny of (*D*) off-midline sections is also warranted. Particular attention should be paid laterally to the soft tissues, facet joints, and marrow.

DIAGNOSIS

Normal cervical spine—T2-weighted spin echo imaging

DISCUSSION

Spinal cord abnormalities, in particular edema, gliosis, demyelination, and neoplasia, are best evaluated on T2-weighted images.[1] For cord tumors as well as some other lesions, T1-weighted images, particularly with contrast enhancement, are also critical. Compromise of the thecal sac, whether bony or soft tissue in origin, is also well depicted on T2-weighted images.

On conventional T2-weighted spin echo imaging, the effects of CSF pulsation are minimized in part by the use of gradient moment refocusing (or nulling), also commonly referred to as flow compensation. This software technique supplements pulse or ECG triggering, lessening the effect of motion that occurs during the time interval TE. A coronal saturation slab or pulse, applied to the anterior soft tissues, is employed with both conventional and fast T2-weighted spin echo techniques, as previously described with T1-weighted techniques, to decrease motion artifacts that might originate from anterior structures.

MR Technique

Conventional T2-weighted spin echo images of the cervical spine are typically acquired with ECG or pulse triggering.[2] A marked improvement in image quality and signal-to-noise ratio is achieved by eliminating spatially mismapped signal from CSF. Triggering can be achieved using either the peripheral pulse or ECG; both approaches are used clinically. T2-weighted fast spin echo images are much less susceptible to image degradation from CSF motion, due to both the short inter-echo interval and even echo rephasing. Thus, fast spin echo images are usually not triggered.

Pitfalls in Image Interpretation

Truncation artifacts (Gibb phenomenon) can be particularly prominent on sagittal T2-weighted images, resulting in an artifactual bright band overlying the cord.[3] The same phenomenon is responsible for edge enhancement at the CSF–cord interface, reducing the apparent cord dimensions. Truncation artifacts are minimized most effectively by increasing the acquisition matrix—for example, by using 256 as opposed to 128 phase-encoding steps.

Clinical References

1. Czervionke LF, Daniels DL. Cervical spine anatomy and pathologic processes: applications of new MR imaging techniques. Radiol Clin North Am 1988;26:921–947.
2. Enzmann DR, Rubin JB, Wright A. Use of CSF gating to improve T2-weighted images; part I: the spinal cord. Radiology 1987;162:763–767.
3. Czervionke LF, Czervionke JM, Daniels DL, Haughton VM. Characteristic features of MR truncation artifacts. AJR 1988;151:1219–1228.

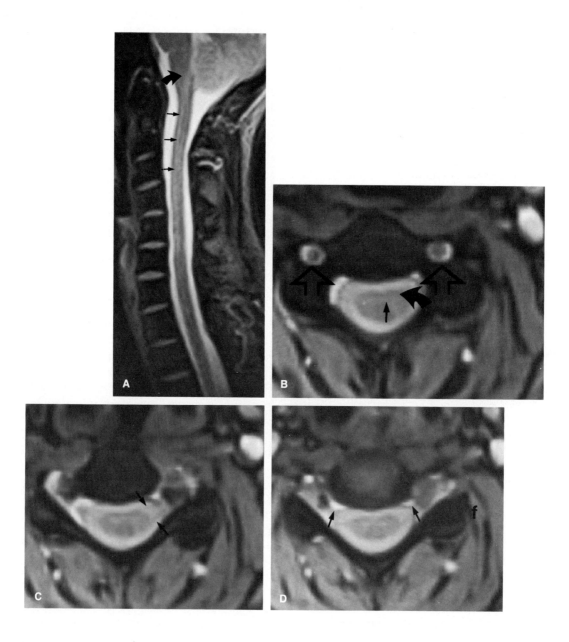

HISTORY

Normal volunteer

FINDINGS

The midline sagittal T2-weighted section (A) from a two-dimensional FLASH gradient echo scan (TR/TE/tip angle = 300/18/10°, one acquisition, 256 × 256 matrix, 4-mm slice thickness, 1 minute scan time) depicts vertebral body marrow as low signal intensity, due to magnetic susceptibility effects, and intervertebral disks and cerebrospinal fluid (CSF) as high signal intensity, due to free water content. A subtle hyperintense line is seen within the cord substance, starting at the obex (*curved arrow*) and continuing within the anterior portion of the cord (*arrows*) in the cervical region. This may represent visualization of normal gray matter, although a truncation artifact would be similar in appearance.

Three axial T2-weighted gradient echo images (*B through D*) from a two-dimensional FISP scan (TR/TE/tip angle = 250/12/20°, four acquisitions, 256 × 256 matrix, 4-mm slice thickness, 30% interslice gap, rectangular field of view, 2 minutes scan time) are presented from the mid-C4 level to the C4–5 interspace. In these axial images, the distinction between gray (*arrow in B*) and white (*curved arrow in B*) matter within the cord is more clearly seen. Gray matter is visualized as a central butterfly or H-shaped region of slight hyperintensity. In *B*, the vertebral arteries (*open arrows*) are noted within their respective foramina in the transverse processes of the fourth cervical vertebral body. In *C*, at the level of the vertebral lamina, a faint ghost of the ventral and dorsal nerve roots (*arrows*) can be seen against the background of high-signal-intensity CSF. In *D*, at the level of the facet joints (*f*) and intervertebral disk (the latter with slight hyperintensity), epidural venous plexus (*arrows*) within the neural foramina appears hyperintense. The interface between the thecal sac and surrounding structures is well seen at all levels. The black lines within the posterior soft tissue structures are artifactual, with signal cancellation occurring at fat–water interfaces due to the TE used.

DIAGNOSIS

Normal cervical spine—gradient echo imaging

DISCUSSION

Gradient echo imaging can be used in both the sagittal and axial planes to provide myelographic-like images with hyperintense CSF.[1] The TR typically chosen is between 250 and 300 msec ("long" for gradient echo techniques); thus, both spoiled (FLASH, SP-GRASS) and rephased (FISP, GRASS) sequences yield similar results. This assumes that imaging is performed using multislice techniques, although an alternative approach is to acquire sequential single-slice images with a short TR (20 to 30 msec). In clinical practice, T2-weighted spin echo techniques have proven superior in the sagittal plane, with gradient echo imaging routinely used only in the axial plane. A compromise exists in the choice of tip angle: smaller values (10° to 15°) provide greater contrast between CSF and the spinal cord but lower signal-to-noise ratio. The choice of tip angle is also influenced by TR and the imaging plane (sagittal versus axial).

The central gray matter of the spinal cord, which can be seen on MR in both the axial and sagittal planes, is best visualized with gradient echo techniques.[2] These may be either proton density or T2 weighted. The use of a high-resolution acquisition matrix (256×256 or greater) minimizes truncation artifacts, which can limit gray/white matter differentiation and produce a central linear artifact (mimicking gray matter) on sagittal images. Gray matter can also be visualized on T1- and T2-weighted spin echo images, although the differentiation of gray and white matter is typically poor. Scan times are longer than with gradient echo imaging.

Pitfalls in Image Interpretation

Although gradient echo techniques are excellent for evaluating foraminal size (and specifically encroachment due to degenerative disease), soft tissue abnormalities within the foramen can be missed. These are best evaluated with T1-weighted spin echo techniques. Gradient echo sequences may also artifactually accentuate canal and foraminal narrowing, particularly when a longer TE is used, due to magnetic susceptibility effects.

Clinical References

1. Enzmann DR, Rubin JB, Wright A. Cervical spine MR imaging: generating high-signal CSF in sagittal and axial images. Radiology 1987;163:233-238.
2. Czervionke LF, Daniels DL, Ho PSP, et al. The MR appearance of gray and white matter in the cervical spinal cord. AJNR 1988;9:557-562.

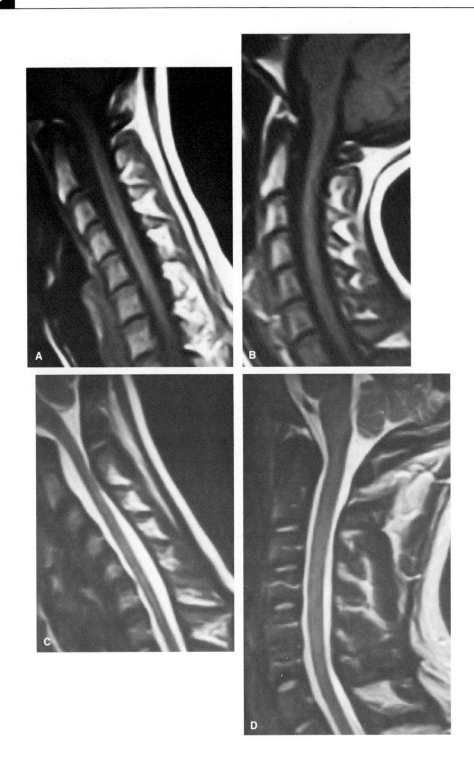

HISTORY

Normal volunteer

FINDINGS

Two views of the cervical spine are presented, each with (*A and B*) T1-weighted and (*C and D*) T2-weighted scan techniques. The neck has been placed in flexion in *A* and *C* and in extension in *B* and *D*. The parameters for the T1-weighted scans were TR/TE = 200/15, with a 128 (phase-encoding steps) × 256 (read-out steps) matrix, giving an acquisition time of 29 seconds. A fast spin echo technique was used for the T2-weighted scans with the parameters TR/TE = 3000/90, with a 196 × 256 matrix giving an acquisition time of 1 minute 23 seconds. The slice thickness was 6 mm. A specialized neck coil with both anterior and posterior elements was used for signal reception.

DIAGNOSIS

Flexion and extension views

DISCUSSION

Although cervical spine MR images are typically acquired with the neck in neutral position, views can also be obtained in flexion and extension. The use of a dedicated neck coil, with both anterior and posterior components, unfortunately limits the degree of flexion and extension that can be achieved. If a greater range of motion is desired, then imaging must be performed with the body coil as a receiver, compromising image quality due to lower signal-to-noise ratio.

Flexion and extension views can demonstrate spinal cord compression not seen with the cervical spine in neutral position. Such views are particularly useful in the evaluation of patients with rheumatoid arthritis.[1] Indications for MR include radiographic instability of the upper cervical spine, myelopathy, and evaluation of the impact of pannus with regard to cord compression. Flexion and extension views allow for selection of operative candidates and determination of levels for fusion. MR has similarly been used preoperatively to evaluate instability at the occipitoatlantal or atlantoaxial levels in other chronic inflammatory diseases.

MR Technique

Due to the difficulty of immobilizing the patient, scan times must be kept short for flexion and extension views. With T1-weighted scan techniques, a typical approach would be to acquire a reduced number of phase-encoding steps (128), using a rectangular field of view and a single data repetition, giving a scan time of 30 seconds for a TR of 500 msec. Adequate signal-to-noise ratio can be achieved by using a larger field of view than normal and thicker (5 to 7 mm) sections. The advent of fast T2 spin echo techniques has permitted acquisition of flexion and extension views with T2-weighted contrast. Use of an eight-echo train, with TR = 3500, 128 phase-encoding steps, and a rectangular field of view results in a scan time of 28 seconds. In the near future, such exams are likely to be performed in a much shorter scan time using echo planar imaging or similar techniques.

Clinical Reference

1. Bell GR, Stearns KL. Flexion-extension MRI of the upper rheumatoid cervical spine. Orthopedics 1991;14:969–974.

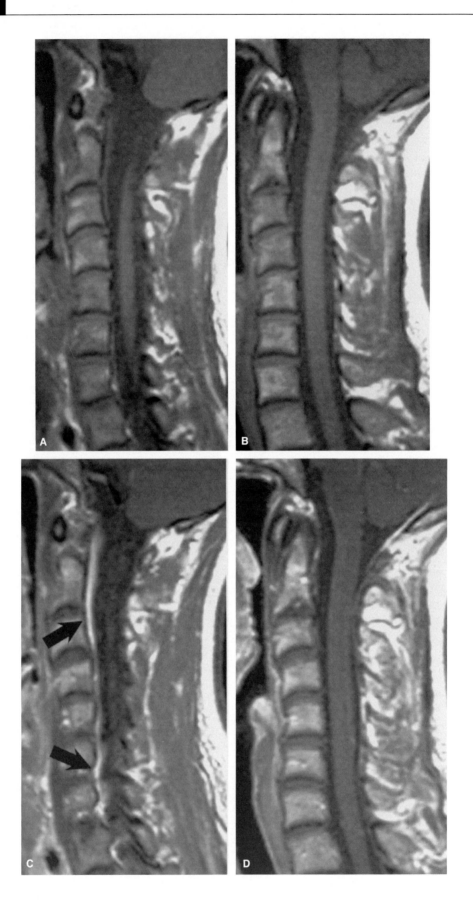

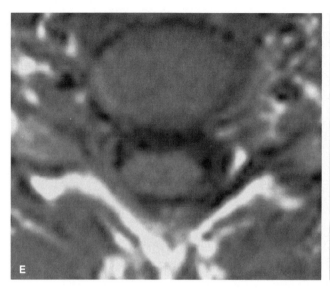
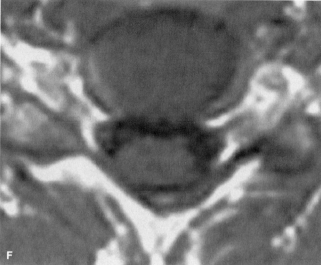

HISTORY

Noncontributory

FINDINGS

Comparison of (*A and B*) precontrast and (*C and D*) postcontrast sagittal T1-weighted images reveals prominent enhancement (*arrows*) posterior to the vertebral bodies and anterior to the thecal sac. This enhancement is most conspicuous laterally in the upper cervical spine and is essentially absent in the midline. Comparison of (*E*) precontrast and (*F*) postcontrast axial T1-weighted images at the C5–6 level demonstrates marked enhancement within the foramina bilaterally, which improves visualization of the bony margins. The outline of the thecal sac, in particular the disk–dural sac interface, is also better defined on the postcontrast image.

DIAGNOSIS

Contrast media—normal enhancing structures, cervical spine

DISCUSSION

In the normal cervical spine, contrast administration leads to venous enhancement on the basis of slow flow (stasis) and T1 shortening. Two venous plexuses, the external and internal, extend the length of the spinal column. The external vertebral plexus consists of a network of veins located over the anterior vertebral body, lami-

nae, and spinous, transverse, and articular processes. The internal vertebral plexus is a network of veins lying in the epidural space, both anteriorly and posteriorly, within the bony vertebral canal. The anterior plexus is larger and consists of longitudinal veins lying on each side of the posterior longitudinal ligament. Blood from the external and internal venous plexuses, as well as from the spinal cord, drains via the intervertebral veins. These accompany the spinal nerves within the intervertebral foramina. The internal (or "epidural") venous plexus is visualized postcontrast in the vast majority of MR exams. It is best seen in the upper cervical spine, with attenuation at lower levels. The plexus tapers at the disk space and appears markedly narrowed or even obliterated over the height of the disk.[1] The basilar plexus, a network of interlacing venous channels lying over the clivus and anterior to the basilar artery, is seen in less than half of cases. This plexus receives blood from the anterior vertebral plexus and drains into the inferior petrosal sinus.

Contrast administration highlights both the normal internal vertebral plexus and changes produced by disease. Such changes—for example, displacement and engorgement of the venous plexus, which often accompanies cervical disk herniation—can be used as indirect evidence of pathology and bring attention to primary disease. Visualization of the vertebral foramina and possible encroachment by degenerative disease is also markedly improved postcontrast.

Clinical Reference

1. Gelber ND, Ragland RL, Knorr JR. Gd-DTPA-enhanced MRI of cervical anterior epidural venous plexus. J Comput Assist Tomogr 1992;16:760–763.

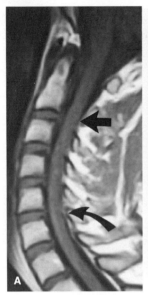
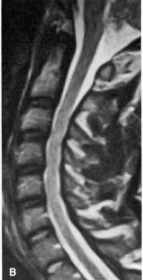
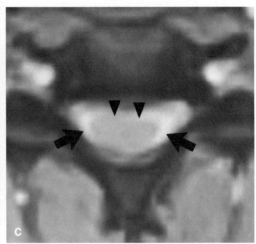

HISTORY

A 33-year-old patient with bilateral arm pain and numbness

FINDINGS

The midline sagittal postinfusion T1-weighted image (*A*) shows a diffusely narrow spinal canal from the C2–3 (*arrow*) through the C5–6 (*curved arrow*) levels. The low signal intensity of cerebrospinal fluid (CSF), in particular posteriorly, tapers at C2–3 and regains its normal dimension only below C5–6. The sagittal fast spin echo T2-weighted image (*B*) demonstrates an interrupted narrow high-signal-intensity line corresponding with the small CSF space anterior and posterior to the intermediate-signal-intensity spinal cord. The axial T2-weighted gradient echo image at the C3–4 level (*C*) reveals flattening of the spinal cord (*arrowheads*). High-signal-intensity CSF (*arrows*) is seen along the lateral margins of the spinal cord, but the CSF space is obliterated anterior and posterior to the cord.

DIAGNOSIS

Congenital stenosis of the cervical spinal canal

DISCUSSION

Congenital stenosis of the cervical spinal canal occurs due to developmentally short pedicles. This may occur alone or may be associated with an underlying syndrome such as Down syndrome or achondroplasia. Myelopathic symptoms, which include extremity weakness, gait abnormalities, reflex changes, and muscle atrophy, are more common than radicular symptoms in patients with spinal stenosis.[1]

The term "relative spinal stenosis" has been used to describe a spinal canal diameter of 13 mm or less. A patient with this amount of narrowing may be symptomatic. Absolute stenosis indicates a measurement of less than 10 mm. Congenital stenosis predisposes the patient to earlier and more severe symptoms when superimposed degenerative changes develop. A disk bulge, osteophytic spurs, or a disk herniation may narrow the anterior canal. The posterior canal can be narrowed by hypertrophy of the facet joints or the ligamentous structures. The narrowed canal also predisposes to traumatic spinal cord injury.

MR Technique

MR is an excellent imaging modality for evaluation of the dimensions of the spinal canal and neural foramina. In addition, abnormalities can be detected in the spinal cord, intervertebral disks, and other soft tissues that may account for the patient's symptoms. T2-weighted spin echo and gradient echo sequences provide a "myelographic" effect without the administration of intrathecal contrast.

Pitfalls in Image Interpretation

Gradient echo images may overestimate the degree of canal or foraminal narrowing. This is particularly true when motion is present.

Clinical Reference

1. Jahnke RW, Hart BL. Cervical stenosis, spondylosis, and herniated disc disease. Radiol Clin North Am 1991;29:777–791.

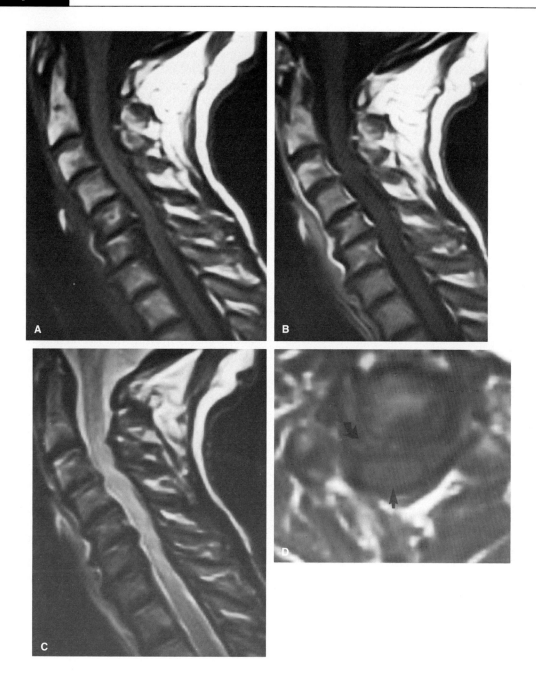

HISTORY

A 69-year-old woman with neck pain and intermittent numbness and weakness in both arms

FINDINGS

(*A*) The sagittal T1-weighted image demonstrates mild reversal of the normal cervical lordosis in the lower cervical spine. Disk space narrowing is identified at the C4–5 through the C6–7 levels. This is accompanied by irregularity of the end plates and inhomogeneity of marrow signal. Posterior osteophytic spurs and disk bulges at C3–4, C4–5, C5–6, and C6–7 produce focal canal narrowing. Cord flattening and deformity is seen, with the cord posteriorly displaced at the stenotic levels. (*B*) The postcontrast T1-weighted image demonstrates thin curvilinear high signal intensity (enhancing epidural venous plexus) along the posterior margins of the vertebrae. The disk bulges and spurs are again identified. (*C*) The T2-weighted image (TE = 45) reveals focal narrowing of the spinal canal from the C3–4 through the C6–7 levels, obliterating the subarachnoid space and causing moderate cord deformity. No abnormal signal is present within the cord. (*D*) The axial T1-weighted image at the upper C5–

6 level illustrates flattening of the spinal cord (*arrow*) in the anteroposterior dimension. Heterogeneous marrow signal in a broad-based posterior spur (*curved arrow*) extends from the lower C5 body, obliterating the ventral subarachnoid space and compressing the spinal cord.

DIAGNOSIS

Degenerative stenosis of the cervical spinal canal

DISCUSSION

Acquired central canal stenosis is usually the result of advanced degenerative disk disease, also termed spondylosis, with multiple factors contributing to canal narrowing. Decreased height of the disk spaces results in thickening, buckling, and redundancy of the intraspinal ligaments. The posterior longitudinal ligament may calcify or ossify, and the ligamentum flavum may calcify. Along the anterior thecal sac, disk bulges or herniations combined with osteophytic spurs contribute to canal narrowing. The osseous canal may be narrowed posteriorly by hypertrophy of the facet joints.

Symptoms associated with acquired cervical canal stenosis typically occur in middle-aged and elderly individuals. The affected population is somewhat older than those affected by disk herniations, although significant overlap exists. Patients with symptoms secondary to disk herniations also tend to have a shorter duration of symptoms, with a more abrupt onset than those with symptoms due to spondylosis. Patients who have a congenitally narrow canal may become symptomatic with relatively mild spondylitic changes; consequently, these patients typically become symptomatic at a younger age.

The normal sagittal diameter of the cervical canal is greater than 13 mm. A canal between 10 and 13 mm is borderline. Some patients may experience symptoms with this degree of narrowing. A diameter less than 10 mm is diagnostic of canal stenosis.[1] Measurements are most accurate on axial images. Volume averaging on sagittal images results in slight underestimation of the actual canal dimensions.

Clinically, significant canal stenosis produces myelopathic symptoms. These patients present with gradually progressive or intermittent numbness and weakness in the upper extremities. Pain and abnormal reflexes are frequently present. Muscle wasting may occur, classically involving the interosseous muscles of the hand, and the patient may walk with a staggering gait. The most commonly affected levels are C4–5, C5–6, and C6–7, with multilevel involvement common.[1] Mild canal stenosis results in effacement of the ventral subarachnoid space. As the disease progresses, the disk protrusions and bulges with associated osteophytic spurs contact the spinal cord. The cord is often deformed and flattened at the most severely narrowed levels, with spinal cord impingement indicated by loss of the ventral subarachnoid space. Complete effacement of the subarachnoid space both anterior and posterior to the cord indicates cord compression.[2]

In some cases of canal stenosis, especially with severe narrowing, increased T2 signal is seen within the spinal cord, indicating edema or gliosis. This may progress to ischemia, infarction, and demyelination in the cord with resultant myelomalacia. In advanced cases, the cord may necrose, with resultant cystic changes or cavitation.[3] Patients with intramedullary signal abnormalities are often symptomatic. The symptoms may be halted or reversed with early surgical decompression of the stenotic canal. However, with irreversible myelomalacia or cystic changes in the cord, symptoms commonly persist.

MR Technique

MR is the modality of choice for the diagnosis of intramedullary lesions, including edema or gliosis associated with severe canal stenosis. T2-weighted spin echo and low flip angle gradient echo scans are used to detect these intrinsic cord abnormalities.

Pitfalls in Image Interpretation

Degenerative disk disease is common, and many persons with significant degenerative changes in the spine are asymptomatic. The imaging findings must be correlated with the clinical symptoms to interpret the significance of the disease.[4]

Clinical References

1. Elghazawi AK. Clinical syndromes and differential diagnosis of spinal disorders. Radiol Clin North Am 1991;29:651–663.
2. Teresi LM, Lufkin RB, Reicher MA, et al. Asymptomatic degenerative disk disease and spondylosis of the cervical spine: MR imaging. Radiology 1987;164:83–88.
3. Al-Mefty O, Harkey LH, Middleton TH, et al. Myelopathic cervical spondylitic lesions demonstrated by MRI. J Neurosurg 1988;68:217–222.
4. Jahnke RW, Hart BL. Cervical stenosis, spondylosis, and herniated disc disease. Radiol Clin North Am 1991;29:777–791.

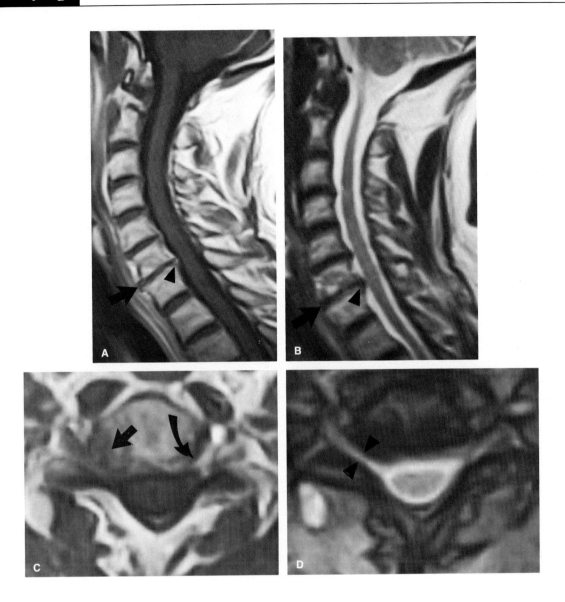

HISTORY

A 54-year-old patient with neck and bilateral arm pain

FINDINGS

(A) The right parasagittal postcontrast T1-weighted image demonstrates narrowing of the C6–7 disk space (*arrow*) with associated degenerative end plate changes. Low-signal-intensity spurs (*arrowhead*) project posterolaterally. (B) The corresponding T2-weighted image confirms these findings. The neural foramina were not well visualized on more lateral sagittal images (*images not shown*). Irregular low signal intensity (*arrow*) is demonstrated on C, the postcontrast axial T1-weighted image.

This finding corresponds to hypertrophic changes and sclerosis of the right C6–7 uncovertebral joint. The spur narrows the right neural foramen. The normal contralateral neural foramen (*curved arrow*) is well delineated on the postcontrast image, due to enhancement of epidural venous plexus within the foramen. (D) The axial T2-weighted gradient echo image again demonstrates, as low signal intensity, the uncovertebral joint spur narrowing the right neural foramen (*arrowheads*).

DIAGNOSIS

Neural foraminal narrowing due to uncovertebral joint spurring

DISCUSSION

The uncovertebral joints, also known as the joints of Luschka, are present along the posterolateral margins of the cervical vertebral bodies. The uncinate processes extend superiorly to articulate with a depression in the inferior end plate of the adjacent vertebral body. These processes are present only at the C3 through C7 bodies and therefore can cause foraminal narrowing at the C2–3 through the C6–7 levels.

Hypertrophic degenerative changes of the uncinate processes result in spurs that narrow the anteromedial border of the neural foramen. This is common in the middle and lower cervical spine, which is also the most common location for cervical disk degeneration. Disk degeneration with disk space narrowing and facet degeneration causes decreased height of the neural foramen. The resulting foraminal stenosis can cause nerve root compression and is a frequent cause of radicular symptoms. This is a more common cause of cervical radiculopathy than disk herniation.[1]

Anatomically, the cervical neural foramina course anterolaterally from the spinal canal at approximately a 45° angle with a slightly inferior course.[2] This is oblique to the sagittal imaging plane and results in volume averaging and poor visualization of the foramina. Oblique MR images give a better demonstration of the foramina and contents than axial or sagittal sections.[3] Newer techniques, including two-dimensional and three-dimensional gradient echo acquisitions, show promise in the evaluation of foraminal disease. Volume acquisition allows imaging of the cervical spine to be accomplished with a single scan, providing considerable time savings over two-dimensional techniques (with each plane requiring a separate scan).[1]

MR Technique

On axial images following contrast administration, the foraminal contents enhance, allowing improved evaluation of foraminal narrowing compared to noncontrast images.

Pitfalls in Image Interpretation

The neural foramina in the cervical spine are not optimally depicted on the sagittal MR images. Foraminal narrowing may be missed without careful evaluation of axial or oblique images. Gradient echo imaging of the cervical spine frequently improves visualization of osseous neural foraminal narrowing but tends to exaggerate the degree of narrowing due to susceptibility artifact.

Clinical References

1. Ross JS, Ruggieri PM, Tkach JA, et al. Gd-DTPA-enhanced 3D MR imaging of cervical degenerative disk disease: initial experience. AJNR 1992;13:127–136.
2. Daniels DL, Hyde JS, Kneeland JB, et al. The cervical nerves and foramina: local-coil MR imaging. AJNR 1986;7:129–133.
3. Modic MT, Masaryk TJ, Ross JS, et al. Cervical radiculopathy: value of oblique MR imaging. Radiology 1987;163:227–231.

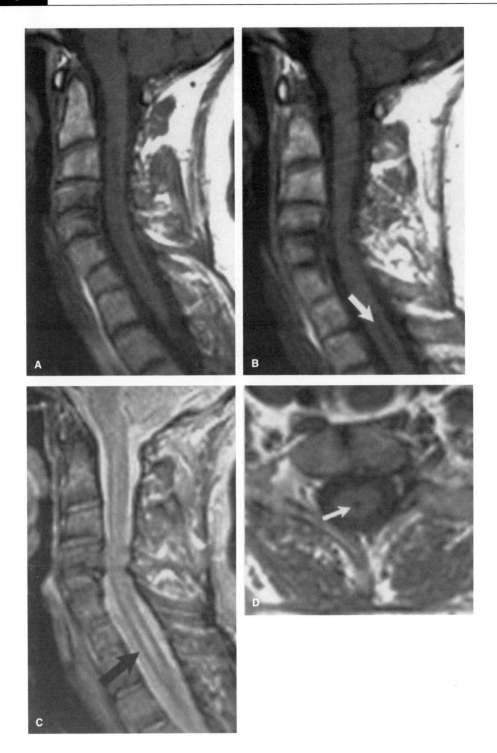

HISTORY

A 51-year-old patient with diffuse neck pain, no long-track signs, normal strength, sensation, and reflexes

FINDINGS

(A and B) Midline sagittal T1-weighted images reveal marked degenerative disease at the C4–5 level, an abnor-

mal shape to vertebral bodies C6, C7, and T1 (height greater than width), and decreased height to the C6–7 and C7–T1 disk spaces. The shape of these vertebral bodies, together with the absence of normal disk material, raises the question of fusion. A syrinx (*arrows in B through D*) is noted on the sagittal T1-weighted exam and is confirmed on (C) the first echo (TE = 45) of the T2-weighted exam and (D) the axial T1-weighted exam. There is cervical spinal stenosis extending from C3 to C5 due to degenerative disease, best seen on the T2-weighted exam. Plain films obtained in (E) flexion and

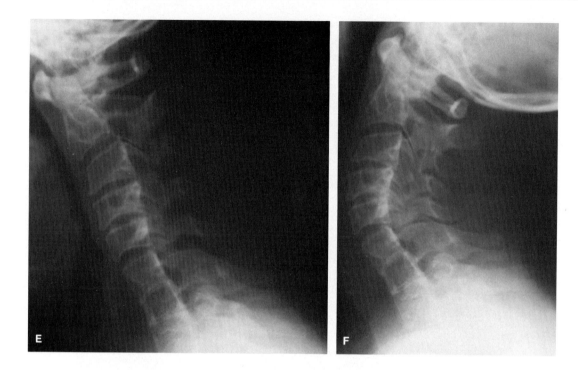

(*F*) extension confirm the fusion of C6–T1 ("block vertebrae") with slight retrolisthesis of C5 on C6 in extension.

DIAGNOSIS

Klippel-Feil syndrome

DISCUSSION

Klippel-Feil syndrome is characterized by fusion of two or more cervical vertebrae, involving most commonly C2–3 and C5–6.[1] At affected levels, the intervertebral disk is absent. Half of patients demonstrate the classic triad of short neck, low posterior hairline, and limited neck motion. Common associated anomalies include deafness, congenital heart disease, Sprengel's deformity (elevation and rotation of the scapula), and urologic abnormalities.

Three types of involvement are described: type I with extensive cervical and thoracic fusion, type II with one or two cervical fusions, and type III, which is type I or II with additional lower thoracic or lumbar fusions. Type II, the most common, may have associated hemivertebrae or occipitoatlantal fusion. In addition to vertebral body fusion, there may be spinous process fusion and vertebral body widening and flattening. Although patients are often asymptomatic, spinal cord or nerve root compression can occur on the basis of the bony anomalies. Patients are predisposed to major neurologic sequelae (specifically spinal cord injury) with seemingly minor trauma. Flexion–extension radiographs are recommended to evaluate potential instability of the unfused segments (with a predisposition to hypermobility at these levels). Subluxation and spinal stenosis are not restricted to adults, in whom these changes have been attributed to degenerative disease and hypermobility, but can also be seen in pediatric patients with Klippel-Feil syndrome.[2]

The advent of MR has made possible recognition of accompanying cord abnormalities, with those reported including syringohydromyelia and diastematomyelia.

Clinical References

1. Smith BA, Griffin C. Klippel-Feil syndrome. Ann Emerg Med 1992;21:876–879.
2. Ritterbusch JF, McGinty LD, Spar J, Orrison WW. MRI for stenosis and subluxation in Klippel-Feil syndrome. Spine 1991;16:S539–S541.

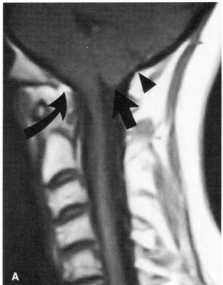 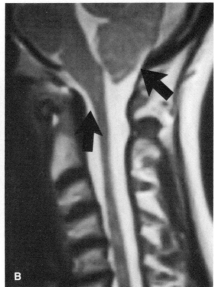

HISTORY

A 54-year-old patient with left arm pain and spasms

FINDINGS

(*A*) The sagittal T1-weighted image demonstrates low-lying cerebellar tonsils (*arrow*). The inferior tip of the tonsil extends 4 mm below the level of the foramen magnum. The opisthion (*arrowhead*) and basion (*curved arrow*), which correspond to the midpoint of the posterior and anterior margins of the foramen magnum (the occiput and clivus) respectively, are identified as low-signal-intensity cortical bone. (*B*) The T2-weighted sagittal image shows high-signal-intensity cerebrospinal fluid (*arrow*) anterior to the brain stem and posterior to the tonsils, producing a myelographic effect. The inferior displacement of the tonsils is again revealed, but the tonsils retain a globular contour with no evidence of crowding or mass effect.

DIAGNOSIS

Cerebellar tonsillar ectopia

DISCUSSION

The position of the cerebellar tonsils is usually measured on sagittal T1-weighted images. This image sequence is commonly obtained with a head study and is nearly always part of a cervical spine examination. Due to signal intensity drop-off at the inferior edge of the head coil,

the cervical spine examination is typically better for assessing the tonsillar position. Anatomically, the tonsils lie just lateral to the midline and are seen best on slightly parasagittal views.

Mild inferior position of the cerebellar tonsils may be seen in asymptomatic normal individuals. Inferior displacement of the tonsils follows a spectrum from tonsillar ectopia to the Chiari I malformation. With tonsillar ectopia, the tonsils retain their normal globular configuration. The tonsils become pointed or peg-like with the Chiari I malformation, but such a deformity is not necessarily symptomatic.[1]

The cerebellar tonsils have a variable position in normal individuals. In the great majority of normal cases, the tonsils lie above the level of the foramen magnum. The tonsils may lie as far as 5 mm below the foramen and still be normal. The degree of inferior displacement does not correlate completely with symptoms. In one study, no asymptomatic persons had inferior displacement of more than 5 mm. However, symptoms were present in some persons with inferior displacement of as little as 3 mm.[1]

Pitfalls in Image Interpretation

The cervicomedullary junction is an often overlooked area on head and cervical spine examinations. This area should be viewed in all patients and incorporated into the reader's routine survey sequence.

Clinical Reference

1. Barkovich AJ, Wippold FJ, Sherman JL, Citrin CM. Significance of cerebellar tonsillar position on MR. AJNR 1986; 7:795–799.

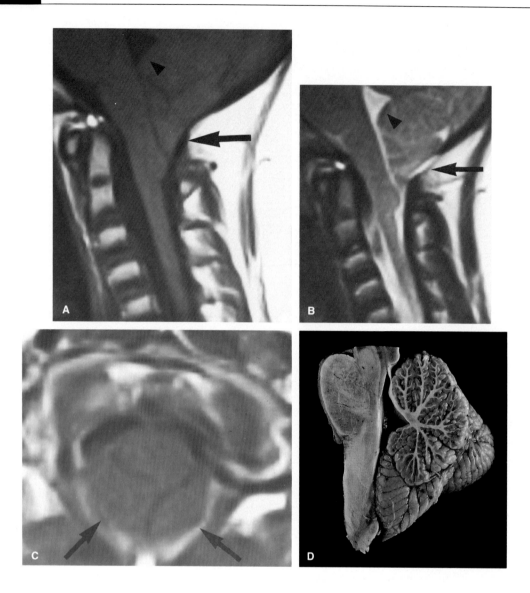

HISTORY

An 11-year-old patient with severe scoliosis

FINDINGS

(*A*) T1-weighted and (*B*) fast spin echo T2-weighted midline sagittal images reveal an abnormally low position of the cerebellar tonsils (*arrows*), which are seen to extend 11 mm beneath the foramen magnum. The tonsils have lost their usual globular configuration and are pointed (or wedge-shaped) in appearance. Because of the patient's scoliosis, the lower cervical spine is seen in a parasagittal plane. The fourth ventricle (*arrowheads*) is normal in position. (*C*) A T1-weighted axial view at the level of the arch of C1 confirms the abnormally low position of the cerebellar tonsils (*arrows*). There is moderate de-

formity of the cervicomedullary junction, right greater than left.

DIAGNOSIS

Chiari I malformation

DISCUSSION

The Chiari I malformation is a congenital hindbrain dysgenesis typified by an abnormally low position of the cerebellar tonsils. Tonsillar ectopia of up to 5 mm below the foramen magnum may be seen in normal individuals. In these subjects, the tonsils will retain their usual globular configuration. The radiographic diagnosis of the Chiari I malformation requires an abnormal wedge shape of the cerebellar tonsils. Associated findings include cervical syrinx, seen in about 50% of cases, and craniovertebral junction abnormalities such as basilar impression, occipitalization of the atlas, and Klippel-Feil deformity.[1] In contrast to the Chiari II malformation, the fourth ventricle should be normally situated. Another point of distinction is the presence or absence of spinal dysraphism, with a myelomeningocele, invariably present in the Chiari II malformation.

Before the advent of MR, diagnosis of a Chiari I malformation required strong clinical suspicion and carefully performed myelographic or computed tomographic (CT) studies. MR's multiplanar imaging capability now allows exquisite noninvasive delineation of anatomic detail in patients with Chiari I malformations. T1-weighted sagittal images are recommended for assessing the degree of cerebellar ectopia, while mass effect on the cervical cord is well seen in either the sagittal or axial plane.

MR Technique

Because of the high incidence of syrinx in Chiari I patients, discovery of a Chiari I malformation on a brain MR examination should prompt investigation of the cervical spine. Conversely, patients with a syrinx should undergo examination of the skull base to rule out a Chiari malformation.

Pitfalls in Image Interpretation

Symptoms in patients with the Chiari I malformation are often vague and may mimic a cervical radiculopathy. Careful attention to the position of the cerebellar tonsils is thus critical in all cervical spine MR examinations.

Pathologic Correlate

A gross midsagittal section of the cerebellum and brain stem (D) demonstrates abnormally low cerebellar tonsils, which are beaked (or wedge-shaped) in appearance. The fourth ventricle is normal in position.

Clinical Reference

1. Poe LB, Coleman LL, Mahmud F. Congenital CNS anomalies. Radiographics 1989;9:801–826.

(D *courtesy of Hauro Okazaki, MD, from the book Fundamentals of Neuropathology, 2nd ed. New York, Igaku-Shoin Medical Publishers, 1989.*)

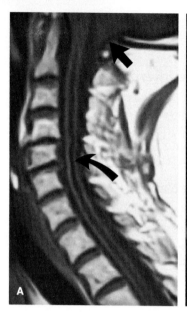
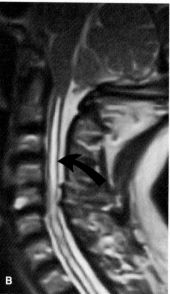
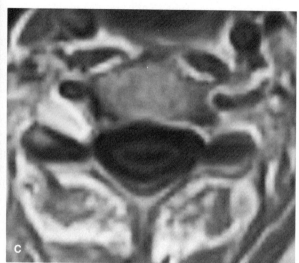

HISTORY

A 69-year-old woman with left arm weakness and atrophy of the left trapezius muscle

FINDINGS

On the T1-weighted midline sagittal image (*A*), the cerebellar tonsils (*arrow*) are noted to be low in position, extending 8 mm below the foramen magnum. The cerebellar tonsils also have an abnormal wedge-shaped configuration. An extensive syrinx (*curved arrow*) is present within the cervical and thoracic spinal cord. Small bony spurs are incidentally noted at C4–5 and C5–6. (*B*) The syrinx (*curved arrow*), with high-signal-intensity cerebrospinal fluid (CSF), is also well demonstrated on the fast spin echo T2-weighted image. A focal area of high signal intensity within the anterior C5 vertebral body is most compatible with an incidental hemangioma. (*C*) The postinfusion axial T1-weighted image at the C6 level also depicts well the central syrinx cavity.

DIAGNOSIS

Chiari I malformation with syringohydromyelia

DISCUSSION

The clinical course in patients with the Chiari I malformation is quite variable. Patients may remain asymptomatic or may present at any time with subtle symptoms related to brain stem compression or a cervical syrinx.[1] Symptoms related to hindbrain compression include headache, cranial nerve deficits, nystagmus, ataxia, and even sudden death. Such patients are more likely to have very low-lying cerebellar tonsils (>10 mm below the foramen magnum). Extremity weakness, back pain, hyperreflexia, and central cord syndrome are among the symptoms that localize the principal abnormality to the spinal cord. In the large majority of these patients, a syrinx is present. Individuals who become symptomatic often benefit from neurosurgical decompression of the foramen magnum or shunting of an associated syrinx. MR allows accurate, noninvasive assessment of these patients in the pre- and postoperative state.

The reason for the variability in presentation of Chiari I patients is debatable. A common belief is that the continual rubbing of the tonsils against the foramen magnum results in arachnoidal adhesions and scarring, which then contribute to brain stem compression. These adhesions may also alter CSF flow dynamics, with the result being syrinx formation.[2] However, adhesions are not invariably present at surgery, and symptoms are not always relieved by decompression of the foramen magnum.

Pitfalls in Image Interpretation

A significant number of asymptomatic patients imaged for unrelated reasons are found to have tonsillar herniations in the range of 5 to 10 mm. Great care should thus be taken in ascribing clinical significance to the incidental Chiari I malformation.

Clinical References

1. Elster AD, Chen MYM. Chiari I malformations: clinical and radiologic reappraisal. Radiology 1992;183:347–353.
2. DeBoulay G, Shah SH, Currie JC, Logue V. The mechanism of hydromyelia in Chiari type I malformations. Br J Radiol 1974;47:579–587.

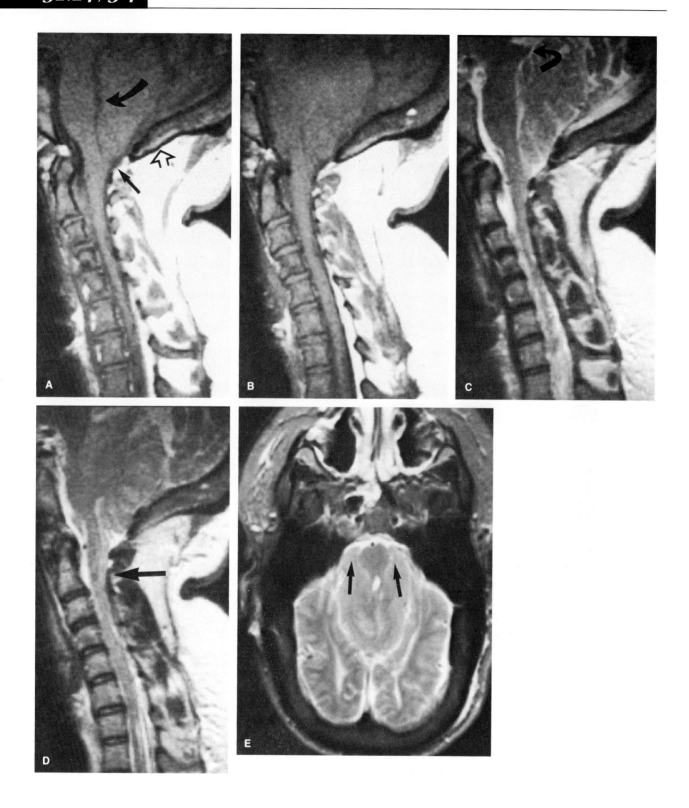

HISTORY

A 21-year-old patient with previous repair of a lumbar myelomeningocele

FINDINGS

(A) The sagittal T1-weighted image of the cervical spine, just off midline, demonstrates an elongated cerebellum

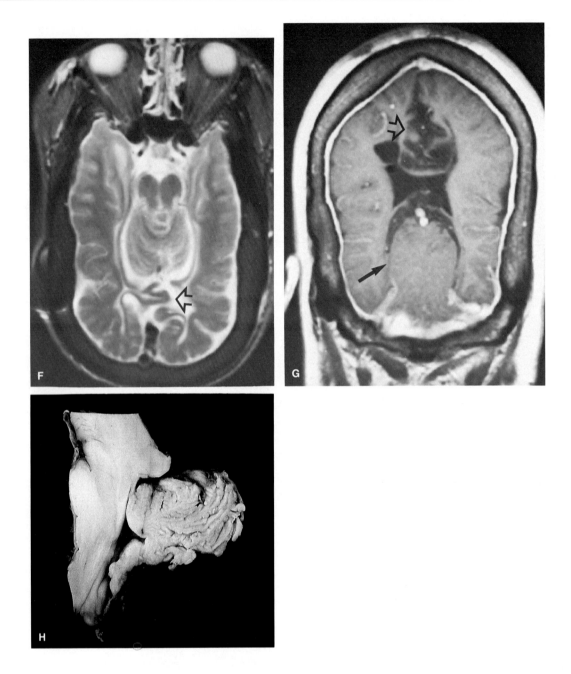

with inferior displacement of the cerebellar tonsils (*arrow*). The fourth ventricle is elongated and slit-like (*curved arrow*). The posterior fossa is small, and the tentorium cerebelli inserts low on the occipital bone (*open arrow*). (*B*) The midline sagittal T1-weighted image shows mild reversal of the normal cervical lordosis but normal segmentation in the cervical spine. The cerebellar tonsils extend inferiorly to the C1–2 level. (*C*) The T2-weighted image, comparable in position to *A*, again illustrates many of these findings. Also well seen is fusion of the colliculi, with resultant "beaking" of the tectum (*curved arrow*). High signal intensity of the cerebrospinal fluid (CSF) outlines the structures of the posterior fossa. (*D*) The midline sagittal T2-weighted image con-

firms the inferior displacement of the cerebellar tonsils (*arrow*). The herniated tonsils and spinal cord are crowded between the odontoid process and the posterior arch of C1. (*E*) An axial T2-weighted image through the midcerebellum demonstrates wrapping of the cerebellar hemispheres (*arrows*) around the brain stem. (*F*) An axial image through the upper cerebellum shows interdigitation of the cerebral gyri (*open arrow*) due to fenestration of the falx. (*G*) A coronal T1-weighted image obtained after intravenous contrast administration reveals that the cerebellum (*arrow*) extends superiorly through the wide incisura of the tentorium cerebelli. The posterior lateral ventricles are dysmorphic, with partial agenesis of the corpus callosum. Interdigitation of the cerebral gyri (*open arrow*) is again noted. Diffuse enhancement of the thickened dura is secondary to long-term ventricular shunt placement.

DIAGNOSIS

Chiari II malformation

DISCUSSION

The Chiari II malformation is a complex abnormality of the posterior fossa. This is the most common major malformation of the posterior fossa with deformity of the calvarium, dura, and hindbrain. Associated abnormalities are present in the spine. This deformity is nearly always associated with hydrocephalus and a myelomeningocele.[1]

Findings in the posterior fossa include low insertion of the tentorium cerebelli on the occipital bone, frequently just above the foramen magnum. The normally large tentorial veins consequently lie near the foramen magnum. This can complicate posterior fossa surgery due to the increased risk of bleeding. The tentorium cerebelli is also hypoplastic, and the poorly developed leaves form a large incisura. Brain growth produces inferior and superior extension of the dysmorphic cerebellum out of the small posterior fossa. The cerebellum commonly extends anteriorly around the brain stem. The pons is somewhat flattened, with scalloping of the clivus and petrous bones. A prominent prepontine CSF space is often present. The midbrain is also elongated, with fusion of the colliculi and beaking of the quadrigeminal plate.[2]

The spinal findings in Chiari II consist of elongation of the brain stem, cerebellum, and fourth ventricle with displacement into the upper cervical canal. The foramen magnum and upper cervical canal are enlarged, but the C1 ring is typically smaller than the foramen magnum and is therefore the level of compression of the caudally displaced brain stem, cerebellar tonsils, and vermis.[3] The posterior arch of C1 may be incompletely fused, but C2 is usually intact. Defects may occur in the posterior arches of the C3 to C7 vertebrae. Occasional fusion of two or more cervical vertebrae may be present. Some abnormalities associated with Chiari I are not seen with Chiari II, including basilar impression and assimilation of C1 to the occiput.

The Chiari III malformation, a much rarer entity, consists of an osseous defect in the occiput and upper cervical spine with cerebellar herniation into a cervico-occipital encephalocele.

MR Technique

Sagittal and axial T1-weighted spin echo images are usually sufficient to demonstrate the anatomic abnormalities of the Chiari II malformation. Magnetic resonance imaging is far superior to computed tomography for evaluation of posterior fossa abnormalities.

Pitfalls in Image Interpretation

On an MR study of the cervical spine, inferior displacement of the cerebellar tonsils is also present with a Chiari I malformation. Evaluation of the posterior fossa, fourth ventricle, cerebellum, and brain stem will help differentiate this entity from a Chiari II malformation. Beaking of the quadrigeminal plate, caudal displacement of the vermis as well as the cerebellar tonsils, elongation of the midbrain, and flattening of the pons indicate a Chiari II malformation.

Pathologic Correlate

A gross midsagittal section of the cerebellum and brain stem (*H*) demonstrates beaking of the tectum (also known as the quadrigeminal plate) and herniation of hypoplastic, midline cerebellar structures beyond the foramen magnum. This infant with a Chiari II malformation died of bacterial infection following meningomyelocele repair.

Clinical References

1. Wolpert SM, Anderson M, Scott RM, et al. Chiari II malformation: MR imaging evaluation. AJNR 1987;8:783–792.
2. El Gammel T, Mark EK, Brooks BS. MR imaging of Chiari II malformation. AJR 1988;150:163–170.
3. Curnes JT, Oakes WJ, Boyko OB. MR imaging of hindbrain deformity in Chiari II patients with and without symptoms of brain stem compression. AJNR 1989;10:293–302.

(H from Okazaki H, Scheithauer B. Atlas of neuropathology. New York, Gower Medical Publishing, 1988, p. 291. By permission of Mayo Foundation.)

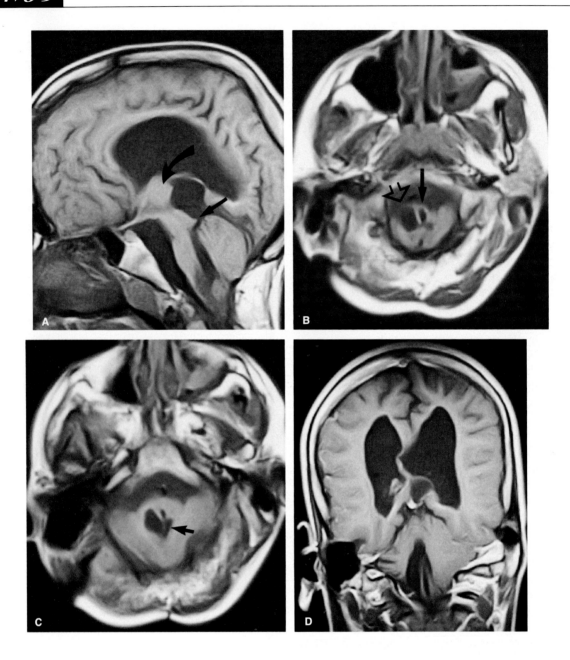

HISTORY

A 14-year-old patient with spina bifida aperta and treated hydrocephalus

FINDINGS

(A) The midline sagittal T1-weighted image reveals findings in the brain stem consistent with a Chiari II malformation. The tectum is fused and beaked (*arrow*). The brain stem is elongated with flattening of the pons and prominence of the prepontine cerebrospinal fluid (CSF) space. The image also demonstrates a large massa intermedia (*curved arrow*). The posterior fossa is small with low insertion of the tentorium cerebelli. A portion of in-

ferior occipital bone is surgically absent from a previous posterior fossa decompression. (B) The axial T1-weighted image demonstrates fluid (CSF) signal intensity in the medulla extending anteriorly in the midline (*arrow*) and ventrolateral to the right (*open arrow*) consistent with syringobulbia. (C) The adjacent, more cephalad, axial T1-weighted image shows the superior extension of the syrinx cavities and leftward displacement of the fourth ventricle (*arrow*). (D) The T1-weighted coronal image through the medulla shows the midline and right-sided cavities in the medulla. (*E and F*) The comparable axial T2-weighted images again demonstrate the antero-lateral (*open arrow*) and midline (*arrow*) syrinx cavities in the medulla. A syrinx cavity was also present in the cervical cord (*images not shown*).

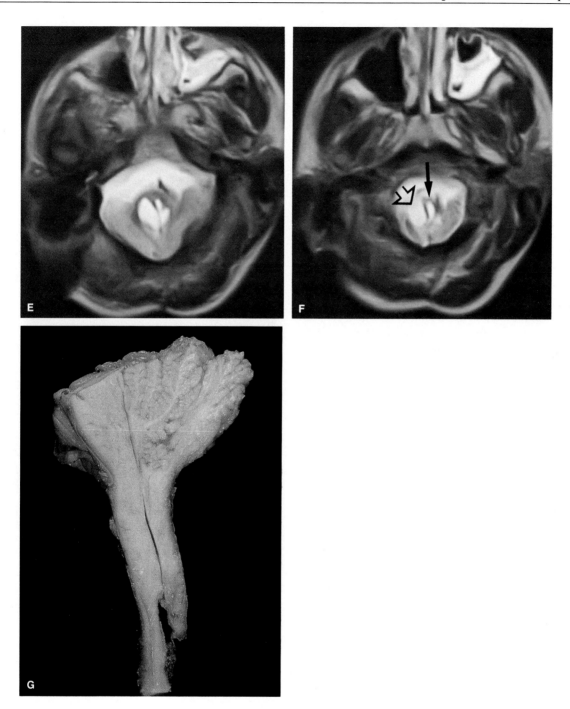

DIAGNOSIS

Chiari II malformation with syringomyelia and syringobulbia

DISCUSSION

The Chiari II malformation is a complex abnormality with a small posterior fossa and low insertion of the tentorium cerebelli. The cerebellar tonsils and vermis, elongated fourth ventricle, and brain stem are caudally displaced into the upper cervical spinal canal. The upper cervical canal demonstrates increased diameter in the anteroposterior dimension. The C1 arch is bifid in 70% of cases. When the posterior arch of the atlas is bifid, a transverse band often bridges the gap between the lamina.[1]

Due to caudal displacement of the spinal cord, the upper cervical nerve roots must ascend to exit through their respective neural foramina. Inferior displacement of the lower brain stem occurs, with a portion of the medulla and even the pons lying below the level of the foramen magnum. The lower cranial nerves must ascend through the foramen magnum. Cerebellar tissue protrudes through the foramen in 90% of cases. Frequently the medulla and upper cervical spinal cord overlap, forming a cervicomedullary kink. The kinking is caused by anchoring of the cervical cord by the dentate ligaments while the brain stem is inferiorly displaced. A kink at or below the C3–4 level has a high association with symptoms attributable to compression of the brain stem or corticospinal tracts.[1]

The fourth ventricle is typically compressed in the Chiari II malformation. A normal-sized fourth ventricle should prompt close inspection of the spinal cord. Syringomyelia is more common in conjunction with a trapped fourth ventricle. Syrinx cavities in patients with the Chiari II malformation are most common in the lower cervical and thoracic spinal cord. The presence of syrinx cavities in the cord has been reported in 15% to 83% of patients with the Chiari II malformation.[2]

Hydrocephalus is frequently present in patients with the Chiari II malformation and is often detected during in utero ultrasound. The aqueduct of Sylvius is stenotic in up to 50% of cases. However, nearly all are patent, but they may show anatomic deformity such as shortening, forking, or even gliosis.[3] The aqueduct may be externally compressed, and some studies have shown a relationship between the degree of hydrocephalus and aqueductal narrowing.[4] Nonvisualization of the aqueduct on direct sagittal thin-section images suggests aqueductal obstruction.[2]

Syringobulbia is a fluid-filled cavity in the brain stem, typically the medulla. The cavity occurs in one of three locations: medially along the median raphe, between the pyramid and olive, or extending ventrolaterally from the floor of the fourth ventricle.[3] Syringobulbia is most commonly the superior extension of a syrinx cavity in the upper cervical cord, but it may originate in the medulla. Symptoms associated with syringobulbia include hemi-facial numbness or facial pain, vertigo, dysphagia, and loss of taste. Syringobulbia is more commonly associated with a Chiari I malformation and syringomyelia.[5]

Pitfalls in Image Interpretation

A syrinx cavity in the brain stem may be mistaken as a normal or dilated fourth ventricle. Careful correlation of orthogonal imaging planes permits differentiation of syringobulbia from a dilated fourth ventricle. Confirmation of syringobulbia should prompt close inspection of the cord for syringomyelia.

Pathologic Correlate

(*G*) Extensive downward herniation of cerebellar tissue is illustrated in this gross midsagittal section from a 7-month-old infant with a Chiari II malformation. The fourth ventricle is slit-like and elongated.

Clinical References

1. Curnes JT, Oakes WJ, Boyko OB. MR imaging of hindbrain deformity in Chiari II patients with and without symptoms of brain stem compression. AJNR 1989;10:293–302.
2. El Gammel T, Mark EK, Brooks BS. MR imaging of Chiari II malformation. AJR 1988;150:163–170.
3. Norman MG, Ludwin SK. Congenital malformations of the nervous system. In: Textbook of neuropathology, 2nd ed. Baltimore, Williams & Wilkins, 1991, 207–280.
4. Wolpert SM, Anderson M, Scott RM, et al. Chiari II malformation: MR imaging evaluation. AJNR 1987;8:783–792.
5. Sherman JL, Citrin CM, Barkovich AJ. MR imaging of syringobulbia. J Comput Assist Tomogr 1987;11:407–411.

(G from Okazaki H, Scheithauer B. Atlas of neuropathology. New York: Gower Medical Publishing, 1988, p. 292. By permission of Mayo Foundation.)

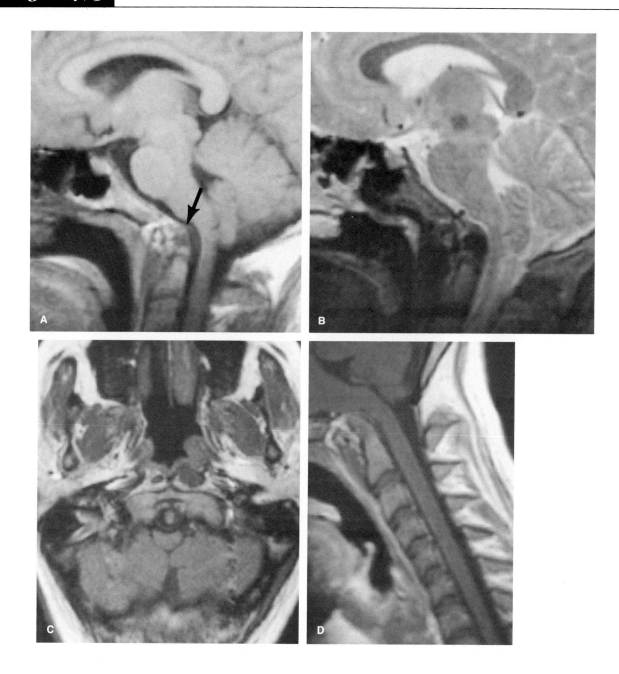

HISTORY

A 27-year-old patient with headaches

FINDINGS

On the midline sagittal T1-weighted scan (*A*), the tip of the odontoid (*arrow*) is noted to lie within the foramen magnum, about 1 cm above Chamberlain's line. This finding is confirmed on the sagittal T2-weighted scan (*B*). The axial T1-weighted scan (*C*) reveals compression and displacement of the medulla by the dens. On the sagittal T1-weighted scan with the neck in flexion (*D*), the pos-

terior arch of C1 is noted to remain immediately adjacent to the occiput. A lateral cervical x-ray (*E*) demonstrates fusion of C1 posteriorly to the occiput.

DIAGNOSIS

Basilar invagination

DISCUSSION

The tip of the odontoid is normally at or just above Chamberlain's line, which is drawn between the posterior margin of the hard palate to the posterior lip of the

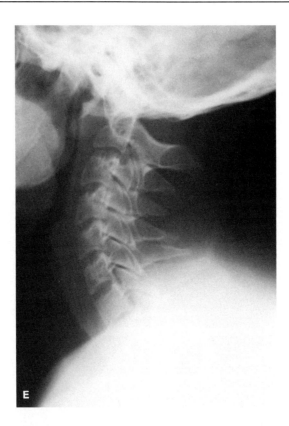

foramen magnum. Location of the tip 5 or more mm above this line defines basilar invagination, which represents an upward migration of the foramen magnum into the cranial cavity.[1] Secondary or acquired types of this malformation are often referred to as basilar impression. The latter can be seen with osteomalacia, osteoporosis, fibrous dysplasia, Paget's disease, achondroplasia and osteogenesis imperfecta.[1]

The bony abnormalities in basilar invagination are well defined by plain radiographs. Although these findings can also be seen on MR, the value of MR lies in the definition of associated deformities of the brain stem and spinal cord.[2] Patients with basilar invagination can present with headaches, neurologic deficits, or symptoms related to vertebrobasilar artery compression.

Basilar invagination is often associated, as in the case presented, with fusion of the atlas and occiput (commonly referred to as occipitalization or assimilation). One fourth of patients with occipitalization of the atlas also have a Chiari I malformation.

Successful surgical treatment of basilar invagination in association with occipitalization of the atlas has been reported.[3] In this subset of patients, common preoperative symptoms include nuchal pain and vertigo. Patients with the Chiari I malformation and syringomyelia may have coexisting basilar impression. Surgical decompression in this instance can also improve symptomatology.[4]

Comparison of pre- and postoperative images has demonstrated a reduction in the size of the syrinx, with the cerebellar tonsils reverting to a more normal rounded appearance.

Platybasia is a separate entity, not to be confused with basilar invagination. The angle formed by the clivus and the floor of the anterior cranial fossa is normally 125° to 140°, with an angle greater than 140° defining platybasia. Such a finding can be isolated, without clinical relevance, or accompanied by other abnormalities, including basilar invagination.

Clinical References

1. Dolan K. Cervicobasilar relationships. Radiol Clin North Am 1977;15:155–166.
2. Smoker W, Deyes W, Dunn V, et al. MRI versus conventional radiologic examinations in the evaluation of the craniovertebral and cervicomedullary junction. Radiographics 1986;6:953–994.
3. Bassi P, Corona C, Contri P, et al. Congenital basilar impression: correlated neurological syndromes. Eur Neurol 1992; 32:238–243.
4. Kohno K, Sakaki S, Nakamura H, et al. Foramen magnum decompression for syringomyelia associated with basilar impression and Chiari I malformation—report of three cases. Neurol Med Chir 1991;31:715–719.

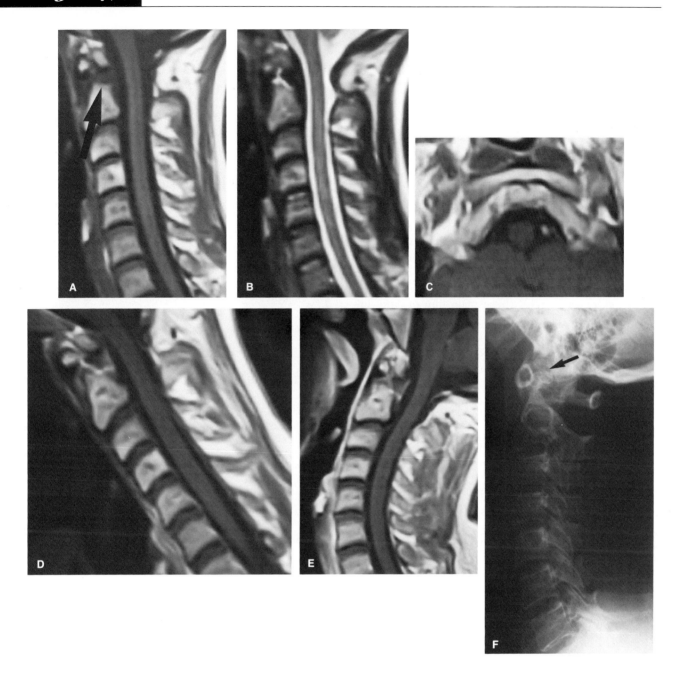

HISTORY

A 46-year-old patient with neck pain following a motor vehicle accident

FINDINGS

(A) A T1-weighted midline sagittal image reveals abnormal separation (*arrow*) between the superior dens and the base of the C2 vertebral body. The superior fragment appears well corticated. The anterior arch of C1 is prominent and has a convex posterior margin. The abnormal separation of the superior dens is confirmed on a fast spin echo T2-weighted midline sagittal image (*B*). The marrow signal intensities of the superior and inferior components of C2 are normal. The cervical spinal canal is normal in caliber, and no evidence for cord injury is seen. (*C*) A T1-weighted axial image at the C1 level reveals normal, close approximation of the superior dens and the anterior arch of C1. Flexion (*D*) and extension (*E*) sagittal images reveal no significant change in the distance between the superior dens fragment and the anterior arch of C1 in either position. No cord compression is identified. (*F*) A lateral radiograph of the cervical spine demonstrates the ununited superior portion of the dens (*arrow*).

DIAGNOSIS

Os odontoideum with stable fibrous union

DISCUSSION

Fractures of the dens are not uncommon following major trauma. Acute dens fractures must be distinguished from an os odontoideum, as the treatment of the two conditions differs markedly. The typical plain film finding of os odontoideum is a corticate ovoid ossicle in the expected location of the dens, which is clearly distinct from the body of C2. Another common appearance, although nonspecific, is enlargement of the anterior arch of C1 with increased cortical thickness and a convex posterior margin of the anterior arch.[1] These plain film findings are readily apparent on the MR images of the current case. Valuable additional information, however, is supplied by the MR. The normal marrow signal intensity of the superior dens fragment and the base of C2 makes an acute traumatic etiology quite unlikely, as significant marrow edema would be expected in an acute fracture. Additionally, MR allows simultaneous evaluation for possible soft tissue and spinal cord injury.

The etiology of os odontoideum is controversial and has been ascribed to both congenital and acquired causes.[2] Familial cases and associations with congenital abnormalities support the congenital etiology, whereas the location of the separation below the epiphyseal plate of the dens and reports of serial development of the abnormality following trauma support an acquired cause. It is likely that both congenital and acquired causes can lead to an appearance of os odontoideum.

MR Technique

Flexion–extension MR views provide clear delineation of the atlanto-occipital and atlantoaxial relationships in cases of os odontoideum. Overlapping shadows are often problematic in plain film evaluation of the dens; MR's ability to obtain thin slices in multiple planes avoids such difficulties. Whereas cord compression or canal stenosis secondary to instability can only be inferred with plain films, MR allows direct visualization of possible mass effect on the cord.

Clinical References

1. Holt RG, Helms CA, Munk PL, Gillespy T. Hypertrophy of C1 anterior arch: useful sign to distinguish os odontoideum from acute dens fracture. Radiology 1989;173:207–209.
2. Morgan MK, Onofrio BM, Bender CE. Familial os odontoideum. J Neurosurg 1989;70:636–639.

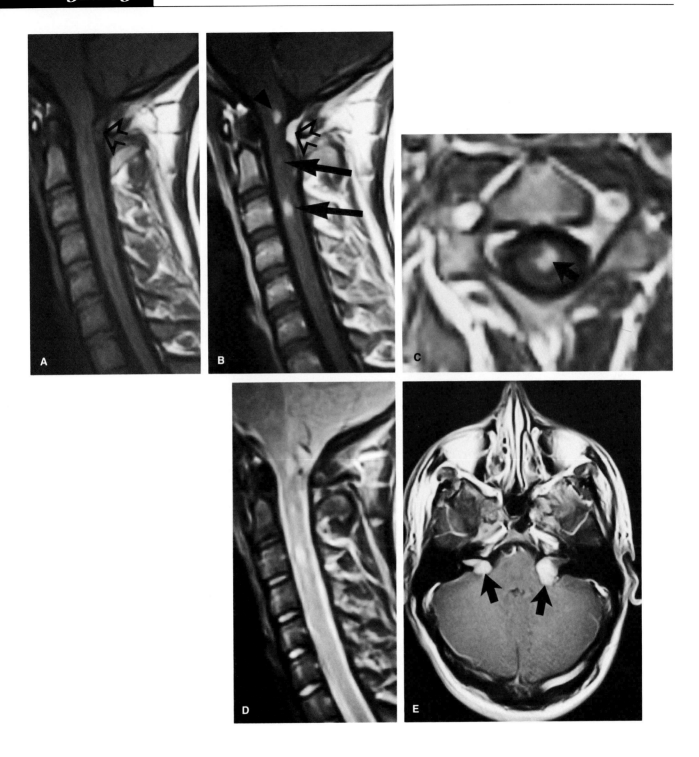

HISTORY

A 25-year-old man with multiple intracranial neoplasms

FINDINGS

(*A*) The midline sagittal T1-weighted image demonstrates abnormal heterogeneous signal in the upper cervical spinal cord with mild expansion of the cord. An extramed-ullary mass with soft tissue signal intensity (*open arrow*) is seen along the posterior margin of the thecal sac, anterior to the posterior arch of the atlas. The mass causes mild deformity of the upper cervical cord. On the post-contrast sagittal T1-weighted image (*B*), two foci of abnormal enhancement (*arrows*) are demonstrated within the cervical spinal cord and one at the cervicomedullary junction (*arrowhead*). The cord shows mild enlargement at the lesion sites. An intradural extramedullary enhancing mass with a broad base against the dura (*open arrow*) is seen along the posterior thecal sac just below the margin of the foramen magnum. (*C*) An axial T1-weighted image, obtained after intravenous contrast administration, confirms the intramedullary location of the enhancing lesion (*arrow*) at the C3 level. (*D*) The sagittal T2-weighted image shows abnormal increased signal in the spinal cord corresponding with the location of the enhancing lesions. (*E*) An axial contrast-enhanced T1-weighted image through the posterior fossa reveals bilateral acoustic schwannomas (*arrows*). Other images through the brain (*images not shown*) demonstrated multiple meningiomas.

DIAGNOSIS

Neurofibromatosis type 2

DISCUSSION

Neurofibromatosis type 2, previously termed central neurofibromatosis, has characteristic cranial findings of bilateral acoustic schwannomas. Other commonly associated intracranial abnormalities include schwannomas, gliomas, and hamartomas. There is also an increased incidence of malignant neoplasms. The spinal findings in neurofibromatosis type 2 consist predominantly of intradural lesions. These may be extramedullary or intramedullary. Most of the intradural extramedullary lesions are neurofibromas or meningiomas. Most of the intramedullary lesions are ependymomas or low-grade astrocytomas.[1]

The differential diagnosis for an intramedullary enhancing lesion in the cervical spinal cord includes a primary neoplasm such as an astrocytoma or ependymoma, a demyelinating process, transverse myelitis, contusion, or metastatic disease. Multiple lesions, as seen in this case, make the diagnosis of a primary neoplasm less likely. Intramedullary metastases are uncommon. This patient had no history of significant prior trauma.

A controversy exists concerning screening of the spine in patients with diagnosed neurofibromatosis type 2. One author proposes screening only symptomatic patients.[2]

Clinical References

1. Egelhoff JC, Bates DJ, Ross JS, et al. Spinal MR findings in neurofibromatosis types 1 and 2. AJNR 1992;13:1071–1077.
2. Elster AD. Radiologic screening in the neurocutaneous syndromes: strategies and controversies. AJNR 1992;13:1078–1082.

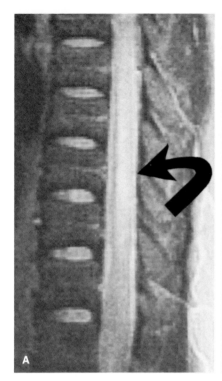
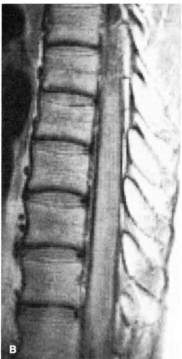
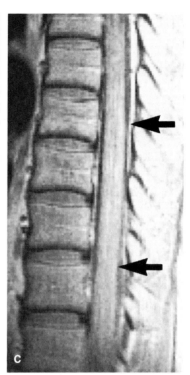

HISTORY

A 35-year-old man presenting with markedly decreased leg strength

FINDINGS

Midline sagittal T2-weighted (*A*) and T1-weighted (*B and C*) images, the latter precontrast (*B*) and postcontrast (*C*), of the lower thoracic spine are presented. There is fusiform enlargement of the thoracic cord, best seen on the precontrast T1-weighted exam. Abnormal high signal intensity is noted on the T2-weighted exam within the area of cord enlargement, compatible with edema (*curved arrow in A*). The postcontrast exam reveals subtle enhancement (*arrows in C*), primarily along the cord surface. The diagnosis was established by CSF studies and skin biopsy. The patient was treated with steroids, with leg strength returning to near normal. A second MR study (*images not shown*) 3 months after presentation demonstrated resolution of both the cord edema and abnormal enhancement.

DIAGNOSIS

Sarcoidosis

DISCUSSION

Sarcoidosis is a noncaseating granulomatous disease of unknown etiology. The central nervous system is involved clinically in 5% of cases, with the most common sites being the basal leptomeninges and the floor of the third ventricle. Involvement of the spinal cord is much less common. However, spinal cord involvement, if untreated or if biopsy is attempted, can lead to severe neurologic sequelae. Fusiform cord enlargement, multiple nodular areas of parenchymal enhancement (which tend to be broad-based along the cord surface), and thin pial enhancement (along the cord surface) have been reported in spinal cord sarcoidosis.[1,2] In the appropriate clinical setting, this appearance is indeed highly suggestive of sarcoidosis. An unusual, but reported, appearance of sarcoidosis on imaging is that of an isolated intramedullary lesion. In the extradural space, sarcoidosis can in rare instances mimic the appearance of diskitis, with both disk and adjacent vertebral body involvement.

Treatment with steroids can result in marked disease improvement, as assessed by imaging; follow-up scans in some instances demonstrate a return to normal appearance.

MR Technique

Meningeal involvement in sarcoidosis may not be apparent on unenhanced scans, mandating the use of IV contrast.

Pitfalls in Image Interpretation

Cord enlargement, nodular parenchymal enhancement, and involvement of the leptomeninges, although suggestive, are not specific for sarcoidosis. This pattern has also been reported in biopsy-proven myelitis and multiple sclerosis.[1]

Clinical References

1. Nesbit GM, Miller GM, Baker HL, et al. Spinal cord sarcoidosis: a new finding at MR imaging with Gd-DTPA enhancement. Radiology 1989;173:839–843.
2. Seltzer S, Mark AS, Atlas SW. CNS sarcoidosis: evaluation with contrast-enhanced MR imaging. AJNR 1991;12:1227–1233.

(Thanks to Barbara Carter, MD, for her assistance.)

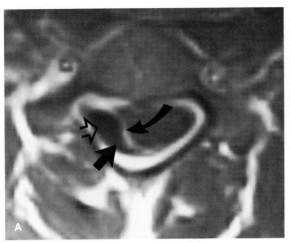 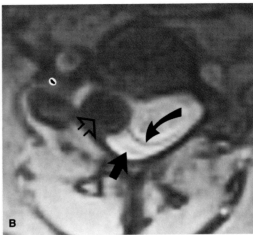

HISTORY

A 29-year-old man with a previous crush avulsion and traumatic amputation of the right arm 3 months before the current exam. The patient experienced phantom limb pain, and an indwelling cervical epidural catheter was inserted at the C6–7 level for pain management. Ten days later the patient presented with neck stiffness, shoulder pain, and low-grade fever.

FINDINGS

(A) The postcontrast axial T1-weighted image shows abnormal fluid (*arrow*) and a gas bubble (*open arrow*) within the epidural space. The enhancing dura (*curved arrow*) appears as a high-signal-intensity curvilinear structure separating the epidural mass from the thecal sac. The epidural mass displaces the thecal sac to the left side of the canal. (B) The axial gradient echo image confirms the epidural location of the gas bubble (*open arrow*) and fluid (*arrow*), with displacement of the curvilinear low-signal-intensity dura (*curved arrow*). The apparent "blooming" (enlargement) of the gas bubble as depicted on the gradient echo image is due to magnetic susceptibility effects.

DIAGNOSIS

Epidural abscess

DISCUSSION

The differential diagnosis for an extradural lesion in the spine includes osteophyte, disk herniation, metastatic disease, primary neoplasm, epidural hematoma, and epidural abscess. The presence of gas in association with a soft tissue mass strongly favors the diagnosis of an epidural abscess. However, this constellation of findings can be seen normally in the immediate postoperative period. In the current case, the air could also have been introduced during injection of medication through the epidural catheter.

Infection in the epidural space can be caused by hematogenous spread, direct extension, or penetrating trauma. With this patient, the epidural space was seeded by the indwelling catheter. The inflammatory process, with granulation tissue and fluid, frequently produces sufficient mass effect to cause cord compression and neurologic symptoms.[1]

MR Technique

Magnetic resonance imaging, with its multiplanar capability and superior soft tissue contrast, is an ideal modality for defining the relationship of a lesion in the spine with regard to the cord and the meninges.[2] This permits improved differential diagnosis.

Clinical References

1. Kricun R, Shoemaker EI, Chovanes GI, Stephens HW. Epidural abscess of the cervical spine: MR findings in five cases. AJR 1992;158:1145–1149.
2. Sharif HS. Role of MR imaging in the management of spinal infections. AJR 1992;158:1333–1345.

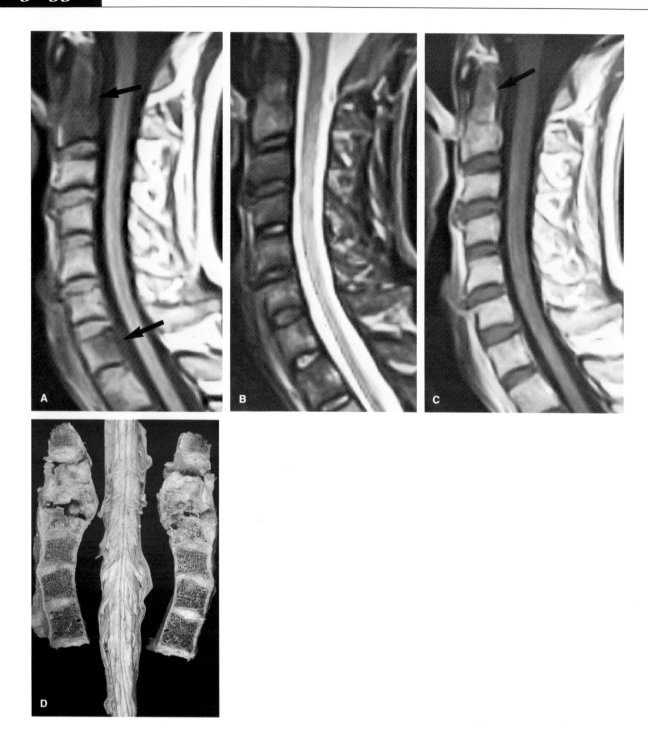

HISTORY

A 43-year-old patient with gastric carcinoma and increasing neck pain

FINDINGS

(A) The T1-weighted midline sagittal image reveals abnormal decreased signal intensity throughout most of C2 (*arrow*). A similar decrease in marrow signal intensity is present within the posterior C7 vertebral body (*arrow*). Additional lesions were present in T1, T2, and T3. On the corresponding T2-weighted sagittal image (*B*), abnormal increased signal intensity is present within C2 and C7. The C7 abnormality appears more extensive on the T2-weighted image. (*C*) Following contrast administration, the lesions become nearly isointense with normal marrow, due to greater relative enhancement. The C7 abnormality is no longer apparent. Mildly decreased signal intensity remains visible within the superior dens (*arrow*). No leptomeningeal or intrinsic cord lesions are noted.

DIAGNOSIS

Cervical metastases

DISCUSSION

Vertebral metastatic disease is a major source of morbidity in cancer patients. Involvement of the vertebrae occurs in as many as 40% of patients dying of disseminated cancer.[1] Plain films are relatively insensitive for detection of vertebral metastases, as at least 50% of the bone must be destroyed before a lesion is well visualized. Bone scans have high sensitivity but low specificity. Infection, trauma, and degenerative disease may result in a false-positive bone scan in the evaluation of metastatic disease. CT provides excellent evaluation of bone destruction, but coverage is limited and soft tissue resolution is relatively poor. Myelography permits cord compression to be evaluated, but lesions are inferred rather than directly visualized. As a result, the various entities that cause epidural disease cannot be differentiated. MR has revolutionized the evaluation of metastatic disease to the spine. Sensitivity and specificity are unparalleled, and the risks of ionizing radiation and intrathecal contrast are avoided. Excellent coverage and soft tissue evaluation are possible, with resultant high utility for the evaluation of epidural and leptomeningeal lesions.

Metastatic vertebral lesions most often demonstrate decreased signal intensity on T1-weighted images and increased signal intensity on T2-weighted scans. Blastic metastases, however, may remain low in signal intensity on T2-weighted images.

Pitfalls in Image Interpretation

The administration of IV contrast is essential to achieve maximum sensitivity for epidural and leptomeningeal metastases. Vertebral lesions, however, can enhance to isointensity with normal marrow on T1-weighted images, and are thus often less conspicuous on postcontrast images.

Pathologic Correlate

(D) A gross midsagittal section of the cervical spine demonstrates a case of metastatic lung carcinoma that involved several upper cervical vertebral bodies. Bony expansion and pathologic fractures are evident.

Clinical Reference

1. Kamholtz R, Sze G. Current imaging in spinal metastatic disease. Semin Oncol 1991;18:158–169.

(D courtesy of Hauro Okazaki, MD, from the book Fundamentals of Neuropathology, 2nd ed. New York, Igaku-Shoin Medical Publishers, 1989.)

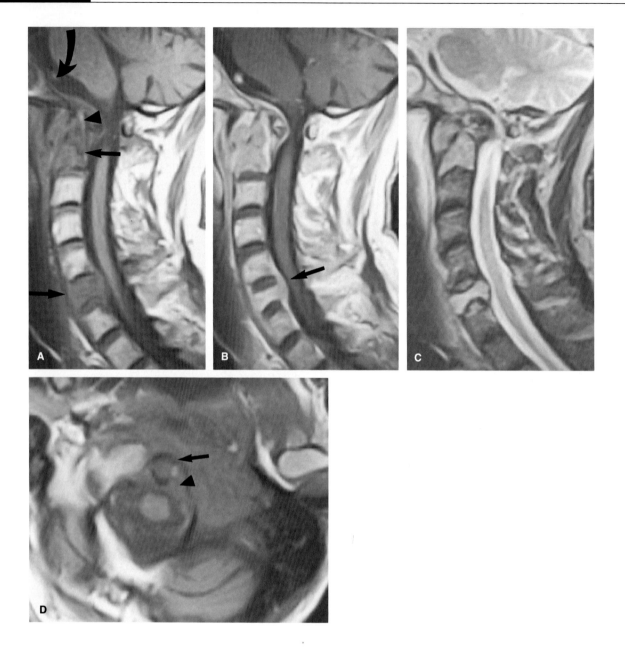

HISTORY

A 61-year-old patient with extensive laryngeal carcinoma and increasing neck pain

FINDINGS

(A) The T1-weighted sagittal image slightly to the left of midline reveals abnormal decreased signal intensity (*arrows*) within the C1, C2, and C6 vertebral bodies. The lesions at C1–2 and at C6 appear expansile. More lateral sagittal images (*images not shown*) revealed contiguity of the vertebral lesions with the patient's extensive laryn-

geal squamous cell carcinoma. The usual high signal intensity of marrow fat within the clivus is also markedly diminished (*curved arrow*). The superior dens (*arrowhead*) lies within the foramen magnum, and was found to lie 1 cm superior to Chamberlain's line (not depicted). (B) Postcontrast, the affected vertebrae and skull base enhance intensely and thus become less distinct from normal marrow fat. Epidural extension of the abnormality at C6 (*arrow*), however, is more clearly depicted. The regions of abnormal marrow demonstrate increased signal intensity on the corresponding T2-weighted sagittal view (C). (D) A T1-weighted axial image at the C1 level confirms the abnormal low signal intensity within the dens (*arrow*) and much of the anterior arch of C1. The abnormal soft tissue that infiltrates the left C1 arch involves the adjacent occipital condyle. Abnormal soft tissue is also present within the anterior spinal canal (*arrowhead*), but no cord compression is visualized at this level.

DIAGNOSIS

Cervical metastases with skull base involvement causing basilar impression

DISCUSSION

High cervical metastatic lesions are a source of great morbidity in cancer patients. Sensory and motor deficits associated with high cervical cord compression are extensive, and severe compression above the C3 level may result in death due to respiratory embarrassment.[1] Spread of tumor to the adjacent skull base may cause patients to present with cranial neuropathies. The fifth cranial nerve is the most commonly affected; tumor involvement of this nerve generally results in numbness or pain along the distribution of its branches.[2] Cranial nerves III, IV, and VI may also be affected by skull base metastatic disease.

Squamous cell carcinomas within the neck primarily spread by local infiltration, and invasion of the adjacent cervical spine or skull base is not uncommon. Involvement of the skull base from distant primary malignancies is also well recognized. The most common etiologies include prostate, lung, and breast carcinoma.[2]

Metastatic disease to the craniocervical junction is an uncommon cause of basilar impression, a term that refers to acquired types of basilar invagination. More typically, primary bone diseases such as osteomalacia, osteoporosis, Paget's disease, or achondroplasia are responsible for basilar impression. However, any cause of abnormal bone softening may result in basilar impression.

MR Technique

Paramagnetic contrast administration has limited utility in routine spin echo evaluation of the skull base, primarily secondary to the large amount of fatty marrow within the mature calvarium. Fat suppression techniques, however, have demonstrated great promise in overcoming this limitation. Postcontrast fat-suppressed images have been found superior to noncontrast images for depiction of the extent of skull base tumor. This technique is also particularly useful in cases of perineural tumor extension.[3]

Pitfalls in Image Interpretation

Venous lakes within the skull base may enhance intensely after contrast administration and could be mistaken for a metastatic lesion. These normal vascular channels are distinguished from neoplastic lesions by their well-defined low signal intensity on T1-weighted images and their lack of bone destruction or adjacent marrow edema.

Clinical References

1. Ratanatharathorn V, Powers WE. Epidural spinal cord compression from metastatic tumor: diagnosis and guidelines for management. Cancer Treat Rev 1991;18:55–71.
2. Laine FJ, Nadel L, Braun IF. CT and MR imaging of the central skull base: part 2. Pathologic spectrum. Radiographics 1991;10:797–821.
3. Barakos JA, Dillon WP, Chew WM. Orbit, skull base, and pharynx: contrast-enhanced fat suppression MR imaging. Radiology 1991;191–198.

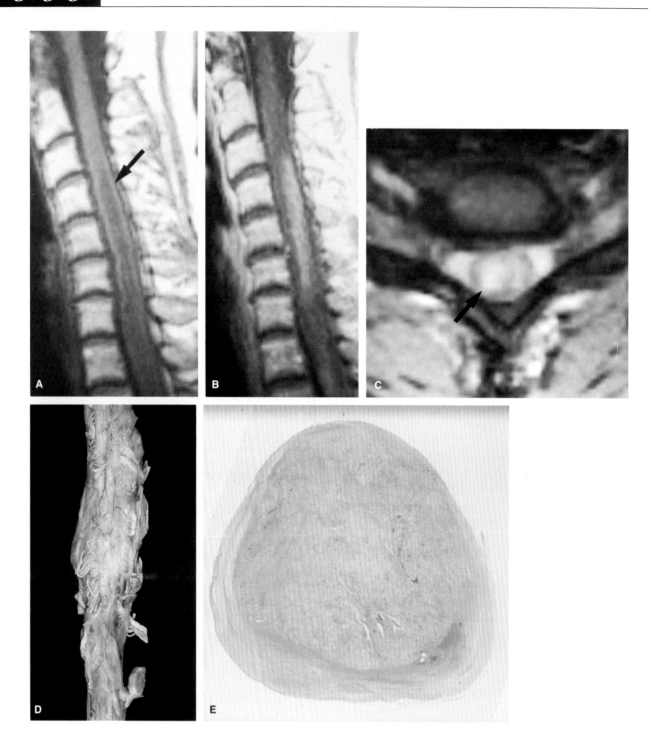

HISTORY

A 48-year-old patient with progressive upper and lower extremity numbness

FINDINGS

(A) The T1-weighted sagittal image reveals abnormally decreased signal intensity within the mid- to lower cervical cord (*arrow*), extending into the superior thoracic region. Mild cord expansion is present. (B) After paramagnetic contrast administration, homogeneous enhancement of the cervical cord abnormality is identified. The enhancement pattern is more irregular in the upper thoracic cord. (C) A gradient echo axial image at the C6–7 level demonstrates abnormal hyperintensity within the spinal cord (*arrow*), more prominent on the right. On T2-weighted images (*images not shown*), the abnormality was also of high signal intensity.

DIAGNOSIS

Grade II astrocytoma

DISCUSSION

Astrocytomas make up the majority of intramedullary tumors in the cervical region. The incidence of astrocytomas declines in the distal spinal cord. This trend is in contrast to ependymomas, which are seen with increased frequency in the distal cord and filum terminale.[1] The peak incidence of cord astrocytomas is in the third and fourth decade, but these tumors are not uncommon in children. Spinal cord astrocytomas tend to be lower-grade malignancies than brain astrocytomas. In general, the younger the patient, the more likely that the cord astrocytoma will be of an aggressive variety. The vast majority of astrocytomas are purely intramedullary, although in rare instances an exophytic extramedullary intradural component is present.

Magnetic resonance's superior soft tissue contrast makes it the modality of choice in evaluation of suspected intramedullary lesions. Most commonly, astrocytomas result in fusiform dilatation of the spinal cord. The lesions typically demonstrate decreased signal intensity on T1-weighted images and increased signal intensity on T2-weighted scans. Associated cysts or hemorrhage, however, may result in variability in signal characteristics. Enhancement is typically seen after paramagnetic contrast administration, although occasionally low-grade astrocytomas will not enhance.

MR Technique

Sagittal T2-weighted images provide an overview of the extent of an intramedullary tumor and its associated edema. Because both tumor and edema are generally hyperintense on T2-weighted images, however, delineation of the exact borders of a tumor is frequently difficult. Postcontrast T1-weighted images provide a more reliable estimation of tumor extent.[2]

Pitfalls in Image Interpretation

An acute cord lesion in patients with multiple sclerosis (MS) may be virtually indistinguishable from an astrocytoma. Like astrocytomas, acute MS lesions may enlarge the cord and often enhance with paramagnetic contrast. MS lesions, however, generally appear more homogeneous than astrocytomas and typically demonstrate a surrounding rim of normal cord signal intensity, which is less common in astrocytomas.[3] Additionally, astrocytomas often involve long segments of the spinal cord, while MS plaques typically affect a small portion of the cord. The key to the diagnosis may lie in demonstration of typical demyelinating lesions in the brain or in the resolution of mass effect on follow-up studies in cases of MS.

Pathologic Correlate

(D) A gross example of a cervical astrocytoma, viewed from its posterior aspect, reveals fusiform enlargement of the spinal cord. (E) A cross section of the lesion demonstrates the near-complete involvement of the width of the cord by neoplastic tissue.

Clinical References

1. Sze G, Twohig M. Neoplastic disease of the spine and spinal cord. In: Atlas SW, ed. MRI of the brain and spine. New York, Raven Press, 1991:921–965.
2. Sze G, Krol G, Zimmerman RD, Deck MDF. Intramedullary disease of the spine: diagnosis using gadolinium-DTPA-enhanced MR imaging. AJR 1988;151:1193–1204.
3. Enzmann DR, DeLaPaz RL. Tumor. In: Enzmann DR, ed. Magnetic resonance of the spine. St. Louis, CV Mosby Company, 1990:301–422.

(D and E from Okazaki H, Scheithauer B. Atlas of neuropathology. New York, Gower Medical Publishing, 1988, p. 88. By permission of Mayo Foundation.)

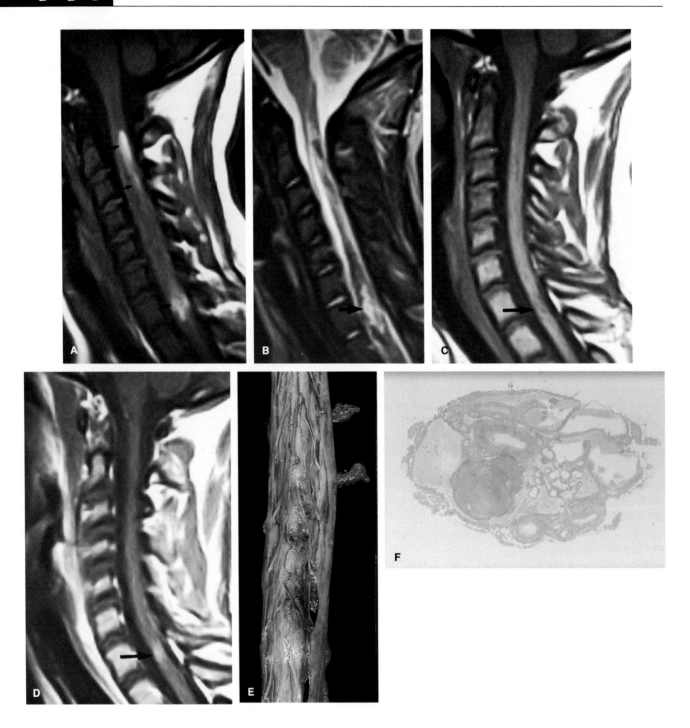

HISTORY

A pregnant patient with a 2-day history of weakness and neck pain

FINDINGS

(A) The midline T1-weighted sagittal image demonstrates abnormally increased signal intensity throughout much of the cervical spinal cord (*arrows*). The lesion was con-

firmed to be intramedullary in location on axial imaging (*images not shown*). Part of the abnormality, at the C7 level (*arrow*), is also of high signal intensity on the T2-weighted sagittal image (*B*). A rim of low signal intensity is also present at this level, and other low signal areas are evident superiorly.

A follow-up examination was performed 6 months later. (*C*) The T1-weighted sagittal image demonstrates resolution of the prior high-signal-intensity abnormality. Subtle foci of low signal intensity (*arrow*) are identified within the cord at the C7 level. After contrast administration (*D*), moderate enhancement (*arrow*) is present in this region. There is no significant cord expansion.

DIAGNOSIS

Arteriovenous malformation causing spontaneous hematomyelia

DISCUSSION

The MR appearance of intramedullary spinal cord hemorrhage is varied. As in the brain, the signal characteristics of cord hemorrhage depend on the age of the hematoma.[1] Very acute hemorrhage may appear isointense to the spinal cord on T1-weighted images. The development of deoxyhemoglobin causes a prominent susceptibility effect on T2-weighted images, with resultant very low signal intensity. Usually within 48 hours, methemoglobin effects begin to dominate. Methemoglobin has a paramagnetic effect similar to IV contrast media, and thus demonstrates increased signal intensity on T1-weighted images. The methemoglobin effect is apparent on the initial scans of this patient. The methemoglobin in this case is predominantly extracellular, as evidenced by the increased signal intensity on T2-weighted images. Intracellular methemoglobin, which is seen earlier, is generally intermediate to low in signal intensity on T2-weighted scans. The region of low signal intensity surrounding the methemoglobin component in this patient is compatible with a hemosiderin or ferritin rim. Both extracellular methemoglobin and hemosiderin/ferritin, but particularly hemosiderin/ferritin, may persist for years after an acute hemorrhage.

In the absence of trauma, intramedullary cord hemorrhage is most likely secondary to a neoplasm or vascular malformation. The lack of cord expansion or edema on the 6-month follow-up scan makes neoplasm unlikely in this case. The round, low-signal areas seen within the cord on the T1-weighted follow-up scan likely indicate flow voids within a small arteriovenous malformation (AVM). An AVM was the presumptive diagnosis in this pa-

tient. Such intramedullary AVMs are usually found in young patients who present with acute hemorrhagic events.[2] In these cases, one should look carefully for an enlarged extramedullary feeding vessel, which is typically located anterior to the cord.

MR Technique

AVMs of significant size are usually easily detectable due to their prominent signal voids. Small AVMs, however, may have few or no obvious signal voids, and frequently have no mass effect. In these cases, paramagnetic contrast agents are quite valuable for detection of the vascular nidus or feeding and draining vessels.[1]

Pitfalls in Image Interpretation

A large spinal cord hematoma may mask a subtle underlying lesion. Follow-up scans are often necessary to clarify the etiology of the cord hemorrhage.

Pathologic Correlate

A gross specimen of a spinal cord AVM (*E*) demonstrates the large, serpiginous vessels that line the cord. An axial section through the lesion (*F*) confirms the multiple abnormal vessels, which appear brown in this image. The normal cord tissue, stained yellow, is severely compromised.

Clinical References

1. Enzmann DR. Vascular diseases. In: Enzmann DR, ed. Magnetic resonance of the spine. St. Louis, CV Mosby Company, 1990:510–539.
2. Minami S, Sagoh T, Nishimura K, et al. Spinal arteriovenous malformation: MR imaging. Radiology 1988;169:109–115.

(E and F from Okazaki H, Scheithauer B. Atlas of neuropathology. New York, Gower Medical Publishing, 1988, p. 34. By permission of Mayo Foundation.)

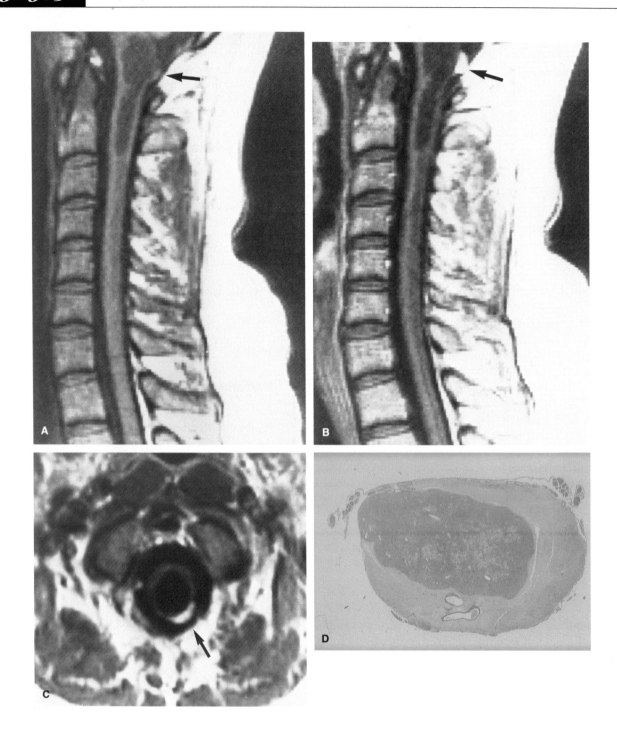

HISTORY

A 42-year-old patient with von Hippel-Lindau disease and a progressive gait disturbance

FINDINGS

On the precontrast sagittal T1-weighted scan (*A*), a syrinx is noted in the upper cervical cord that extends into the brain stem (syringobulbia). The fluid within the syrinx is of slightly greater signal intensity than CSF, suggesting a neoplastic origin. On (*B*) sagittal and (*C*) axial postcontrast T1-weighted scans, an enhancing mural nodule (*arrows*) can be identified. In retrospect, a portion of the nodule (*arrow in A*) is visualized on the precontrast scan.

DIAGNOSIS

Hemangioblastoma

DISCUSSION

Features seen on MRI in spinal cord hemangioblastoma include enlarged draining veins, an enhancing intramedullary nodule, a sharply marginated intramedullary cyst, and diffuse cord enlargement.[1] Tumor nodules demonstrate intense enhancement. The cyst wall does not enhance.

Hemangioblastomas are benign tumors most frequently found in the posterior fossa and much less commonly in the spinal cord. The tumor can be solitary or multiple, with the latter typically associated with von Hippel-Lindau disease. Treatment is by surgical removal of the tumor nodule, which can lead to dramatic resolution of gross cord enlargement (edema) and the associated cyst.

MR Technique

Postcontrast TI-weighted scans prove superior to all other sequences for tumor margin definition and cyst characterization in cases of spinal cord tumor.[2] Contrast use is thus highly recommended, combined with attention in scan interpretation to postcontrast images. In spinal hemangioblastoma specifically, precise tumor delineation is impossible without contrast administration.[3]

Pitfalls in Image Interpretation

Close inspection of postcontrast surface coil images is required for identification of enhancing lesions that lie near or adjacent to normal paraspinal fat. Comparison of pre- and postcontrast scans and implementation of image normalization programs (to compensate for signal intensity drop-off) further facilitate lesion recognition.

Pathologic Correlate

(*D*) A gross axial section of a spinal cord hemangioblastoma demonstrates a solid eccentric lesion. Two large feeding vessels are noted ventral to the tumor. The typical gross appearance of a hemangioma is that of a globular, firm lesion, with mottled red-yellow color due to intrinsic vascularity and lipid content.

Clinical References

1. Colombo N, Kucharczyk W, Brant-Zawadzki M, et al. MRI of spinal cord hemangioblastoma. Acta Radiol Suppl 1986; 369:734–737.
2. Chamberlain MC, Sandy AD, Press GA. Spinal cord tumors: gadolinium-DTPA-enhanced MR imaging. Neuroradiology 1991;33:469–474.
3. Isu T, Abe H, Iwasaki Y, et al. Diagnosis and surgical treatment of spinal hemangioblastoma. No Shinkei Geka 1991; 19:149–155.

(A through C *from Runge VM. Clinical magnetic resonance imaging. Philadelphia, JB Lippincott, 1990, p. 154. D from Okazaki H, Scheithauer B. Atlas of neuropathology. New York, Gower Medical Publishing, 1988, p 140. By permission of Mayo Foundation.*)

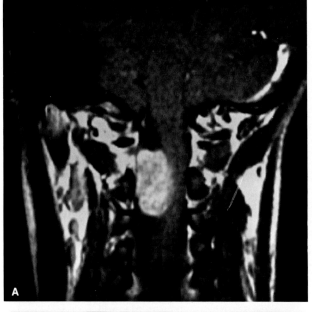

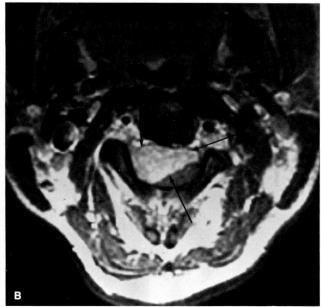

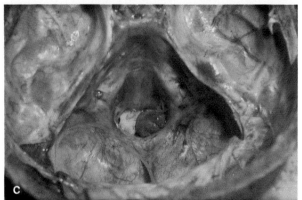

HISTORY

A middle-aged woman with upper and lower extremity weakness

FINDINGS

Coronal (*A*) and axial (*B*) T1-weighted postcontrast scans are presented. The lesion was isointense relative to the spinal cord on precontrast T1-weighted images (*images not shown*). Postcontrast, there is intense lesion enhancement (*arrows in B*). The spinal cord is deformed and displaced posteriorly and to the left. The adjacent neural foramen is normal in size.

DIAGNOSIS

Meningioma

DISCUSSION

Meningiomas represent 25% of all intraspinal tumors, second in incidence only to neurinomas (29%). Meningiomas are usually solitary (with multiple lesions seen in neurofibromatosis), with a peak age of incidence of 45 years. These tumors are usually histologically benign and slow-growing and cause symptoms due to cord and nerve root compression. With a sufficiently large lesion, the cord will be displaced with widening of the subarachnoid space both above and below the lesion, as seen in the coronal image in this case. Meningiomas enhance intensely following gadolinium chelate administration. MR is substantially safer than myelography or CT-myelography because lumbar puncture can acutely worsen symptoms in cases of subarachnoid block.

One to three percent of all meningiomas occur at the foramen magnum. Of benign extramedullary tumors at the foramen magnum, three fourths are meningiomas and one fourth neurofibromas. Frequent clinical symptoms in the case of a benign tumor of the foramen magnum include suboccipital neck pain, upper and lower extremity weakness, and dysesthesias.[1]

MR Technique

With intra- and extramedullary spinal tumors (and in particular meningiomas and neurinomas), contrast-enhanced T1-weighted scans offer substantial advantages over other imaging techniques for lesion detection and delineation.[2,3] Acquisition of postcontrast scans in all three orthogonal planes is recommended.

Pitfalls in Image Interpretation

The adjacent neural foramen should be closely inspected, with growth into and widening of the foramen favoring the diagnosis of a neurinoma or neurofibroma. Both lesions can mimic a meningioma.

Pathologic Correlate

(*C*) A foramen magnum meningioma is shown compressing the cord on a gross view of the skull base with the brain removed. This lesion was associated with chronic neck pain and was not the cause of death.

Clinical References

1. Meyer FB, Ebersold MJ, Reese DF. Benign tumors of the foramen magnum. J Neurosurg 1984;61:136–142.
2. Parizel PM, Baleriauz D, Rodesch G, et al. Gd-DTPA-enhanced MR imaging of spinal tumors. AJR 1989;152:1087–1096.
3. Schroth G, Thron A, Guhl L, et al. MRI of spinal meningiomas and neurinomas—improvement of imaging by paramagnetic contrast enhancement. J Neurosurg 1987;66:695–700.

(A and B *from Runge VM. Clinical magnetic resonance imaging. Philadelphia, JB Lippincott, 1990, p. 224. C courtesy of Hauro Okazaki, MD, from the book Fundamentals of Neuropathology, 2nd ed. New York, Igaku-Shoin Medical Publishers, 1989.*)

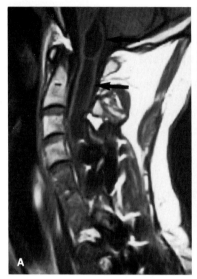
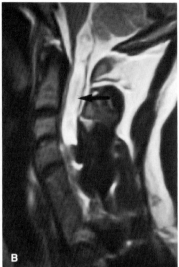
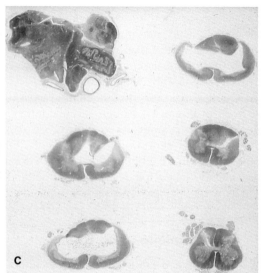

HISTORY

A 31-year-old patient status post–cervical fusion 8 years ago for multiple fractures

FINDINGS

(A) The T1-weighted midline sagittal image reveals postoperative changes at C5–6, including decreased signal intensity within the C5 and C6 vertebral bodies and indistinctness of the intervening disk. A large amount of metallic susceptibility artifact is present in the region of the posterior elements, compatible with known stainless steel fixation wires. A septated fluid collection (*arrow*) is identified within the spinal cord above the site of fusion, extending superiorly to near the inferior extent of the fourth ventricle. The abnormal fluid collection (*arrow*) is again noted on the fast spin echo T2-weighted sagittal image (*B*). The abnormality is isointense to CSF on T1- and T2-weighted images.

DIAGNOSIS

Syringobulbia

DISCUSSION

Longitudinally oriented fluid cavities within the spinal cord are commonly described as syringomyelia. When the fluid space extends into the brain stem, syringobulbia is present. The causes of syringobulbia can be generally grouped into two classes.[1] The most common patients are those with obstruction of CSF pathways at the foramen magnum, usually secondary to a Chiari malformation. Syringobulbia in these patients is usually slit-like. The mechanism of syringobulbia formation in this group of patients is thought to be related to obstruction of the normal caudad flow of CSF through the foramen magnum. As a result, CSF is forced through the inferior fourth ventricle into the central canal of the spinal cord. In the second group of patients, a preexisting syrinx of any etiology extends superiorly to involve the brain stem. Syringobulbia in these patients tends to be more tubular or saccular in appearance.[2] The superior movement of CSF within the syrinx is probably a response to episodes of increased intra-abdominal pressure, as may occur with coughing. The increased pressure from below is transmitted to the epidural venous plexus and subsequently to the dura. CSF then ascends through the path of least resistance, the central gray matter.[1] Clinical findings of ascending neurologic symptoms following a cough or sneeze may be present in this patient group.

Small syringobulbic cavities often form asymmetrically within the brain stem, with resultant unilateral symptoms.[2] The most common symptoms include facial numbness, dsyphagia, vertigo, facial pain, and loss of taste. In severe cases, swallowing and respiratory problems may be life-threatening.

MR Technique

Sagittal MR images allow accurate estimation of the extent of large syringobulbic cavities. With small cavities, axial images are necessary to evaluate the extent of and possible lateralization of the syringobulbia.

Pathologic Correlate

(C) Gross axial sections through the medulla and upper spinal cord, stained with Weil's method, demonstrate a case of syringomyelia with syringobulbia. The variable contour of the cavity and the gliotic tissue lining the cavity are well seen.

Clinical References

1. Morgan D, Williams B. Syringobulbia: a surgical appraisal. J Neurol Neurosurg Psychiatry 1992;55:1132–1141.
2. Sherman JL, Citrin CM, Barkovich AJ. MR imaging of syringobulbia. J Comput Assist Tomogr 1987;11:407–411.

(C from Okazaki H, Scheithauer B. Atlas of neuropathology. New York, Gower Medical Publishing, 1988, p. 294. By permission of Mayo Foundation.)

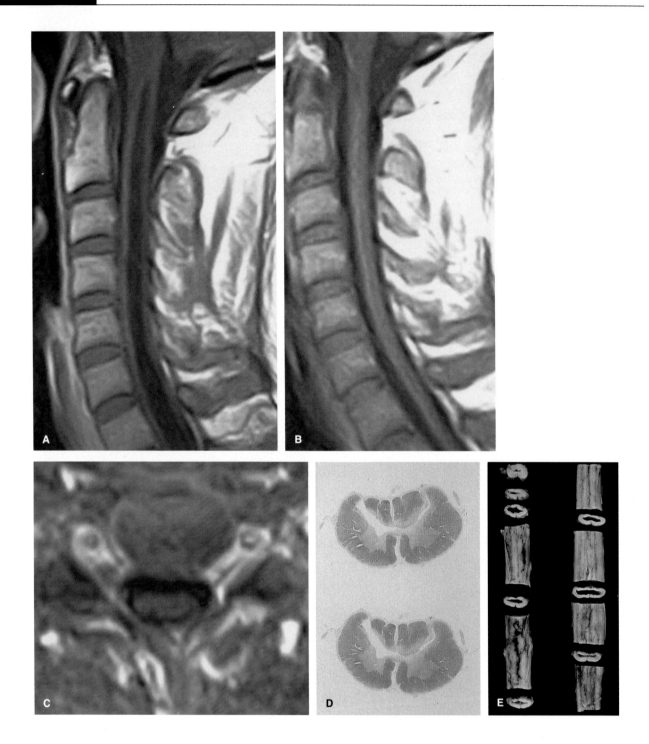

A | B

C | D | E

HISTORY

A 44-year-old white man with a history of a T9 fracture treated by laminectomy and fusion 12 years ago. The patient presents with delayed, progressive neurologic deficit.

FINDINGS

The preoperative study demonstrates fluid signal extending down the central portion of the spinal cord from the cervicomedullary junction through the visualized upper thoracic cord. This is seen as low signal intensity within the cord on the sagittal postcontrast T1-weighted image (*A*). No abnormal enhancement is detected. This is a posttraumatic syrinx secondary to a severe wedge compression fracture of T9 (*image not shown*). Corresponding high-signal-intensity fluid was seen within the cord on the sagittal T2-weighted image (*image not shown*). The spinal cord is expanded with effacement of the surrounding subarachnoid space.

The patient underwent a thoracic laminectomy with placement of a syringoperitoneal shunt. Postoperative (*B*) sagittal and (*C*) axial T1-weighted images of the cervical spine demonstrate collapse of the syrinx. The spinal cord is mildly atrophic, with cerebrospinal fluid (CSF) now present surrounding the cord. The sagittal T2-weighted image (*image not shown*) revealed high signal intensity in the central cord. This was thought to represent gliosis. Postoperatively, the patient's muscle strength and sensation improved.

DIAGNOSIS

Posttraumatic syringohydromyelia with interval shunting and collapse

DISCUSSION

By definition, syringomyelia describes a cavity in the spinal cord that is separate from but may communicate with the central canal. Hydromyelia is a dilatation of the central canal, lined by ependymal cells. In long-standing hydromyelia, however, the ependymal cells may be replaced by gliosis. If a syringomyelic cavity communicates with the central canal, it may develop an ependymal lining. In addition, the two entities may coexist. Therefore, it is difficult for the pathologist to distinguish syringomyelia from hydromyelia. The two entities are indistinguishable on imaging studies, and the terms syringohydromyelia and syrinx are often used to describe such cavities.

Syringohydromyelia has multiple etiologies that include trauma, cord neoplasm, arachnoiditis, surgery, and hindbrain malformations such as the Chiari malformations.[1] A posttraumatic syrinx may not be evident at the time of the initial trauma and may develop over months or years, presumably due to altered CSF flow dynamics. The clinical presentation of a cervical syrinx usually consists of progressive upper extremity weakness and muscle wasting, decreased upper extremity reflexes, and loss of sensation of pain and temperature but preservation of light touch and proprioception. With a posttraumatic syrinx, the sensory and motor findings are usually referable to a level above the cord injury site. An expanding spinal cord syrinx with progressive symptoms occurs in about 5% to 10% of traumatic spinal cord injuries.[2]

In patients with posttraumatic neurologic deterioration, MR can distinguish a possible treatable cause such as an enlarging syrinx compromising the cord from an untreatable cause such as myelomalacia. The decision to surgically shunt the syrinx depends on clinical symptomatology and progression of symptoms. Surgical correction of a syrinx may consist of shunting into the subarachnoid, pleural, or peritoneal space. A syrinx associated with a hindbrain malformation can additionally be treated with posterior fossa decompression, allowing the fourth ventricle to communicate with the subarachnoid space. The symptoms or neurologic deficit may not be reversed, but surgery frequently improves symptoms and halts progression.

MR Technique

MR is noninvasive and has rendered myelography obsolete in the diagnosis of syringohydromyelia. The syrinx can be directly visualized along with possible cord compression. The underlying etiology, such as a tumor, inferiorly displaced cerebellar tonsils, or trauma, is often also evident.

Pitfalls in Image Interpretation

Pulsation artifact or other patient motion can superimpose low signal over the spinal cord on sagittal images, simulating a syrinx. Comparison with axial images should disprove or confirm the presence of a cord abnormality.

Pathologic Correlate

Pathologically, syringomyelia appears to begin as a slit within one dorsal horn that connects behind the central canal to the other dorsal horn. This is illustrated in two stained cross sections of the spinal cord (*D*). As the slit enlarges, more and more of the adjacent tissue is destroyed, including the anterior horn. A more extensive syrinx in shown on gross section of the cervical (left) and thoracic (right) cord (*E*).

Clinical References

1. Sherman JL, Barkovich AJ, Citrin CM. The MR appearance of syringomyelia: new observations. AJR 1987;148:381–391.
2. Madsen PW, Green BA, Bowen BC. Syringomyelia. In: Rothman RH, Simeone FA, ed. The spine, 3rd ed. Philadelphia, WB Saunders, 1992;1575–1604.

(D and E *from Okazaki H, Scheithauer B. Atlas of neuropathology. New York, Gower Medical Publishing, 1988, p. 293. By permission of Mayo Foundation.*)

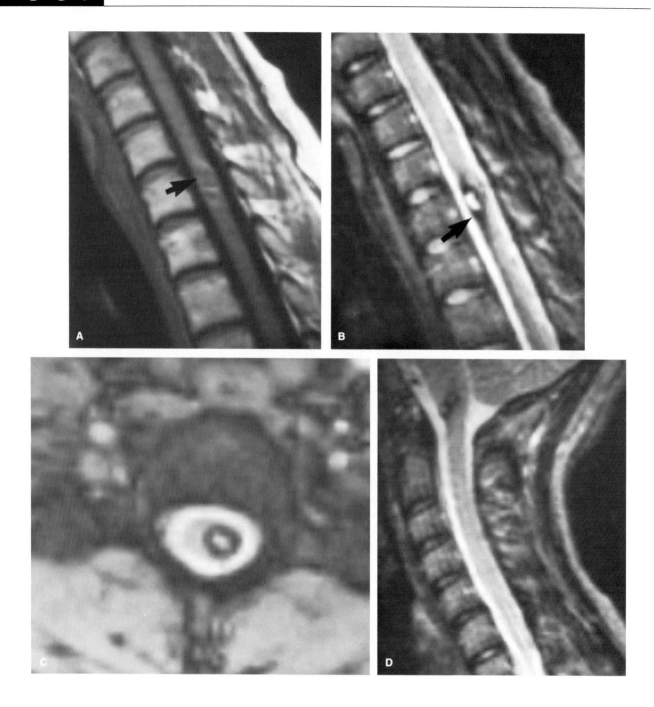

HISTORY

A 34-year-old woman with neck pain

FINDINGS

(A) There is a vague focus of high signal intensity within the spinal cord at the C7–T1 level (*arrow*), on the sagittal noncontrast T1-weighted image. (B) A central focus of high signal intensity with a surrounding smoothly marginated rim of hypointensity (*arrow*) is demonstrated at the corresponding level on the heavily T2-weighted image, consistent with hemorrhage. The axial gradient echo scan (*C*) demonstrates the central hyperintense fluid collection (methemoglobin), together with the smooth peripheral rim of hypointensity (hemosiderin/ferritin). (*D*) A second lesion with similar characteristics is present within the medulla (the slice adjacent to *B* on the T2-weighted sagittal scan is presented).

DIAGNOSIS

Multiple cavernous angiomas

DISCUSSION

Cerebrovascular malformations can be classified into four major categories: capillary telangiectasia, cavernous angioma, venous angioma, and arteriovenous malformation. Capillary telangiectasia and cavernous angioma cannot be distinguished by any imaging modality. Because they are usually angiographically occult, they are collectively referred to as occult cerebrovascular malformations (OCVM). Capillary telangiectasias most commonly occur in the pons as small solitary lesions. The overwhelming majority are clinically silent. Cavernous angiomas can occur anywhere in the central nervous system (CNS) and are multiple in up to one third of cases.[1-3] Up to 80% are familial. Seizure is the most common presentation, although many are clinically silent.

The appearance of OCVMs on MR imaging is characteristic and is related to hemosiderin and ferritin deposition within the parenchyma after hemorrhage. They are small, smoothly marginated lesions with borders that are mildly hypointense on T1-weighted images and markedly hypointense on T2-weighted images. This appearance results from hemosiderin/ferritin granule accumulation within macrophages that have phagocytosed extravasated blood. In the brain and spinal cord, macrophages cannot be removed, with subsequent accumulation around abnormal blood vessels. These findings are in distinction to the lesion centrally, which consists of a honeycomb of vascular spaces separated by fibrous strands. Irregularly marginated mild hypointensity may also be seen centrally due to calcium deposition.

Our case is a presumptive diagnosis based on characteristic MR findings. OCVMs are often a radiographic diagnosis, as most are asymptomatic and are discovered as incidental findings on exams performed for unrelated reasons.

Clinical References

1. Atlas SW. Intracranial vascular malformations and aneurysms. In: Magnetic resonance imaging of the brain and spine. New York, Raven Press, 1991;379–409.
2. Gomori JM, Grossman RI, Goldberg HI, et al. Occult cerebral vascular malformations: high field MR imaging. Radiology 1986;158:707–713.
3. Rigamonti D, Spetzler RF. Cerebral cavernous malformations—incidence and familial occurrence. N Engl J Med 1988;319:343–347.

(Parts of this case, as well as 31.412, 31.492, 31.498, 31.811, 32.3662, and 33.1521, were contributed by Robert Yeager, MD.)

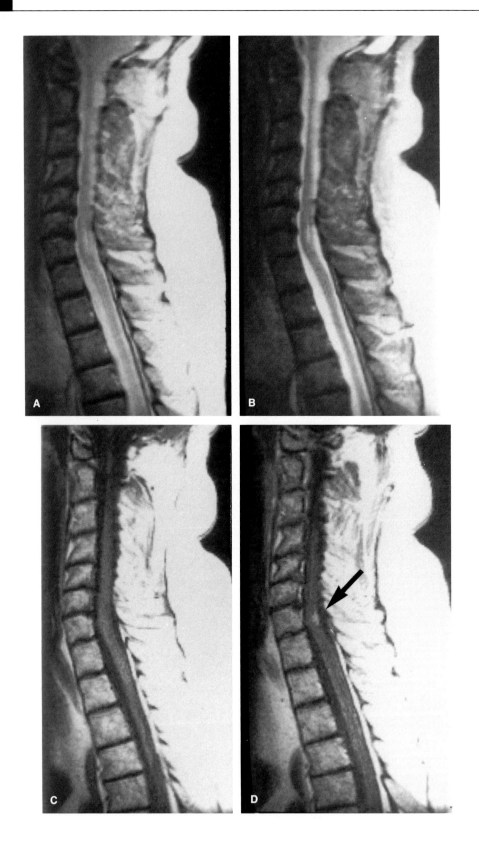

HISTORY

A 55-year-old patient with left arm weakness

FINDINGS

Sagittal (*A and B*) T2-weighted (TE = 45, 90) and (*C*) precontrast and (*D*) postcontrast T1-weighted images are presented. The precontrast exam is grossly normal. After contrast administration, an enhancing focus (*arrow*) is noted within the cord at the C7 level. In retrospect, a high-signal-intensity abnormality can be noted in the same general location on the T2-weighted exam. Two additional cord lesions were noted on adjacent sagittal postcontrast T1-weighted images (*images not shown*).

DIAGNOSIS

Spinal cord metastasis

DISCUSSION

In this instance, tumor appears to have metastasized to the cord substance itself. The cerebrospinal fluid was positive for neoplastic cells, and a lesion elsewhere was biopsied with the pathology revealing metastatic adenocarcinoma (unknown primary).

One in 20 cases (5%) of metastatic carcinoma to the central nervous system will demonstrate intramedullary spinal metastases. This occurs in most instances in conjunction with widespread metastatic disease to the central neuraxis. The thoracic cord is most often involved, with bronchogenic carcinoma the most frequent primary. Two patterns of cord involvement have been described: one in which the metastasis is confined within the cord, unassociated with leptomeningeal disease, and a rarer form in which a leptomeningeal deposit has grown to involve the cord parenchyma.

MR Technique

A recent clinical trial revealed that postcontrast scans were more informative than precontrast scans in 68% of all spine cases.[1] The most common type of additional information gained postcontrast was improved lesion visualization, as demonstrated in this case. IV contrast is advocated when intramedullary disease is suspected.

Pitfalls in Image Interpretation

The principal differential diagnosis in this instance would be a primary cord tumor (astrocytoma). However, these lesions tend to be quite large on presentation. The multiplicity of involvement in the present case also virtually excludes this diagnosis.

Clinical Reference

1. Runge VM, Bradley WG, Brant-Zawadzki MN, et al. Clinical safety and efficacy of gadoteridol: a study in 411 patients with suspected intracranial and spinal disease. Radiology 1991;181:701–709.

(A through D from Runge VM, Bradley WG, Brant-Zawadzki MN, et al. Clinical safety and efficacy of gadoteridol: a study in 411 patients with suspected intracranial and spinal disease. Radiology 1991; 181:701–709.)

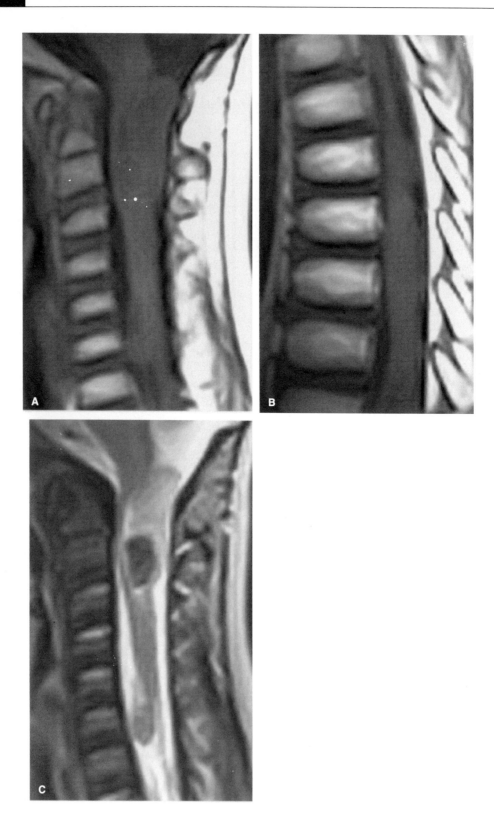

HISTORY

Two years before the present exam, this 9-year-old boy presented with persistent headache and vomiting. Imaging revealed obstructive hydrocephalus, with a mass in the pineal region that proved (by subtotal resection) to be a pineoblastoma. The patient subsequently received brain and spinal axis radiation, as well as chemotherapy. At this time, he presents with intractable vomiting, ataxia, and back pain.

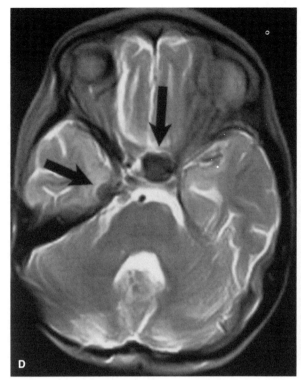

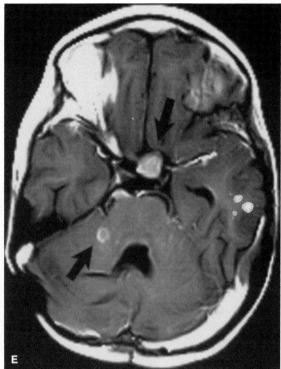

FINDINGS

A bulky soft tissue mass is noted at the C1–2 level, causing marked cord compression on the sagittal T1-weighted exam (*A*). (*B*) In the midthoracic region on the same exam, multiple additional soft tissue masses are seen within the thecal sac. These are immediately adjacent to the cord and produce an irregular surface contour. (*C*) The T2-weighted (TE = 90) exam in the cervical region identifies an additional lesion at the C6 level, which was poorly seen on the T1-weighted exam. A portion of the larger lesion at C1–2 is of low signal intensity, suggesting tumoral hemorrhage. (*D and E*) A head MR obtained 2 weeks later reveals intracranial metastases. Two low-signal-intensity foci (*arrows*) can be identified precontrast on the T2-weighted exam (*D*). At least two enhancing lesions (*arrows*) are identified postcontrast on the T1-weighted exam (*E*).

DIAGNOSIS

Leptomeningeal metastases from pineoblastoma

DISCUSSION

Tumors of the pineal region can arise from either pineal cells or germ cells. With regard to the former category, there are two main cell types: parenchymal cells (pinealocytes) and astrocytes. The more primitive tumors of pinealocyte origin are termed pineoblastomas, the more differentiated type pineocytomas. Tumors of astrocyte origin range from astrocytomas to glioblastomas. Most pineoblastomas occur in children in the first decade of life, with a 2:1 male:female ratio. These tumors are highly primitive and thus malignant, with frequent wide dissemination via cerebrospinal fluid (CSF). The prognosis is poor; this patient died 1 month after the head MR exam due to progression of metastatic disease. Pineocytomas occur in late adult life. Those with evidence of neuronal differentiation are relatively benign.

Although not illustrated in this case, IV contrast administration improves the sensitivity of MR for detection of subarachnoid tumor seeding. Its use should be considered in particular in pediatric patients with primary intracranial neoplasms, who frequently develop CSF-borne metastases.[1] Contrast-enhanced MR is thought to be superior to CT-myelography, with intramedullary tumor involvement in particular impossible to detect on CT. In a small pediatric clinical trial, contrast-enhanced MR was shown to be superior to both CSF evaluation and CT-myelography.[2] Nodular tumor growth and coating of the spinal cord by tumor were better delineated by MR than CT-myelography, with enhanced MR recommended as the initial screening modality for evaluation of possible subarachnoid metastatic disease spread.

Clinical References

1. Blews DE, Wang H, Kumar AJ, et al. Intradural spinal metastases in pediatric patients with primary intracranial neoplasms: Gd-DTPA-enhanced MR vs CT myelography. J Comput Assist Tomog 1990;14:730–735.
2. Kramer ED, Rafto S, Packer RJ, Zimmerman RA. Comparison of myelography with CT follow-up versus gadolinium MRI for subarachnoid metastatic disease in children. Neurology 1991;41:46–50.

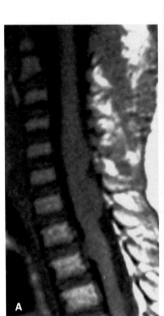

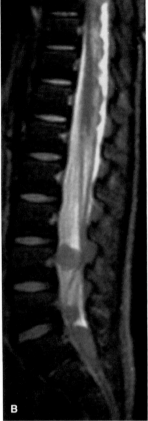

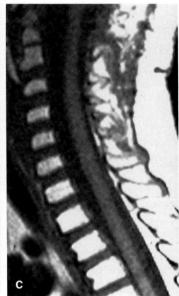

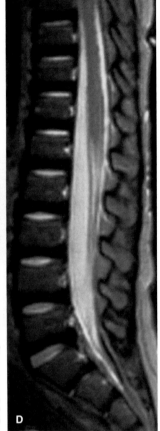

A   B   C   D

HISTORY

A 4-year-old child with headaches for 9 months who now presents with diminished coordination. Head MR (*images not shown*) revealed a midline enhancing posterior fossa mass with obstructive hydrocephalus. An initial spine MR was obtained (*A and B*). Treatment included resection of the posterior fossa mass, followed by whole brain and spinal axis radiation. A follow-up exam (*C and D*) was performed 2 months later.

FINDINGS

On the sagittal T1-weighted precontrast exam (*A*), multiple large soft tissue nodules are noted adjacent to the cervical cord. These demonstrated only very slight enhancement postcontrast (*exam not shown*). On the lumbar T2-weighted exam (*B*), additional soft tissue nodules are noted adjacent to the conus, adherent to the cauda equina, and near the termination of the thecal sac. On the follow-up exam 2 months later (*C*, sagittal T1 of the cervical spine; *D*, sagittal T2 of the lumbar spine), the thecal sac and its contents in both the cervical and lumbar regions appear normal. The effects of radiation therapy can be noted on the precontrast T1-weighted exam (*C*),

with homogeneous high marrow signal intensity. Detection of this change is aided by comparison with the previous exam and examination of the relative signal intensity of the cord, disk spaces, and marrow. The increase in marrow signal intensity and uniformity of signal is caused by radiation-induced replacement of normal red marrow by fat.

DIAGNOSIS

Leptomeningeal ("drop") metastases from medulloblastoma

DISCUSSION

Medulloblastomas are highly malignant neoplasms with a propensity for early cerebrospinal fluid dissemination. Postoperative radiation therapy applied to the entire neuraxis has markedly improved prognosis, with 10-year survival rates in the vicinity of 50%. Improved survival rates have correlated with the extent of surgical resection and magnitude of radiation therapy. Scans of the patient in this case were also normal at 6 months after therapy.

In the head, contrast enhancement has been dem-

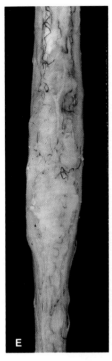
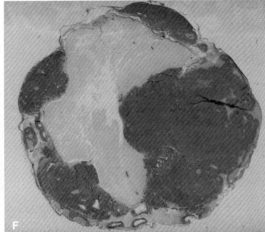
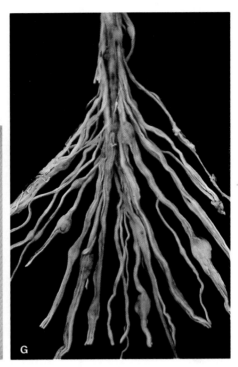

onstrated to reveal lesions (leptomeningeal seeding from medulloblastoma) not apparent without contrast, thus mandating the postcontrast exam.[1] However, not all recurrent medulloblastoma cases demonstrate abnormal enhancement, raising caution with respect to interpretation of spinal images.[2]

MR Technique

The entire spinal axis (cervical, thoracic, and lumbar) should be studied to rule out leptomeningeal tumor spread. Attention should be paid specifically to the dorsal aspect of the cord and the lumbar region, with the predominance of deposits in the latter likely to be on the basis of gravity.

Pitfalls in Image Interpretation

In the first few weeks after cranial surgery, the presence of methemoglobin can cause CSF to have abnormally high signal intensity on T1-weighted scans. If only postcontrast spine scans are obtained, this appearance could potentially be mistaken for leptomeningeal tumor spread.[3]

Pathologic Correlate

Three autopsy specimens are illustrated, each from a patient with dissemination of medulloblastoma within the subarachnoid space. (*E*) Diffuse subarachnoid spread can encase the spinal cord, causing an appearance resembling "icing." (*F*) A cross section of the cord reveals the deformity that may result from such encasement. (*G*) Subarachnoid seeding may also produce studding of caudal nerve roots.

Clinical References

1. Rippe DJ, Boyko OB, Friedman HS, et al. Gd-DTPA-enhanced MR imaging of leptomeningeal spread of primary intracranial CNS tumor in children. AJNR 1990;11:329–332.
2. Rollins N, Mendelsohn D, Mulne A, et al. Recurrent medulloblastoma: frequency of tumor enhancement on Gd-DTPA MR imaging. AJR 1990;155:153–157.
3. Wiener MD, Boyko OB, Friedman HS, et al. False-positive spinal MR findings for subarachnoid spread of primary CNS tumor in postoperative pediatric patients. AJNR 1990;11: 1100–1103.

(E through G *from Okazaki H, Scheithauer B. Atlas of neuropathology. New York, Gower Medical Publishing, 1988, pp. 113 and 114. By permission of Mayo Foundation.*)

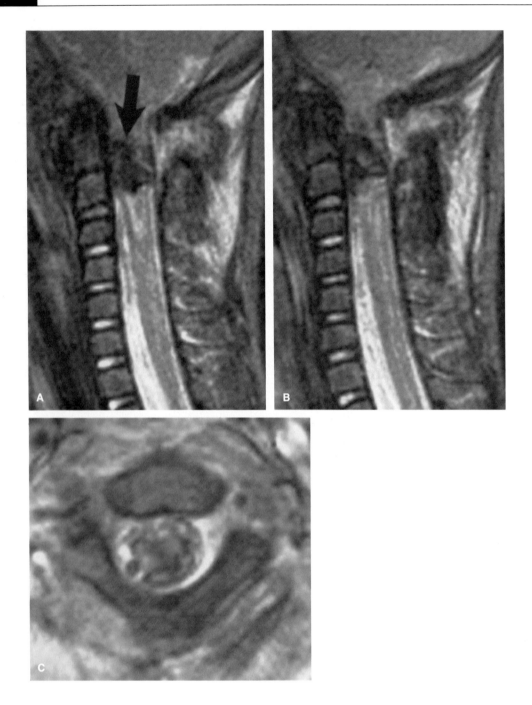

HISTORY

A 4-year-old girl following a motor vehicle accident

FINDINGS

(*A and B*) Two adjacent slices from the T2-weighted sagittal exam of the cervical spine reveal an intramedullary low-signal-intensity mass at the C1–2 level. The signal characteristics of the mass are consistent with deoxyhemoglobin. The caliber of the adjacent spinal cord is in-creased due to edema, which also extended into the medulla. (*C*) The axial gradient echo image through the body of C2 confirms the cord expansion, which is due at this level to intramedullary hemorrhage. There is substantial posterior soft tissue edema, best appreciated on the sagittal T2-weighted exam.

DIAGNOSIS

Acute spinal cord hemorrhage secondary to trauma

DISCUSSION

Acute injury to the spinal cord may result in one of several MR patterns that are best evaluated on T2-weighted images.[1,2] Type I pattern is a central area of hypointensity with a thin rim of hyperintensity, corresponding to deoxyhemoglobin with a methemoglobin periphery. Type II is a uniform area of hyperintensity, corresponding to spinal cord edema. Type III is isointense centrally with a thick rim of hyperintensity and is believed to represent a combination of hemorrhage and edema. Type I has a very poor prognosis. Patients presenting with spinal cord hemorrhage can expect very little recovery of neurologic function. A type II pattern, on the other hand, has an excellent prognosis. Patients with cord edema usually have significant improvement in neurologic function, often with complete recovery. Type III pattern patients show a variable course, usually with at least some recovery of function. Patients with a normal MR in the setting of acute injury and neurologic deficit have an excellent prognosis, usually with full recovery of neurologic function.

MR Technique

T2-weighted images should be used to assess acute spinal cord injury. Both hemorrhage and edema are well visualized.

Clinical References

1. Kulkarni MV, Bondurant FJ, Rose SL, Narayana PA. 1.5 Tesla MRI of acute spinal trauma. Radiographics 1988;8:1059–1082.
2. Mirvis SE, Geisler FH, Jelineck JJ, et al. Acute cervical spine trauma: evaluation with 1.5 T MR imaging. Radiology 1988;166:807–816.

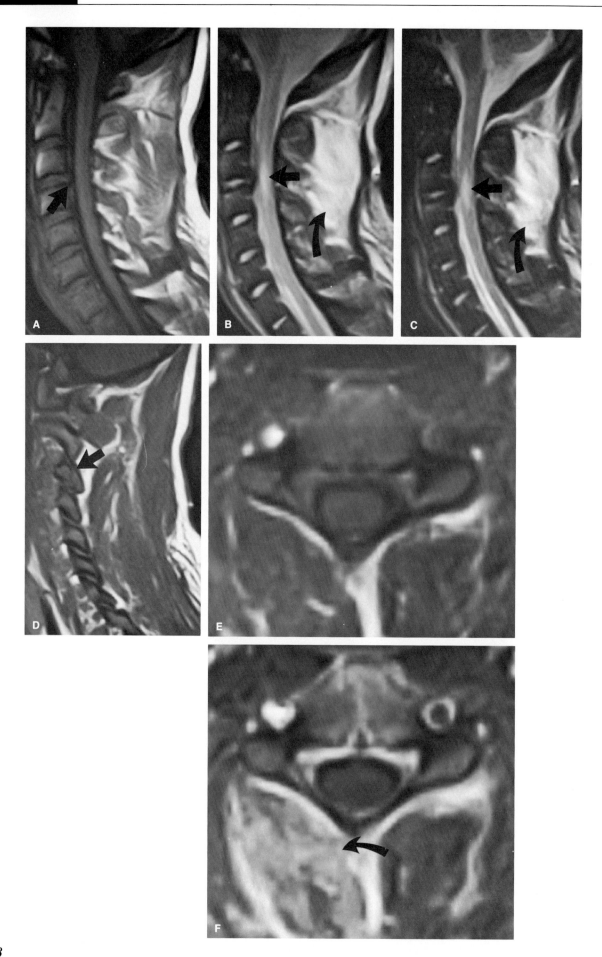

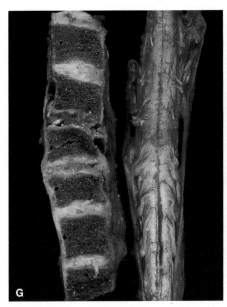
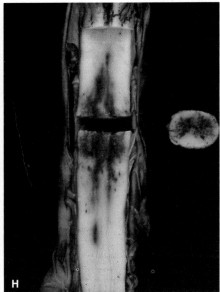

HISTORY

A 28-year-old man with central cord syndrome 3 days after a motor vehicle accident

FINDINGS

(A) The noncontrast T1-weighted sagittal image demonstrates a small central disk herniation (*arrow*) and small end plate spurs at the C3–C4 level, causing mild canal stenosis. The vertebral bodies are grossly normal in height and alignment. The (B) first (TE = 45) and (C) second (TE = 90) echoes of the sagittal T2-weighted exam demonstrate mild increased signal in the C3 and C4 vertebral bodies suggestive of microfractures. The C3–4 disk herniation and small spurs are again shown. Increased signal is present within the spinal cord at the C3–4 level (*arrow*), consistent with edema and cord contusion. No abnormal signal intensity that would suggest hemorrhage is present in the cord. The posterior musculature (*curved arrow*) shows abnormal high signal intensity. (D) The precontrast T1-weighted parasagittal image reveals discontinuity and deformity of the left C3 pedicle (*arrow*), consistent with a fracture. The (E) precontrast and (F) postcontrast T1-weighted axial images demonstrate asymmetric abnormal enhancement within the injured right paraspinous muscles (*curved arrow*).

Plain cervical spine films (*images not shown*) revealed a fracture–dislocation of C3–C4 with about 3 mm anterior listhesis of C3 on C4. No vertebral fracture was detected. Computed tomography (*images not shown*) revealed a linear fracture through the left pedicle at C3. Mild anterior listhesis of C3 on C4 was present with 20%

compromise of the spinal canal but no direct impingement on the spinal cord. Traction was applied before the MR, accounting for the normal alignment revealed on this study.

DIAGNOSIS

Flexion–rotation injury of the cervical spine

DISCUSSION

Flexion–rotation injuries of the cervical spine result in abnormalities attributable to a combination of these mechanisms. Bilateral facet fracture or dislocation is categorized as a flexion injury, with the unilateral facet fracture in this case resulting from flexion plus rotation. The subradiographic vertebral body fractures result from compression forces caused by hyperflexion of the spine. Injury of the posterior musculature and ligaments also results from a flexion mechanism, but the unilaterality is from rotation of the cervical spine causing preferential hyperextension and injury of the affected muscles.

This patient presented with a central cord syndrome. This syndrome is characterized by weakness in the upper extremities greater than the lower extremities, with or without sensory loss and loss of bladder control. Injury is thought to be due to compression of the central cervical spinal cord, with possible compression of the anterior spinal artery. A recent study with pathologic correlation found predominant involvement of the white matter in the lateral columns of the spinal cord in the region of the corticospinal tracts. Hemorrhage in the cord was not a common finding in this study.[1] This is in deference to the widely taught principle of damage in the central gray matter and cord hemorrhage.

Although it is important to evaluate the entire image when viewing all MR studies, this is particularly important in trauma cases. The spinal cord, marrow spaces, paraspinous soft tissues, and pedicles must be carefully evaluated. Abnormal signal in the spinal cord has been shown to correlate with significant neurologic injury.[2] The parasagittal images give a unique opportunity to evaluate the contour, alignment, and signal characteristics of the pedicles.

MR Technique

MR is valuable in evaluation of the posttraumatic spine, with the ability to detect intrinsic abnormalities of the spinal cord and soft tissue injury. The cord abnormalities can be inferred by a myelogram or CT, but direct visualization of cord injury is possible only with MR.

Pitfalls in Image Interpretation

Although MR is valuable in evaluating soft tissue trauma, cord injuries, and vertebral body fractures, CT is the method of choice for evaluation of posterior element fractures and canal narrowing due to retropulsed bone

fragments.[3] The patient must also be clinically stable and able to remain still for 30 to 45 minutes to obtain a high-quality MR study.

Pathologic Correlate

As is often the case, the external appearance of the spinal cord reveals little evidence of trauma in a gross specimen from a patient with a (*G*) C4–C5 fracture–dislocation. By sectioning the cord (*H*), the rostral and caudal extent of hemorrhagic necrosis is well depicted.

Clinical References

1. Quencer RM, Bunge RP, Egnor M, et al. Acute traumatic central cord syndrome: MRI-pathological correlations. Neuroradiology 1992;34:85–94.
2. Flanders AE, Schaefer DM, Doan HT, et al. Acute cervical spine trauma: correlation of MR imaging findings with degree of neurologic deficit. Radiology 1990;177:25–33.
3. Beale SM, Pathria MN, Masaryk TJ. MRI of spinal trauma. Top Magn Reson Imag 1988;1:53–62.

(G and H from Okazaki H, Scheithauer B. Atlas of neuropathology. New York, Gower Medical Publishing, 1988, p. 276. By permission of Mayo Foundation.)

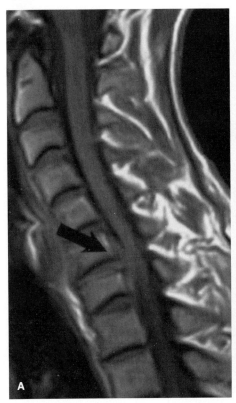 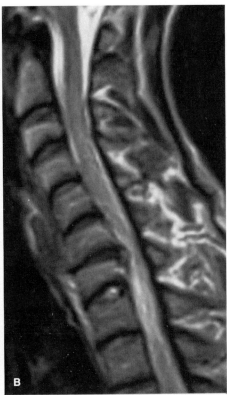

HISTORY

A 36-year-old patient with severe right arm and neck pain following a whiplash injury

FINDINGS

(A) The T1-weighted sagittal image, just to the right of midline, reveals a prominent extradural defect (*arrow*) at the C6–7 level. Abnormal soft tissue intensity extends well above and below the level of the disk. (B) The corresponding fast spin echo T2-weighted sagittal image redemonstrates the abnormality, which again appears contiguous with the C6–7 disk. Following contrast administration (C), it is evident that much of the lesion is made up of enhancing epidural venous plexus (*arrows*). (D) A postinfusion axial image at the C6–7 level confirms the abnormal extradural lesion (*arrow*), which fills the right C6–7 neural foramen. Mild mass effect on the right side of the spinal cord is also noted.

DIAGNOSIS

Posttraumatic right foraminal disk herniation at C6–7

DISCUSSION

Posttraumatic disk herniation is more common in the cervical region than in the thoracic or lumbar spine. As in this example, cervical disk herniation may occur following relatively minor trauma. As one might expect, the incidence of posttraumatic disk herniation increases as the degree of traumatic injury increases. Disk herniations are present in as many as half of patients with cervical spine fractures or a demonstrable neurologic deficit.[1] Posttraumatic disk herniations are most common in patients with hyperextension injuries, although they are by no means uncommon in flexion injuries. In flexion trauma, disk herniations are highly associated with facet dislocations.[2] Overall, posttraumatic disk herniations are most common at C5–6, followed by C6–7 and C4–5 in order of frequency.[1]

Acceleration hyperextension injuries, commonly referred to as whiplash injuries, are common, often secondary to motor vehicle accidents. In such patients, acute posterolateral disk herniations are prevalent.[3] These patients usually present with immediate onset of neck and arm pain. With milder trauma, delayed onset of pain is more typical and usually indicates ligamentous injury.

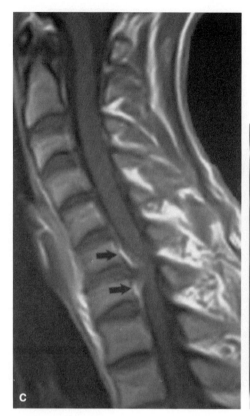

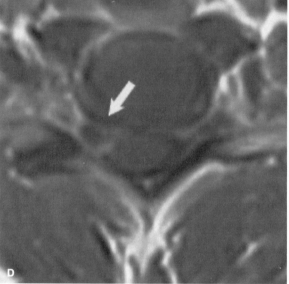

MR Technique

In patients with cervical spine fractures, disk herniations are most common immediately below the fracture site and somewhat less common just above the fracture.[1] Axial images at levels adjacent to the fracture site are thus mandatory in the evaluation of the posttraumatic cervical spine.

Clinical References

1. Flanders AE, Schaefer DM, Doan HT, et al. Acute cervical spine trauma: correlation of MR imaging findings with the degree of neurologic deficit. Radiology 1990;177:25–33.
2. Rizzolo SJ, Piazza MR, Cotler JM. Intervertebral disc injury complicating cervical spine trauma. Spine 1991;16:S187–189.
3. Davis SJ, Teresi LM, Bradley WG, et al. Cervical spine hyperextension injuries: MR findings. Radiology 1991;180:245–251.

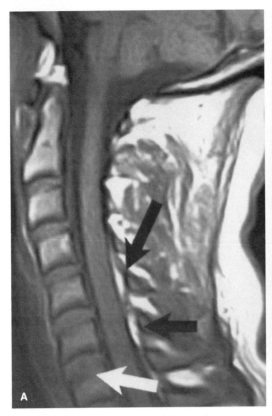

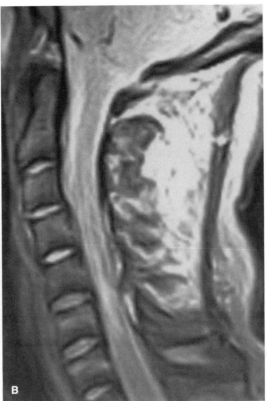

HISTORY

A 25-year-old man who was involved in a motor vehicle accident 12 hours earlier and now complains of bilateral upper extremity and shoulder pain

FINDINGS

(A) The sagittal T1-weighted exam on first inspection appears unremarkable, with perhaps only subtle loss of definition of the superior end plate of C7 (*white arrow*). On (B) the first and (C) the second echoes of the T2-weighted exam, abnormal high signal intensity is identified within the cord from C5 to C6, consistent with edema (cord contusion). There is obliteration from C4 to C6 of the CSF space that normally surrounds the cord. Posteriorly in the extradural space, abnormal soft tissue (with mixed high and low signal intensity) is identified (*white arrow in C*), causing thecal sac compression. Viewing the T1-weighted scan in retrospect, this abnormality can be seen and demonstrates high signal intensity (*black arrows in A*). Without comparison to the T2-weighted scan, this small extradural hematoma might have been mistaken for normal epidural fat. High signal intensity is identified on the T2-weighted images within the bodies of C6 and C7, due to microfractures and resultant marrow edema. This finding is consistent with the poor visualiza-

tion of the superior end plate of C7, which suggests gross bony damage. Extensive high signal intensity in the soft tissues posteriorly (*labeled "E" in C*) on the T2-weighted exam points to substantial soft tissue and ligamentous injury.

DIAGNOSIS

Cord contusion with small posterior extradural hematoma

DISCUSSION

In spinal trauma, both extraspinal soft tissue injury and intraspinal damage are common.[1] In the latter category, the abnormalities most frequently encountered on MR, when performed within 3 weeks of trauma, include extradural hematomas and spinal cord contusion. In the acute phase of injury, potentially correctable causes of neurologic impairment such as disk herniation or extradural hematomas can be identified by MR. Cervical spinal epidural hematoma, when large, requires emergency decompression.[2] In the case presented, the lesion did not require surgical intervention due to its small size and the stability of the patient's neurologic dysfunction, which was also only minor in degree.

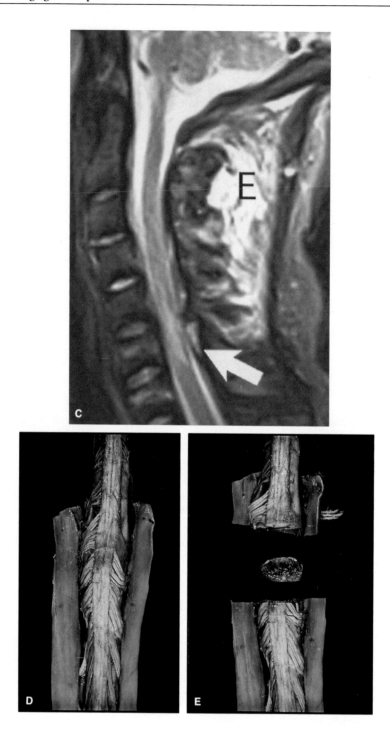

CT is superior to MR for the demonstration of osseous injury. However, in a recent comparison of CT and MR for evaluation of acute cervical spinal column injury, MR successfully demonstrated cord injuries in 13 of 33 patients, while CT was negative in all.[3] MR was also superior for demonstration of traumatic disk herniation. Thus, CT and MR should be used in conjunction for the assessment of spinal column injury.

MR Technique

As demonstrated in this case, on T1-weighted images it may be difficult to differentiate blood (methemoglobin) from fat. Newer fat-suppression techniques may thus play an important role in the assessment of trauma patients.

Pitfalls in Image Interpretation

T1-weighted scans, as in this patient, can underestimate the extent of thecal sac compromise. Soft tissue injury and marrow edema, the latter due to vertebral body microfractures, also are not well visualized on T1-weighted scans. It is thus important to examine the T2-weighted images closely for the detection of these abnormalities.

Pathologic Correlate

A gross specimen of a spinal cord from a C6–C7 fracture dislocation (D) demonstrates discoloration externally at the site of injury. Hemorrhagic necrosis is best illustrated with the specimen cut in cross section (E) through the point of maximum impact.

Clinical References

1. Kerslake RW, Jaspan T, Worthington BS. MRI of spinal trauma. Br J Radiol 1991;64:386–402.
2. Olshaker JS, Barish RA. Acute traumatic cervical epidural hematoma from a stab wound. Ann Emerg Med 1991; 20:662–664.
3. Levitt MA, Flanders AE. Diagnostic capabilities of MRI and CT in acute cervical spinal column injury. Am J Emerg Med 1991;9:131–135.

(D and E *from Okazaki H, Scheithauer B. Atlas of neuropathology. New York, Gower Medical Publishing, 1988, p. 276. By permission of Mayo Foundation.*)

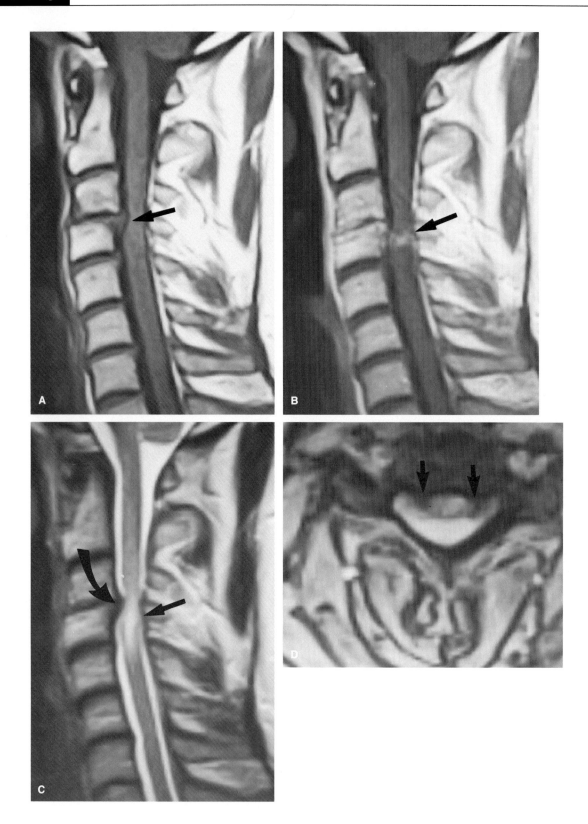

HISTORY

A 44-year-old patient with increasing pain and numbness in the upper extremities

FINDINGS

Mild retrolisthesis of C3 on C4 is identified on the midline T1-weighted sagittal image (*A*). The C3–4 intervertebral disk is narrowed, and a large extradural defect (*arrow*) is seen posterior to the disk. The cervical cord is moderately flattened by the extradural lesion but is normal in signal intensity. (*B*) The corresponding postcontrast T1-weighted image reveals prominent enhancement (*arrow*) within the flattened cervical cord. Abnormal enhancement is also apparent about the C3–4 disk. On the fast spin echo T2-weighted sagittal image (*C*), abnormally increased signal intensity is seen within the cord (*arrow*), extending from approximately mid-C3 to C4–5. The large extradural defect (*curved arrow*) at C3–4 is again noted; on this T2-weighted image, the abnormality is seen to be associated with prominent osteophytes. (*D*) A gradient echo axial image at the C3–4 level confirms the large extradural defect, which has high signal intensity compatible with disk material. Associated low-signal-intensity osteophytes (*small arrows*) are also apparent. The spinal cord is flattened and demonstrates abnormally increased signal intensity.

DIAGNOSIS

Early compressive myelomalacia secondary to a large hard disk herniation at C3–4

DISCUSSION

Myelomalacia is a general term used to describe a spectrum of findings that may be seen with chronic cord compression. The earliest form of myelomalacia is characterized by cord edema. Histologically, compression and stasis within postcapillary venules are present at this time. Disruption of the blood–cord barrier is also present, as evidenced by focal enhancement within the cord

in cases of early myelomalacia.[1] Precontrast T1-weighted images are usually normal at this time. T2-weighted images reveal increased signal intensity at the site of compression, usually with involvement of the width of the cord. With intermediate stages of myelomalacia, long-term cord edema results in cystic necrosis within the central gray matter. High signal intensity on T2-weighted images within the cord may then acquire a "snake eyes" appearance on axial images. In the intermediate setting, low signal intensity may be present within the cord on T1-weighted images. Late in the disease process, progressive cystic degeneration occurs within the central spinal cord. The central cyst fills with CSF that migrates through enlarged Virchow-Robin spaces or is produced by gliotic cells lining the cavity.[1] The central cyst may then progress to a frank syrinx that extends above and below the site of original compression, with eventual cord atrophy.

Abnormal signal intensity within a compressed spinal cord appears to have prognostic significance.[2] Mehalic and colleagues found that in patients who underwent decompression, decreased hyperintensity within the cord on T2-weighted images postoperatively correlated highly with improved clinical status. Additionally, patients with intense T2 signal abnormalities preoperatively fared better than patients with mild T2 abnormalities, perhaps indicating a more active process in the former patient group.

Pitfalls in Image Interpretation

Increased signal intensity within the spinal cord on T2-weighted images is a nonspecific finding. Causes other than myelomalacia include neoplasm, demyelinating disease, hemorrhage, gliosis, and contusion. Clinical evidence of myelopathy and imaging evidence of chronic cord compression assist in making the diagnosis of compressive myelomalacia.

Clinical References

1. Ramanauskas WL, Wilner HI, Metes JJ, et al. MR imaging of compressive myelomalacia. J Comput Assist Tomogr 1989; 13:399–404.
2. Mehalic TF, Pezzuti RT, Applebaum BI. MRI and cervical spondylotic myelopathy. Neurosurgery 1990;26:217–226.

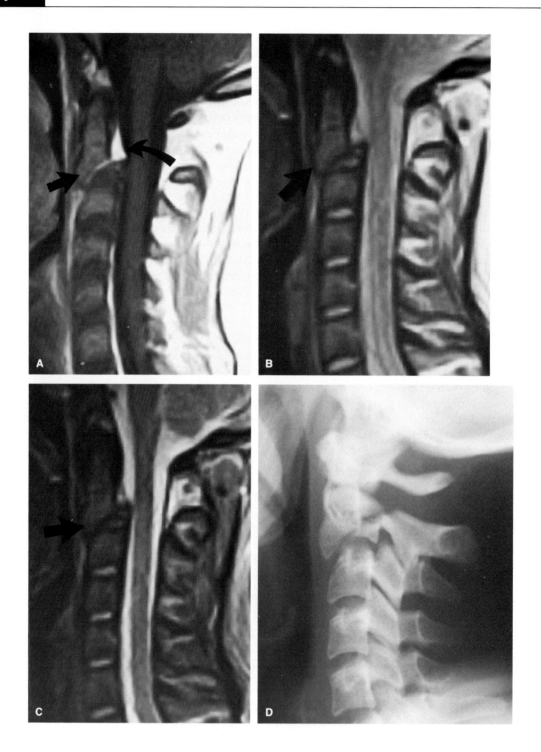

HISTORY

A 19-year-old woman 1 month after an unrestrained motor vehicle accident

FINDINGS

(*A*) T1-weighted sagittal image (obtained following contrast administration) and (*B and C*) dual echo T2-weighted sagittal images demonstrate a fracture (*arrows*) through the base of the dens. Mild anterior listhesis of the superior fracture fragment relative to the C3 vertebral body is present. A small amount of enhancing granulation tissue or venous plexus (*curved arrow*) is identified posterior to the dens. No evidence for cord compression or contusion is seen. (*D*) A plain lateral radiograph of the cervical spine confirms the dens fracture and the offset of the C2 and C3 vertebral bodies.

DIAGNOSIS

Type II dens fracture

DISCUSSION

Dens fractures may result from either hyperflexion or hyperextension injuries. These fractures are classified by Anderson based on the anatomic location of the fracture line.[1] Type I fractures involve the upper dens, type II fractures involve the junction of the dens and body, and type III fractures extend into the body of C2. More recently, it has been proposed that type I fractures represent occipitoatlantal disassociation and should thus be considered separately.[2] In clinical practice, it is common to discuss dens fractures as being high or low. High dens fractures are usually confined to the dens and frequently course transversely or obliquely through the dens. Because of the large amount of cortical bone in the dens, high dens fractures suffer from a high rate of nonunion. The low dens fracture represents a fracture through the superior body of the atlas. Because the body of the atlas is composed of high amounts of cancellous bone, complete healing of these fractures is the rule. Both high and low dens fractures are mechanically unstable. In either case, the dens and the atlas can move as a single unit on the body of C2.

MR Technique

Computed tomography (CT) can be superior to MR in detection of cervical spine fractures. The advantage of MR lies in improved contrast resolution, which allows simultaneous detection of disk herniations, ligamentous injury, and other soft tissue abnormalities. Assessment of the spinal cord is particularly important. T2-weighted images are highly sensitive for cord contusions and hemorrhage. Such findings are key factors in judging patient prognosis and often affect decisions regarding surgical intervention.[3]

Pitfalls in Image Interpretation

A transverse dens fracture may not be apparent on axial images, as the fracture line frequently parallels the imaging plane. This is a common pitfall with CT. In MR, the acquisition of sagittal correlative views obviates this problem.

Clinical References

1. Anderson LD, D'Alonzo RT. Fractures of the odontoid process of the axis. J Bone Joint Surg [Am] 1974;56:1663–1674.
2. Ellis G. Imaging of the atlas (C1) and axis (C2). Emerg Med Clin North Am 1991;9:719–732.
3. Flanders AE, Schaefer DM, Doan HT, et al. Acute cervical spine trauma: correlation of MR imaging findings with degree of neurologic deficit. Radiology 1990;177:25–33.

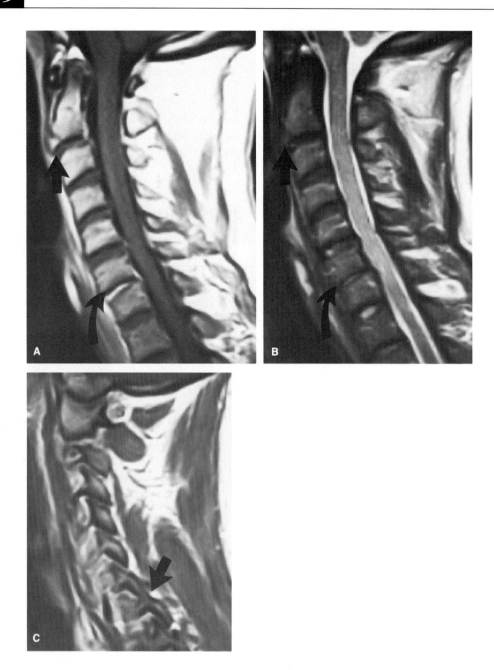

HISTORY

Left arm pain 6 months after a motor vehicle accident

FINDINGS

The midline T1-weighted (*A*) and fast spin echo T2-weighted (*B*) sagittal images demonstrate a teardrop fracture (*arrow*) at the base of C2, which had been previously noted. A very mild anterior listhesis of C6 on C7 (*curved arrow*) is also apparent. (*C*) T1-weighted sagittal images to the left of midline reveal a facet dislocation at C6–7 (*arrow*). The alignment of the facets on the right was normal (*image not shown*).

DIAGNOSIS

C2 teardrop fracture and unilateral perched facet at C6–7

DISCUSSION

MR is often useful for determining the cause of persistent pain after trauma. Disk herniations, which may present months after initial trauma,[1] are well visualized, and MR's superior soft tissue contrast allows detection of subtle cord and ligamentous injuries. The role of MR in evaluation of bony abnormalities is less clear. Computed tomography (CT) appears more sensitive than MR for detection of cervical spine fractures.[2] However, MR is quite useful in cases of persistent malalignment, where views of vertebral relationships are of foremost importance. Plain films are notoriously suboptimal for visualization of the lower cervical spine, particularly in patients who are immobilized because of their initial trauma. Oblique films may be impossible to obtain in these patients. Misalignments of the facets, such as the perched facet in this case, are largely inapparent on CT unless sagittal reconstructions are performed. MR easily images the lower cervical spine, and direct sagittal views reliably delineate vertebral alignment.

MR Technique

T1-weighted images are most useful for evaluating the anatomic relationships of the vertebral bodies, interver-

tebral disks, and the spinal cord. T2-weighted images are the most sensitive for intrinsic spinal cord abnormalities and soft tissue or ligamentous injury.

Pitfalls in Image Interpretation

Lateral sagittal images often receive little attention from novice MR readers. Facet dislocations are surprisingly common and are easily diagnosed when these images are carefully reviewed.

Clinical References

1. Davis SJ, Teresi LM, Bradley WG. Cervical spine hyperextension injuries: MR findings. Radiology 1991;180:245–251.
2. Mirvis SE, Geisler FH, Jelinek JJ, et al. Acute cervical spine trauma: evaluation with 1.5 T MR imaging. Radiology 1988; 166:807–816.

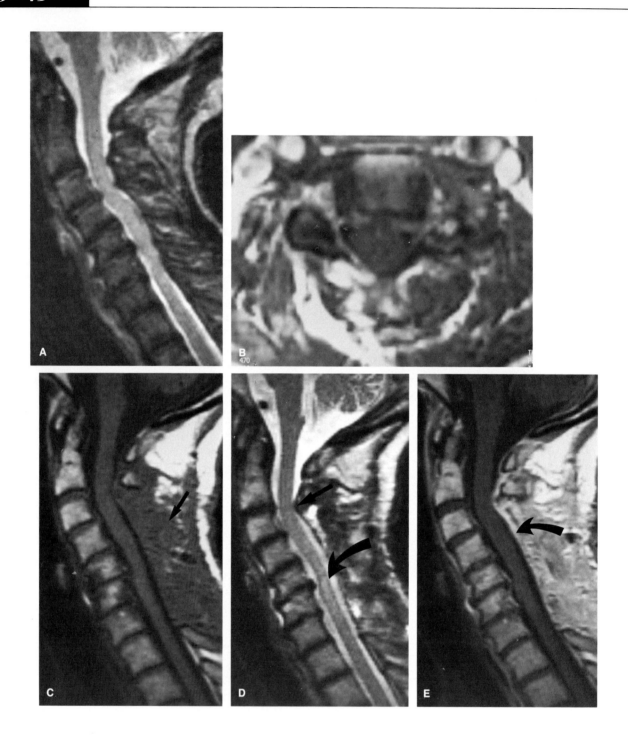

HISTORY

A 69-year-old patient with neck and bilateral arm pain

FINDINGS

(A) The T2-weighted sagittal image demonstrates mild congenital canal narrowing. Superimposed degenerative disease has resulted in mild to moderate cervical steno-sis, most prominent at C3–4, C4–5, and C5–6. Loss of the usual high-signal-intensity CSF space anterior and poste-rior to the cord is apparent in this region. The signal characteristics of the spinal cord are normal. (B) A post-contrast T1-weighted axial image at the C3–4 level reveals a small central disk herniation covered with a bony ridge. The resultant spinal stenosis causes mild cord flattening. The cord has an abnormal, somewhat triangular contour.

The patient underwent multilevel laminectomies 4 months after the original MR. Because of bilateral hand weakness postoperatively, a follow-up MR was performed. (*C*) The T1-weighted sagittal image reveals marked soft tissue edema and absence of the spinous processes from C3 to C7 (*arrow*), compatible with the recent laminectomies. On the fast spin echo T2-weighted sagittal image (*D*), the cervical canal appears substantially larger (compared with the preoperative exam), as evidenced by the presence of high-signal-intensity CSF anterior and posterior to the cord. The most significant area of relative canal narrowing at this time is at C2–3 (*arrow*), where no laminectomy was performed. Also noted is a small area of abnormally increased signal intensity within the cord at C5–6 (*curved arrow*). (*E*) A postcontrast T1-weighted sagittal image redemonstrates the bony hypertrophic changes at the posterior vertebral margins (C3–4 to C5–6). As a result of the laminectomies, however, ample CSF space is now present posterior to the cord (*curved arrow*). The cord has assumed a more normal, rounded configuration. The posterior soft tissues at the site of surgery demonstrate enhancement, which is due to postoperative inflammation and is not suggestive of infection.

DIAGNOSIS

Multilevel laminectomy for degenerative spinal stenosis

DISCUSSION

Cervical spondylosis is perhaps the most common cause of spinal cord disease in the elderly. Damage to the spinal cord and the resultant myelopathy are likely secondary to progressive cord compression with ischemic changes. Repetitive minor trauma as a result of the small dimensions of the canal may also play a role in cord pathology.[1] Results of surgery in patients with cervical stenosis have been somewhat disappointing. In general, the aim of surgery is to prevent further deterioration in cord function. Only 60% to 75% of patients will actually experience improvement in neurologic status postoperatively.[2]

The choice of anterior versus posterior approaches in the neurosurgical treatment of cervical stenosis remains somewhat controversial. Typically, anterior approaches are preferred in patients with one or at most two levels of stenosis. Patients with congenital canal narrowing or extensive contiguous levels of spondylotic narrowing generally fare better with multiple laminectomies.

MR is useful in both the pre- and postoperative assessment of patients with cervical stenosis. If significant cord atrophy or myelomalacia is present preoperatively, clinical improvement following surgery is unlikely.[1] If surgery is contemplated, MR provides excellent visualization of areas of significant canal compromise, thereby guiding the surgical approach. Postoperatively, causes of poor outcome such as inadequate decompression, spinal instability, or intrinsic cord damage are well visualized. In the current case, the patient developed worsening upper extremity symptoms despite apparently adequate decompression. The increased signal intensity within the cord on the postoperative study was a new finding, and thus a diagnosis of postoperative cord contusion was suggested.

Pitfalls in Image Interpretation

In patients who have undergone surgery for spinal stenosis, increased signal intensity on T2-weighted images within the cord is a nonspecific finding. The abnormality may represent myelomalacia or gliosis secondary to the prior stenosis. However, postoperative complications, including cord contusion and infarction, also have this appearance. Knowledge of clinical findings and comparison with prior studies assist in determining the true significance of these lesions.

Clinical References

1. Clifton AG, Stevens JM, Whitear P, Kendall BE. Identifiable causes for poor outcome in surgery for cervical spondylosis: postoperative CT and MR imaging. Neuroradiology 1990;32:450–455.
2. Batzdorf U, Flannigan BD. Surgical decompressive procedures for cervical spondylotic myelopathy: a study using MRI. Spine 1991;16:123–127.

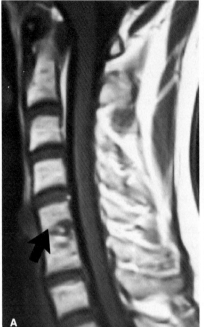 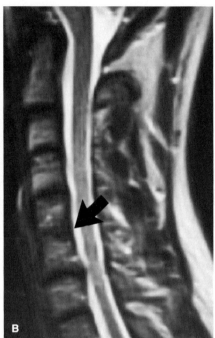

HISTORY

Left arm pain 4 months post–anterior diskectomy and fusion for a C5–6 herniated disk

FINDINGS

(*A*) The sagittal T1-weighted image (obtained following contrast administration) demonstrates fusion of the C5 and C6 vertebral bodies. Mildly decreased signal intensity is evident within the central portion of the fusion (*arrow*). Decreased signal intensity at the fusion site (*arrow*) is also present on the T2-weighted sagittal image (*B*). No normal intervertebral disk is identified at C5–C6. The alignment of the cervical spine is normal.

DIAGNOSIS

Normal late appearance of anterior cervical diskectomy and fusion

DISCUSSION

Anterior diskectomy and fusion is the most commonly performed neurosurgical procedure in patients with cervical disk disease. The procedure usually involves removal of the abnormal disk and portions of the adjacent vertebral bodies, followed by insertion of a bone graft. Immediately following this procedure, the bone graft is readily apparent as a rectangular area of abnormal signal intensity at the level of the disk space. The signal intensities of grafts vary widely due to the variability of marrow within the grafts.[1] Months after the operation, abnormal signal at the level of the disk is still present, although the bone graft is no longer identified as a discrete entity. The signal characteristics of the graft remain variable, although decreased signal intensity on T1- and T2-weighted images is usually seen. After 2 years or more, continuous marrow signal at the site of fusion is the rule. At this point, no signs of the bone graft or the native intervertebral disk should be apparent.

Pitfalls in Image Interpretation

In the early postoperative period, increased signal intensity on T2-weighted images is commonly seen in the prevertebral space. This appearance is usually secondary to edema from the anterior approach. Edema should be isointense to muscle on T1-weighted images. Areas of high signal intensity on T1-weighted images suggest the presence of a hematoma.

Clinical Reference

1. Ross JS, Masaryk TJ, Modic MT. Postoperative cervical spine: MR assessment. J Comput Assist Tomogr 1987;11:955–962.

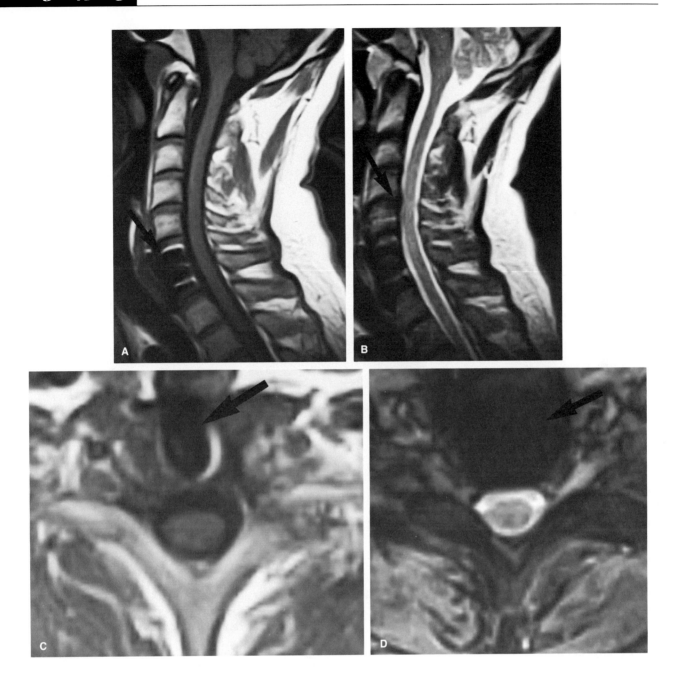

HISTORY

A 48-year-old patient with continued neck pain following anterior diskectomy and fusion for a C6–7 disk herniation

FINDINGS

The T1-weighted midline sagittal image (*A*) reveals a prominent metallic susceptibility artifact (*arrow*) anterior to and within the C6 and C7 vertebral bodies. The alignment of the cervical vertebral bodies is normal. No significant canal stenosis is present. The artifact is again apparent on the fast spin echo T2-weighted sagittal image (*B*). A minimal osteophyte (*arrow*) causes effacement of the ventral subarachnoid space at C4–5. The T1-weighted axial image at C6–7 (*C*) redemonstrates the metallic artifact (*arrow*) and confirms the normal dimensions of the spinal canal. On the corresponding gradient echo axial image (*D*), the susceptibility artifact (*arrow*) is much more severe, resulting in distortion of the normal dimensions of the vertebral bodies. A lateral plain radiograph of the cervical spine (*E*) demonstrates a metallic plate and three screws that fuse the C6 and C7 vertebral bodies.

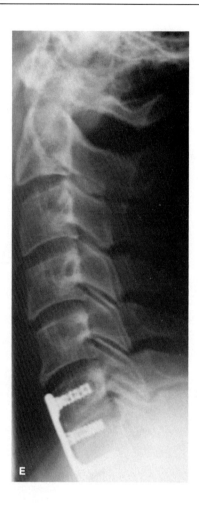

DIAGNOSIS

Normal appearance post–anterior diskectomy and titanium plate fusion at C6–7

DISCUSSION

A wide variety of techniques of anterior diskectomy and fusion are currently used in the treatment of cervical disk herniation.[1] Common to virtually all of these techniques is removal of the offending intervertebral disk and subsequent bone grafting to achieve stable union of the adjoining vertebral bodies. The technique most commonly used in the United States is the Smith-Robinson method, in which a horseshoe-shaped graft is placed between the vertebral bodies following diskectomy. The vertebral end plates are usually preserved with this technique. The Bailey and Badgley technique and the Cloward technique are alternative methods in which portions of the adjacent vertebral bodies are removed and a bone graft is placed that attempts to match the surgically created defect. In patients in whom multiple anterior diskectomies and fusions are performed, increased rates of graft failure, graft collapse, and pseudoarthrosis formation are seen. To avoid such difficulties, many surgeons prefer subtotal corpectomies and fusion using a long fibular strut graft. This type of procedure is recommended for cases in which three or more levels of disease are present.

Recently there has been increased interest in the use of anterior cervical plate fixation to facilitate cervical fusion. This technique allows for cervical decompression and stable fixation in a single stage.[2] The titanium supports provide immediate stability, with theoretical advantages for optimal bony union. Fixation of the bone graft to the anterior plate provides protection against graft extrusion, a significant source of morbidity in conventional cervical fusion patients.

MR Technique

Gradient echo techniques are often used for evaluation of the cervical spine. In patients with metallic fixation devices, however, the lack of a 180° refocusing radio-frequency pulse in gradient echo sequences leads to markedly increased susceptibility artifacts as compared with spin echo techniques. Spin echo imaging is thus essential in the evaluation of these patients.

Pitfalls in Image Interpretation

Titanium's strength, malleability, and endurance have led to its increased use for internal fixation procedures of the spine. MR artifacts from titanium, while apparent, are relatively minor. Stainless steel alloys are also commonly used for spinal fixation and for the most part are considered nonmagnetic. In the strong magnetic fields used for MR, however, stainless steel exhibits considerable magnetism, and the resultant artifacts often preclude adequate assessment of the spinal canal.[3]

Clinical References

1. Wood EG, Hanley EN. Types of anterior cervical grafts. Orthop Clin North Am 1992;23:475–486.
2. Suh PB, Kostuik JP, Esses SI. Anterior cervical plate fixation with the titanium hollow screw plate system: a preliminary report. Spine 1990;15:1079–1081.
3. Mirvis SE, Geisler F, Joslyn JN, Zrebeet H. Use of titanium wire in cervical spine fixation as a means to reduce MR artifacts. AJNR 1988;9:1229–1231.

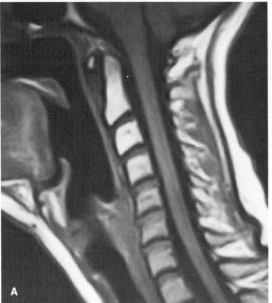
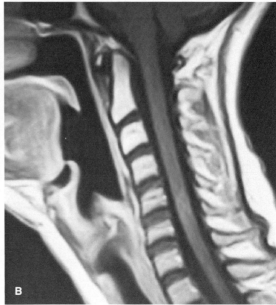

HISTORY

A 45-year-old woman with a previous left radical neck dissection and radiation therapy for squamous cell carcinoma of the mouth

FINDINGS

The midline sagittal T1-weighted image (A) demonstrates diffuse homogeneous high signal intensity throughout the marrow spaces of the C2 through the C4 vertebral bodies. The high signal intensity in the marrow spaces shows an abrupt transition to the normal marrow signal intensity of the adjacent lower cervical vertebral bodies. The postcontrast image reveals no focal enhancement (B).

DIAGNOSIS

Radiation therapy changes with fatty replacement of bone marrow

DISCUSSION

Radiation therapy is a common treatment for malignant diseases in many locations of the body. The radiation port may therefore include the spine, from the cervical region to the coccyx. Radiation changes are confined to the treatment area and are sharply demarcated from the adjacent normal marrow signal, corresponding with the radiation port.[1] Fatty replacement of bone marrow is a sequela of irradiation that can occur as early as 2 weeks after initiation of radiation therapy, with a gradual increase in signal intensity over time. In a prospective study, the fatty changes persisted for at least 2 years, with no evidence of reconversion.[2] Recurrent disease will present as low T1 signal intensity.

The high signal of fatty marrow is accentuated in young patients. The normal marrow spaces in these individuals have low T1 signal intensity due to hematopoietic elements in the marrow. With normal aging, gradual replacement of the hematopoietic elements by fat results in decreased contrast between the normal marrow and areas of fatty infiltration secondary to the radiation treatment.

MR Technique

T1-weighted sagittal images best demonstrate fatty marrow changes. These images show high signal in the affected vertebrae and normal signal in the unaffected levels.

Pitfalls in Image Interpretation

In a patient with fatty marrow replacement due to radiation therapy, enhancing metastatic lesions may be difficult to differentiate from the high signal of the fatty marrow on postcontrast images. Precontrast images are usually more sensitive for detection of metastatic foci, even in the absence of fatty marrow.

Clinical References

1. Remedios PA, Colletti PM, Raval JK, et al. MRI of bone after radiation. Magn Reson Imag 1988;6:301–304.
2. Yankelevitz DF, Henschke CI, Knapp PH, et al. Effect of radiation therapy on thoracic and lumbar bone marrow: Evaluation with MR imaging. AJR 1991;157:87–92.

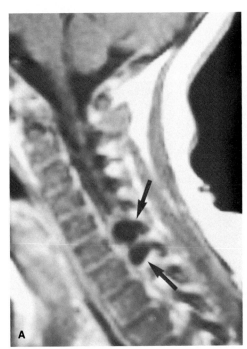
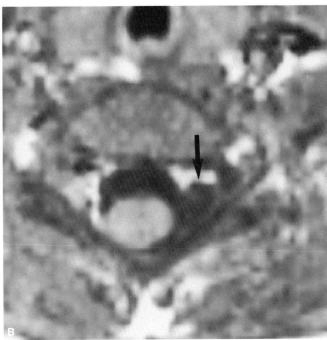

HISTORY

A 15-month-old infant with left upper extremity spasticity since birth

FINDINGS

(A) The T1-weighted left parasagittal view of the cervical spine reveals two low-signal-intensity extradural fluid collections (*arrows*) within the C6–7 and C7–T1 neural foramina. These two abnormalities remained isointense with CSF on T2-weighted scans (*images not shown*). (B) An axial T1-weighted spin echo scan confirms, at one level, the extradural location of the lesion (*arrow*) and the association with the exiting nerve root sleeve.

DIAGNOSIS

Meningocele secondary to birth trauma

DISCUSSION

Supraclavicular traction of the brachial plexus may occur during breech deliveries or, as in this case, shoulder dystocia (difficult shoulder delivery). This can result in a variety of pathologic conditions, including posttraumatic neuromas, focal or diffuse fibrosis, and traumatic meningocele with or without nerve root avulsion.[1,2] Neuromas appear as a fusiform mass contiguous with or adjacent to the brachial plexus, and have been described (in this setting) to be isointense to normal nerve tissue on all pulse sequences. Fibrosis is also isointense to nerve tissue, appearing as focal or diffuse thickening of the roots or trunk. Meningoceles will follow the course of the nerve root as it enters the neural foramen and are isointense to CSF on all pulse sequences. The role of MR in assessing nerve root avulsion appears limited to date, with this condition best evaluated by cervical myelography.

Clinical References

1. Gupta R, Mehta V, Banerji A, Jain R. MR evaluation of brachial plexus injuries. Neuroradiology 1989;31:377–381.
2. Popovich M, Taylor F, Helmer E. MR imaging of birth-related brachial plexus avulsion. Am J Neuroradiol 1989; 10:S98.

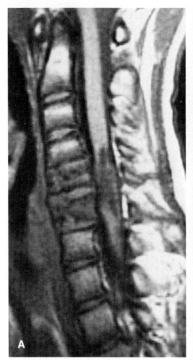
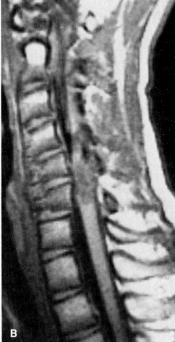
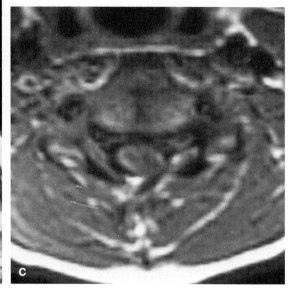

HISTORY

A 13-year-old boy, 1 year after a sledding accident

FINDINGS

Sagittal (*A and B*) and axial (*C*) T1-weighted scans reveal abnormal low signal intensity within the cord substance from C4 to C6. There is slight cord expansion. Associated findings include abnormal marrow signal intensity and loss of height of C5 and C6. There is also indentation of the thecal sac anteriorly by bone and disk at C5–6.

DIAGNOSIS

Myelomalacia in chronic cord injury

DISCUSSION

Chronic injuries of the spinal cord have a variety of appearances on MR imaging. Five patterns have been described: (1) normal signal intensity; (2) normal signal on T1-weighted images and high signal intensity on T2-weighted images; (3) hypointensity on T1-weighted and hyperintensity on T2-weighted images; (4) cord atrophy; and (5) syrinx formation with signal intensity that approximates CSF on all pulse sequences.[1] These patterns correlate well with the severity of spinal cord injury and the spectrum of pathologic changes. Patients with normal T1- and T2-weighted images have only slight neurologic injury and an excellent prognosis, while those with hypointensity on T1-weighted and hyperintensity on T2-weighted images have severe injury and the least favorable prognosis.

Cord edema may be the only pathologic change when injury is mild, with an excellent prognosis for recovery and scant MR findings. Increasingly greater forces will result in cord contusion and, finally, frank hemorrhage with rupture of cellular membranes, liquefaction, and necrosis. Myelomalacia is the result of tissue necrosis and is manifested on MR images as hypointensity on T1-weighted images. This may or may not progress to development of a syrinx.[2] A syrinx is believed to result from central cores of necrotic tissue that coalesce to form a cavity that communicates with the central canal. The syrinx may increase in size over time, resulting in a progressive loss of neurologic function. Atrophy of the spinal cord, defined as a cord diameter of less than 6 mm in the cervical spine and less than 5 mm in the thoracic spine, may occur in patients with a long-standing myelopathy. Atrophy may be limited to the local site of injury or involve a variable length of cord distally.

MR Technique

The presence or absence of a syrinx and its extent are best determined on T1-weighted axial images. Sagittal or coronal images may miss a small syrinx or underestimate its extent due to partial volume imaging. Although in the past T2-weighted images have been inferior for delineation and/or recognition of a syrinx, due to image degradation from CSF pulsation, newer fast spin echo T2-weighted techniques show promise and may in certain instances be superior to T1-weighted images.

Clinical References

1. Yamashita Y, Takahashi M, Matsuno Y, et al. Chronic injuries of the spinal cord: assessment with MR imaging. Radiology 1990;175:849–854.
2. Curati WL, Kingsley DP, Kendall BE, Moseley IF. MRI in chronic spinal cord trauma. Neuroradiology 1992;35:30–35.

(Images courtesy of Mark Osborne, MD)

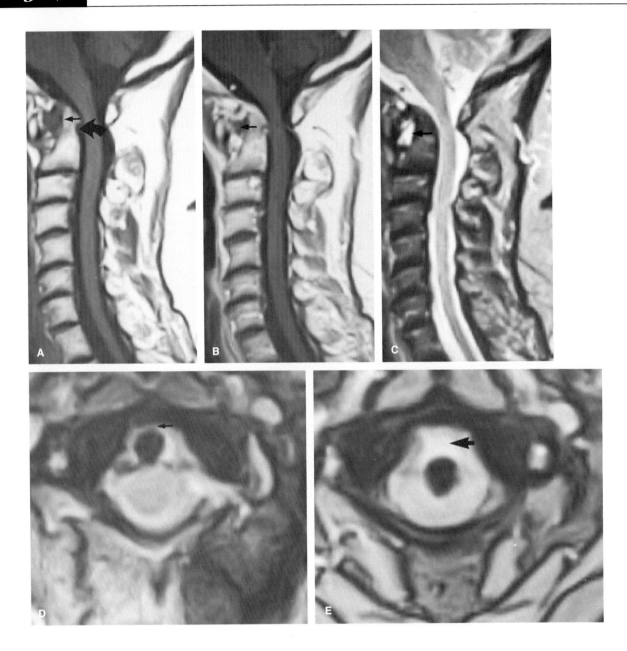

HISTORY

A 72-year-old woman with advanced rheumatoid arthritis who now presents with neck and left arm pain

FINDINGS

(A) The sagittal T1-weighted precontrast image demonstrates a large soft tissue mass (*small arrow*) predominantly anterior to the odontoid process. The cortex of the dens is mildly irregular (*curved arrow*). (B) Enhancement of the soft tissue mass (*small arrow*) is seen on the postcontrast sagittal T1-weighted image. (C) The sagittal T2-weighted image shows high signal intensity within the soft tissue mass (*small arrow*), representing fluid and inflammation. Areas of low signal intensity consistent with fibrosis and chronic reactive changes are also present. (D) A normal space (*arrow*) is present between the dens and the anterior arch of C1 on the axial gradient echo image. (E) The axial gradient echo image in flexion demonstrates increased space (*arrow*) measuring 8 mm between the dens and C1, indicating atlantoaxial subluxation. The upper cervical cord is compressed between the dens and the posterior arch of C1. Atlantoaxial subluxation is confirmed on the lateral plain radiograph of the cervical spine (F). The distance between the anterior arch of C1 and the dens measured 11 mm.

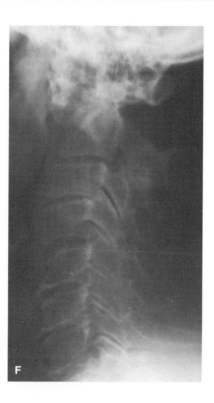

DIAGNOSIS

Rheumatoid arthritis with atlantoaxial subluxation

DISCUSSION

Rheumatoid arthritis begins as a synovitis and can occur in any synovial-lined joint of the body. The disease typically presents with polyarticular involvement of the appendicular skeleton. It can also involve the axial skeleton, and the upper cervical spine is commonly affected in patients with long-standing rheumatoid arthritis. This occurs most frequently at the articulation between the atlas and the dens, but may also affect other levels in the cervical spine.

Rheumatoid involvement of the craniocervical junction and upper cervical spine may result in numerous abnormalities. Inflammatory changes at the articulation between the atlas and the dens may result in increased atlantodental space due to atlantoaxial subluxation and instability. An inflammatory pannus often surrounds and erodes the odontoid process. Involvement of the transverse ligament or synovium can produce a retrodental soft tissue mass. Long-standing involvement may produce settling of the skull on the atlas. Atlantoaxial subluxation and settling at the craniovertebral junction may result in neurologic symptoms due to compression of the spinal cord or cervicomedullary junction.

Magnetic resonance imaging is valuable in fully identifying the abnormalities at the craniovertebral junction including abnormal angulation and compression at the cervicomedullary junction.[1] The anatomy of the cranio-vertebral junction is accurately depicted on the sagittal images. The high soft tissue contrast of MR also permits demonstration of inflammatory tissues. The detection of spinal cord impingement may indicate the need for surgical intervention and stabilization of the atlantoaxial articulation.[2]

MR Technique

Images obtained with the neck flexed may show evidence of atlantoaxial subluxation and spinal cord or brain stem compression not detected with the neck in neutral position.

Pitfalls in Image Interpretation

Cortical bone destruction and erosion of the odontoid process in rheumatoid arthritis may be overestimated by MR due to associated osteopenia, as well as senile osteoporosis.[3]

Clinical References

1. Bundschuh C, Modic MT, Kearney F, et al. Rheumatoid arthritis of the cervical spine: surface coil MR imaging. AJR 1988;151:181–187.
2. Aisen AM, Martel W, Ellis JH, McCune WJ. Cervical spine involvement in rheumatoid arthritis: MR imaging. Radiology 1987;165:159–163.
3. Pettersson H, Larsson EM, Holtas S, et al. MR imaging of the cervical spine in rheumatoid arthritis. AJNR 1988;9:573–577.

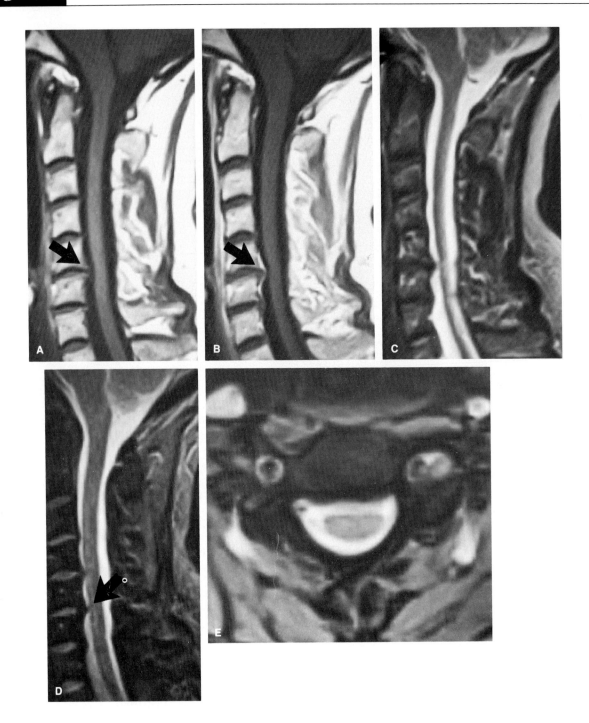

HISTORY

A 57-year-old female with right-sided neck and arm pain

FINDINGS

T1-weighted sagittal images before (*A*) and after (*B*) contrast administration and the precontrast sagittal T2-weighted image (*C*) demonstrate a ventral extradural defect (*arrow in A and B*) along the anterior margin of the

thecal sac at the C5–6 level. (*A*) The precontrast sagittal T1-weighted image shows pointed extensions of bone marrow signal intensity along the posterior end plates adjacent to the C5–6 disk. (*B*) Postcontrast, enhancement of the dilated venous plexus is noted immediately above and below the C5–6 level. (*D*) The sagittal T2*-weighted gradient echo image demonstrates the low-signal-intensity spurs at C5–6 (*arrow*), as well as small spurs at C4–5 and C6–7 that partially efface the ventral subarachnoid space. Mild irregularities of the posterior margin of the vertebral end plate are present on the axial T2*-weighted gradient echo image (*E*). The signal intensity of these projections is very low, indicative of cortical bone. These findings are consistent with osteophytes extending from the posterior vertebral end plates.

DIAGNOSIS

Hypertrophic osteophytic end plate spurs

DISCUSSION

Hypertrophic spurs may be asymptomatic or may produce significant canal stenosis with cord impingement and compression. Symptoms can be indistinguishable clinically from a disk herniation. Radiographic findings, however, may not correlate well with the patient's symptoms.[1]

Osteophytic spurs are the end result of a disk bulge or disk herniation that elevates the ligamentous attachments to the end plates. During the healing process, bone is laid down, forming an osseous projection. The spurs frequently have a curved contour corresponding with the adjacent disk herniation. These projections have low signal intensity on MRI consistent with cortical bone.

One goal of MRI is to distinguish an osteophyte from an acute disk herniation. Gradient echo images are quite helpful in this regard. On gradient echo images, disk material is usually of high signal intensity, even in degenerated disks.[2] In contrast, osseous spurs are nearly void of signal. Cerebrospinal fluid (CSF) has very high signal intensity, outlining the spur with low signal intensity.

Postinfusion images are also helpful in defining a spur on spin echo sequences. The intense enhancement of the epidural venous plexus profiles the low signal intensity of the spur. T1-weighted images may also show a pointed projection at the vertebral end plates that is contiguous with and follows the signal intensity of bone marrow. Marrow extension into the osteophyte is more common with larger spurs.

MR Technique

Gradient echo images are particularly beneficial in delineating osseous margins. Osteophytic spurs are low signal intensity outlined by the high signal intensity of adjacent CSF contained within the thecal sac.

Pitfalls in Image Interpretation

Posterior osteophytes may be difficult to differentiate from a calcified disk.

Clinical References

1. Ross JS, Modic MT, Masaryk TJ, et al. Assessment of extradural degenerative disease with Gd-DTPA-enhanced MR imaging: correlation with surgical and pathologic findings. AJNR 1989;154:1151–1157.
2. Hackney DB. Degenerative disk disease. Top Magn Reson Imag 1992;4:12–36.

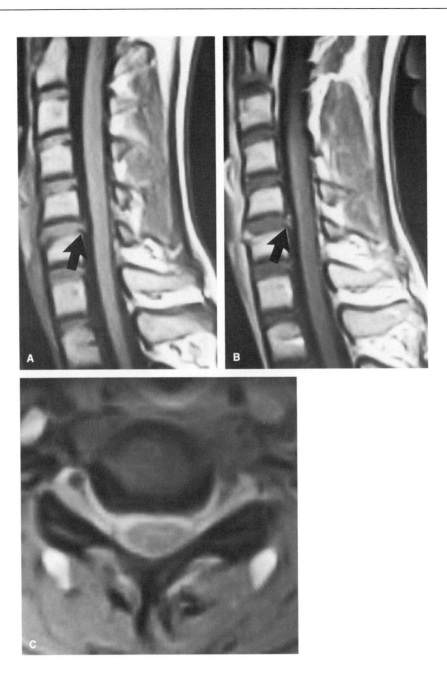

HISTORY

A 20-year-old woman with neck pain

FINDINGS

(A) The sagittal preinfusion T1-weighted image demonstrates a broad-based disk bulge (*arrow*) at the C5–6 level. The disk protrusion flattens the adjacent thecal sac and spinal cord. These findings (*arrow*) are confirmed on the postcontrast T1-weighted sagittal image (B). Enhancement of the epidural venous plexus aids in delineating the disk features. (C) The axial gradient echo T2*-weighted image shows a smoothly contoured posterior disk margin with no focal disk protrusion.

DIAGNOSIS

Concentric bulge of the annulus fibrosus

DISCUSSION

A disk bulge, also termed a bulge of the annulus fibrosus or annular bulge, is present when the disk margin extends past the posterior edge of the adjacent vertebral body end plates. This occurs early in the spectrum of disk degeneration. A simple broad-based disk bulge indicates decreased elasticity of the annulus fibrosus and laxity of the annular fibers. The fibers of the annulus are frequently torn with centrifugal expansion of the disk.

The goal of magnetic resonance imaging is to differentiate a simple disk bulge from a herniation of the nucleus pulposus. A disk herniation is a focal protrusion of disk material. A disk bulge is a circumferential, broad-based expansion of the disk. Frequently, a disk bulge is asymptomatic.[1] With a severe bulge or in the setting of a congenitally narrow osseous spinal canal, however, a disk bulge can produce canal narrowing with compression of the thecal sac or spinal cord. If the bulge causes sufficient narrowing of the neural foramina, radicular symptoms may result due to nerve root impingement. However, symptoms may be unrelated to radiographic findings.[2]

MR Technique

Multiplanar MR is useful in differentiating a broad-based disk bulge from a focal disk herniation. Correlation of the shape of the posterior disk border and its relationship to the adjacent vertebral body end plates in the sagittal and axial planes will increase diagnostic accuracy. The use of contrast enhancement can also increase the conspicuity of the abnormality and may help in some cases.[3]

Clinical References

1. Modic MT, Masaryk TJ, Ross JS, Carter JR. Imaging of degenerative disk disease. Radiology 1988;168:177–186.
2. Teresi LM, Lufkin RB, Reicher MA, et al. Asymptomatic degenerative disk disease and spondylosis of the cervical spine: MR imaging. Radiology 1987;164:83–88.
3. Ross JS, Modic MT, Masaryk TJ, et al. Assessment of extradural degenerative disease with Gd-DTPA-enhanced MR imaging: correlation with surgical and pathologic findings. AJNR 1989;154:1151–1157.

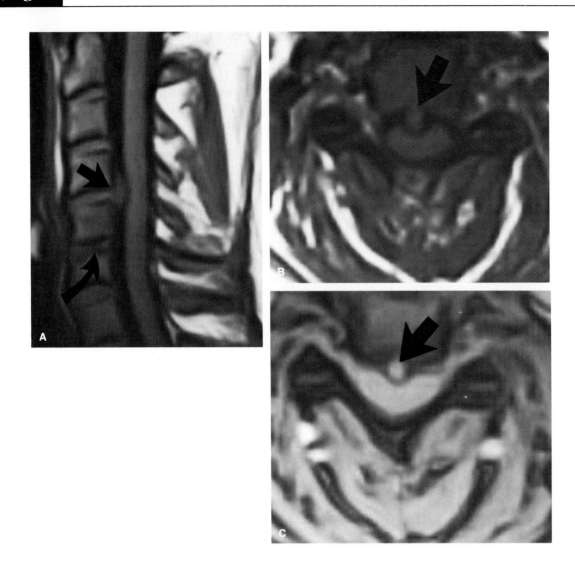

HISTORY

A 42-year-old patient with prior diskectomy and fusion for a C5–6 disk herniation, now with recurrent neck pain

FINDINGS

(A) The T1-weighted midline sagittal image reveals a prominent anterior extradural soft tissue mass (*arrow*) posterior to the C4–5 intervertebral disk. The abnormality is of relatively low signal intensity, similar to the intervertebral disks, on this T1-weighted scan. On T2-weighted images (*images not shown*), the abnormality remained isointense to disk material. The C5–6 disk space (*curved arrow*) is narrowed and indistinct, compatible with the prior anterior diskectomy and fusion. (B) A T1-weighted axial view through the C4–5 disk confirms the extradural lesion (*arrow*), and the resultant central cord deformity is well demonstrated. The lesion is contiguous with and isointense to the C4–5 disk. (C) A cor-

responding axial gradient echo scan, in which the intervertebral disks are of high signal intensity, reveals the abnormality (*arrow*) as a high-signal-intensity lesion.

DIAGNOSIS

Central disk herniation at C4–5

DISCUSSION

The cervical spine is most mobile at the C4–5, C5–6, and C6–7 levels. As a result, the vast majority of cervical disk herniations occur at these locations.[1] Patients commonly present with cervical disk herniation in the third and fourth decades. Symptoms from cervical disk herniation are generally insidious in nature, and the degree of disability often appears independent of imaging findings. Coexisting degenerative abnormalities such as bony canal stenosis, hypertrophic foraminal narrowing, and ligamentous hypertrophy or ossification frequently complicate the clinical picture.

MR allows noninvasive evaluation of the entire cervical region from the foramen magnum to the thoracic spine. The sensitivity of MR for degenerative cervical disk and bony disease appears at least equal to that of post-myelography CT and is continually improving.[1] Of course, the risks and hardships of intrathecal contrast administration are avoided. Additionally, MR allows unsurpassed evaluation of the character of the spinal cord itself, and multiple imaging planes are easily obtainable.

In patients who have had prior anterior diskectomy and fusion, bony stenosis at the operative site is a not uncommon cause for recurrent symptoms. Even more prevalent is the development of new disk herniations above or below the site of a prior fusion.[2] Such herniations may occur in as many as 80% of cervical fusion patients, and are likely secondary to the added stress placed on levels about the fusion.

MR Technique

Sagittal images provide an excellent overview of the cervical region for detection of possible extradural lesions and canal stenosis. Axial images, however, are necessary for optimal evaluation of mass effect on the spinal cord. In patients who have had prior cervical fusions, axial images should be selected at the fusion site to evaluate possible bony stenosis. Additional axial views are necessary above and below the site of fusion in light of the high incidence of disk herniation at these levels.

Pitfalls in Image Interpretation

On gradient echo images, a thin rim of low signal intensity is often present along the posterior aspect of a disk herniation. This appearance is usually secondary to a combination of dura and the posterior longitudinal ligament[3] and should not be confused with calcification.

Clinical References

1. Jahnke RW, Hart BL. Cervical stenosis, spondylosis, and herniated disk disease. Radiol Clin North Am 1991;29:777–791.
2. Ross JS, Masaryk TJ, Modic MT. Postoperative cervical spine: MR assessment. J Comput Assist Tomogr 1987;11:955–962.
3. Enzmann DR. Degenerative disc disease. In: Enzmann DR, DeLaPaz RL, Rubin JB, eds. Magnetic resonance of the spine. St. Louis, CV Mosby, 1990;437–509.

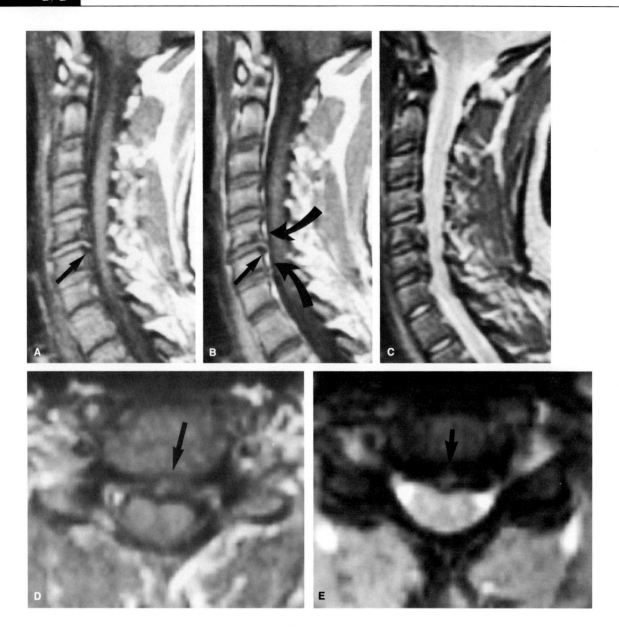

HISTORY

A 39-year-old patient with neck pain and bilateral arm pain and numbness worse on the left, with progression over the past few months

FINDINGS

The sagittal T1-weighted image just to the left of midline (*A*) reveals soft tissue contiguous with the C5–6 disk impinging (*arrow*) on the thecal sac. Pointed extensions of the adjacent end plates, representing osteophytic spurs, are seen above and below this abnormal soft tissue. Similar, but less prominent, findings are present at the C4–5 and C6–7 levels. The comparable sagittal T1-weighted im-

age following contrast administration (*B*) again demonstrates posterior herniation of disk material at C5–6 (*arrow*). The enhancing epidural venous plexus appears as vertical linear high signal intensity posterior to the vertebral bodies (*curved arrows*). The osteophytic spurs remain low signal intensity adjacent to the protruding disks. The sagittal T2-weighted image (*C*) also demonstrates the bony spurs projecting into the canal at C5–6 and C6–7, causing focal canal narrowing and mild cord deformity at these levels. No abnormal signal is present in the cord. The axial T1-weighted image at the C5–6 level (*D*) demonstrates intermediate signal intensity in the left paracentral region of the ventral epidural space (*arrow*) consistent with disk material. The cord displays mild flattening and deformity. Curvilinear low signal separates the disk material from the cord. The axial gradient echo image at

C5–6 (*E*) again demonstrates the high-signal disk protrusion in the left paracentral region (*short arrow*). High-signal-intensity CSF fills the lateral portions of the thecal sac, but no CSF signal is present anterior or posterior to the cord. An irregular curvilinear area of low signal intensity separates the disk protrusion from the spinal cord. This may represent the displaced posterior longitudinal ligament and outer annular fibers or the posterior margin of the osteophytic projections. Irregular low signal is also revealed along the posterior and posterolateral margins of the vertebral body causing narrowing of the left neural foramen.

DIAGNOSIS

Old left paracentral disk herniation covered by spurs

DISCUSSION

A calcified disk herniation or "hard disk" is the result of a longstanding disk herniation, which becomes covered by spurs from the vertebral body end plate due to bone remodeling.[1] Protrusion of disk material elevates the periosteum of the adjacent vertebral bodies. A periosteal reaction ensues, with deposition of bone and formation of osteophyte. The ossification or calcification can be quite irregular or can form a smooth curvilinear projection.

It is important to identify bony spurs or calcification associated with a herniated disk. This finding may change surgical plans to an anterior approach, as opposed to the posterior approach commonly used for an acute "soft" disk herniation.[2] Patients with narrowing of the central spinal canal on the basis of longstanding disk disease present with myelopathic symptoms more often than radicular symptoms.

Pitfalls in Image Interpretation

The posterior longitudinal ligament and outer annular fibers are low signal intensity on all pulse sequences. This appearance may mimic spurs or a calcified disk herniation on the axial images. Careful correlation with sagittal images will often identify the accompanying spurs of a "hard disk."

Clinical References

1. Ducker TB, Zeidman SM. The posterior operative approach for cervical radiculopathy. Neurosurg Clin North Am 1993; 4:61–74.
2. Hunt WE, Miller CA. Management of cervical radiculopathy. Clin Neurosurg 1986;33:485–502.

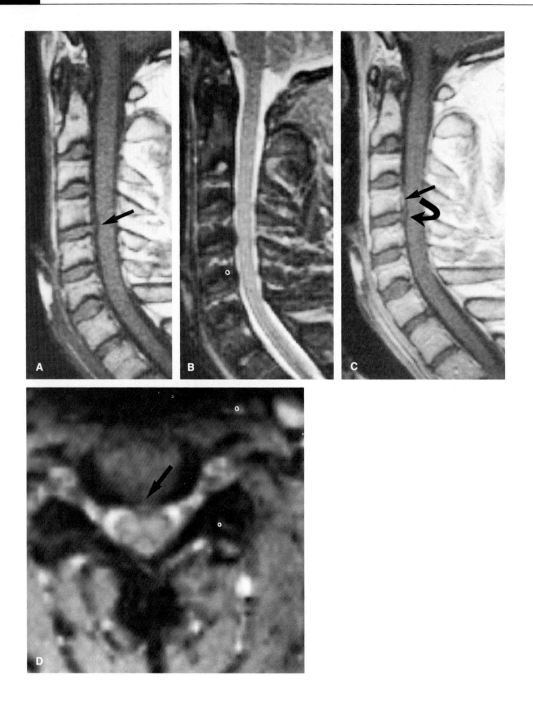

HISTORY

A 41-year-old patient with neck pain and occasional arm numbness

FINDINGS

(A) The T1-weighted midline sagittal image demonstrates a subtle, extradural lesion (*arrow*) that contacts the cord at the C4–5 level. The lesion is contiguous with and isoin-tense to the C4–5 intervertebral disk. On the heavily T2-weighted sagittal image (*B*), the abnormality is barely perceptible. On the postcontrast T1-weighted sagittal im-age (*C*), enhancement of the adjacent epidural venous plexus (*arrow*) results in increased conspicuity of the ex-tradural abnormality (*curved arrow*). An axial gradient echo image at the C4–5 level (*D*) confirms the small cen-tral lesion (*arrow*), which remains isointense to disk ma-terial. The lesion effaces the high-signal-intensity CSF an-terior to the cervical cord and causes mild mass effect on the cord. The neural foramina are widely patent bi-laterally.

DIAGNOSIS

Small central disk herniation at C4–5

DISCUSSION

Symptoms in cervical disk herniation may be secondary to either nerve root compression or cord compression. The former is usually a result of lateral or foraminal disk herniations compressing an exiting nerve root. Myelopathic symptoms generally require a large disk herniation, usually with a significant midline component.[1] Occasionally, small central disk herniations may result in myelopathy, but in these cases either congenital canal narrowing or coexisting ligamentous or bony hypertrophic changes are also present.

The clinical significance of small disk herniations, particularly when central, is a subject of controversy. Teresi and colleagues demonstrated disk herniations in 20% of asymptomatic individuals aged 45 to 54.[2] In patients over age 64, the incidence of asymptomatic cervical disk herniation approached 60%. In light of these findings, caution must be exercised in attributing clinical symptoms to morphologic abnormalities detected on MR.

Pitfalls in Image Interpretation

On axial images, partial volume averaging of an osteophyte may result in an intermediate signal abnormality that mimics a disk herniation. Thin slices and careful correlation with sagittal images are important for minimizing this pitfall.

Clinical References

1. Enzmann DR. Degenerative disk disease. In: Enzmann DR, DeLaPaz RL, Rubin JB, eds. MRI of the spine. St. Louis, CV Mosby, 1990;437–509.
2. Teresi LM, Lufkin RB, Reicher MA, et al. Asymptomatic degenerative disk disease and spondylosis of the cervical spine: MR imaging. Radiology 1987;164:83–88.

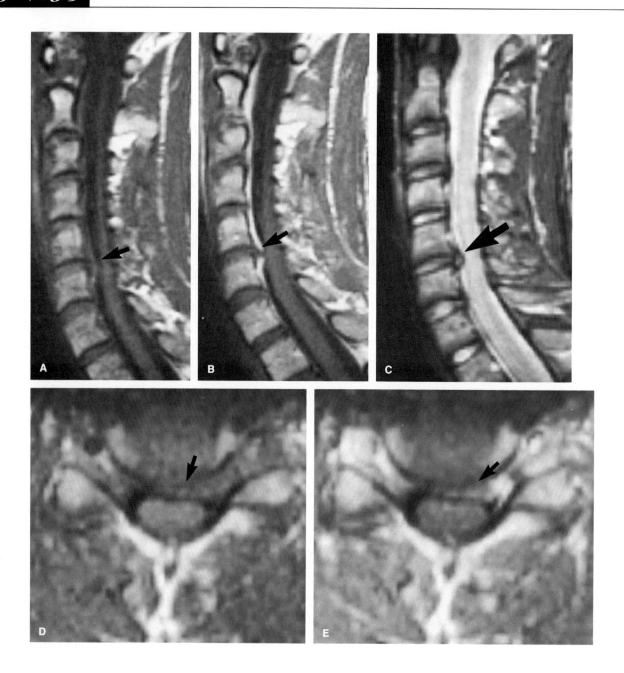

HISTORY

A 35-year-old patient with left neck and shoulder pain

FINDINGS

(*A*) The T1-weighted sagittal image to the left of midline demonstrates a prominent, extradural soft tissue lesion (*arrow*) indenting the cord posterior to the C5–6 level. (*B*) Following paramagnetic contrast administration, much of the abnormality enhances. A central non-enhancing component (*arrow*) is present at the disk space level. (*C*) On the intermediate T2-weighted scan, the central component (*arrow*) appears contiguous to

and isointense with the C5–6 intervertebral disk. (*D*) A T1-weighted axial image at the C5–6 level demonstrates abnormal soft tissue (*arrow*) anterior to the spinal cord, causing mild cord deformity. The lesion is difficult to separate from the contents of the left neural foramen. (*E*) The corresponding postcontrast axial image provides much clearer delineation of the abnormal extradural soft tissue (*arrow*). The lesion abuts the exiting left C6 nerve root sleeve, which is well seen within the normally enhancing foraminal contents.

DIAGNOSIS

Left paracentral disk herniation at C5–6

DISCUSSION

The use of paramagnetic contrast in the cervical spine provides valuable information in the evaluation of degenerative disk disease. Postcontrast T1-weighted images have shown promise for increasing diagnostic confidence in the cervical region.[1] This effect is primarily a result of the increased conspicuity of small disk herniations following enhancement of surrounding epidural venous plexus or granulation tissue. The postcontrast images also provide a more accurate depiction of the size of a disk herniation. On noncontrast T1-weighted images, surrounding epidural venous plexus or granulation tissue is generally isointense to the intervertebral disk. Noncontrast images may thus result in significant overestimation of the size of a herniated disk.

Perhaps the most valuable information provided by postcontrast imaging of degenerative cervical disk disease is the improved visualization of the neural foramina. Low flip angle gradient echo imaging, which provides high-signal-intensity CSF, is used by most MR sites for evaluation of foraminal disease. However, these sequences have a relatively low signal-to-noise ratio and often overestimate the degree of foraminal narrowing.[2] With postcontrast T1-weighted images, enhancement of the epidural and foraminal venous plexus allows clear definition of the boundaries of the neural foramina, and, as in this case, the nonenhancing foraminal nerve root sleeve is often apparent. The relatively low soft tissue intensity of herniated disk material contrasts well with enhancing foraminal structures in cases of lateral or foraminal disk herniation.

MR Technique

A drawback to the use of postcontrast spin echo imaging in evaluating foraminal disease is the increased imaging time required as compared to routine gradient echo techniques. One potential solution is the use of a three-dimensional T1-weighted gradient echo acquisition such as three-dimensional MP RAGE. With this technique, a relatively high signal-to-noise, postcontrast volume acquisition is obtained that can subsequently be reformatted into any desired imaging plane. Axial, sagittal, and even oblique images may be reformatted from a single, approximately 6-minute acquisition.[2]

Pitfalls in Image Interpretation

Symptoms in cervical disk disease are nonspecific, and as a result multiple disease entities may mimic the symptoms of disk herniation. In general, inflammatory and neoplastic conditions that may be mistaken clinically for disk disease are better characterized with the use of paramagnetic contrast. For example, enhancement of a foraminal neurofibroma may be the only means of distinguishing this entity from a lateral disk herniation.

Clinical References

1. Ross JS, Modic MT, Masaryk TJ, et al. Assessment of extradural degenerative disease with Gd-DTPA-enhanced MR imaging: correlation with surgical and pathologic findings. AJNR 1989;10:1243–1249.
2. Ross JS, Ruggieri PM, Tkach JA, et al. Gd-DTPA-enhanced 3D MR imaging of cervical degenerative disk disease: initial experience. AJNR 1992;13:127–136.

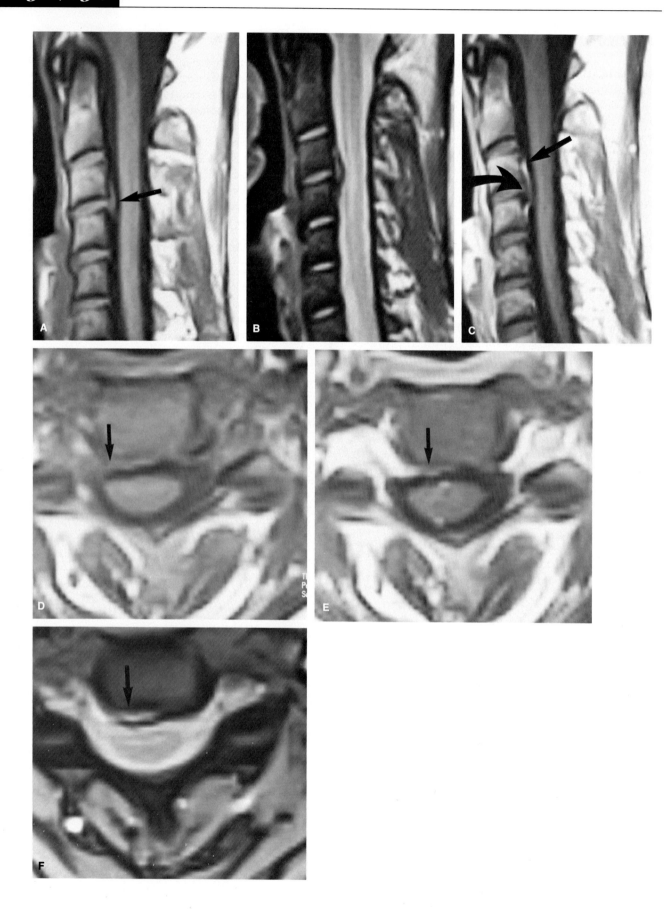

HISTORY

A 35-year-old patient with neck and right arm pain following a motor vehicle accident

FINDINGS

(*A*) The sagittal T1-weighted image to the right of midline demonstrates an extradural mass (*arrow*) at the C3–4 disk level. There is mild compression of the cervical spinal cord. The mass is isointense to disk material on both T1-weighted and (*B*) T2-weighted sagittal images. Following contrast administration (*C*), enhancing epidural venous plexus (*arrow*) can be distinguished from the mass, and the borders of the mass become more obvious. Axial pre- and postcontrast T1-weighted images (*D and E*), together with a precontrast gradient echo axial image (*F*), confirm the right paracentral extradural mass (*arrows*).

DIAGNOSIS

C3–4 right paracentral disk herniation

DISCUSSION

Disabilities associated with cervical disk disease are a leading cause of morbidity in the working years. Determining the exact level of disease based on history and clinical signs is often difficult, thus making accurate radiologic assessment critical. Cervical myelography in a patient with severe neck and arm pain is painstaking to perform and involves the risks of C1–2 puncture and iodinated contrast administration.[1] MR provides noninvasive evaluation of cervical disk disease with multiplanar capability and superior soft tissue contrast.

Disk herniations in the cervical spine usually present as an anterior epidural mass. Unless an extruded fragment is present, the abnormality is contiguous with the disk space and usually similar in signal intensity to the native disk on both T1- and T2-weighted images. Correlation of axial and sagittal images is important for determining the position of the disk herniation and detecting possible encroachment on the neural foramina.

MR Technique

Cervical disk disease is generally well demonstrated using a combination of T1- and T2-weighted images in the sagittal and axial planes. On gradient echo images, cerebrospinal fluid is high signal intensity, providing a myelographic effect that improves the conspicuity of an extradural lesion.[2] However, detection of intramedullary lesions with this technique is inferior to spin echo imaging. A similar increase in lesion conspicuity is obtained with the use of paramagnetic contrast agents,[3] principally as a result of persistent enhancement of the epidural venous plexus. Additionally, enhancement of veins within the neural foramina allows better delineation of the relationship of the herniated disk to the neural foramen.

Pitfalls in Image Interpretation

Compare the T1-weighted sagittal images before (*A*) and after (*C*) contrast administration. The size of the disk herniation could easily be overestimated on the noncontrast exam, as adjacent epidural venous plexus has similar signal intensity to disk. With enhancement of the epidural venous plexus, the precise borders of the disk herniation become more evident.

Clinical References

1. Nakstad PH, Hald JK, Bakke SJ, et al. MRI in cervical disk herniation. Neuroradiology 1989;31:382–385.
2. Enzmann DR, Rubin JB. Cervical spine: MR imaging with a partial flip angle, gradient-refocused sequence. Radiology 1988;166:473–478.
3. Modic MT. Degenerative disorders of the spine. In: Modic MT, Masaryk TJ, Ross JS, eds. MRI of the spine. Chicago, Year Book Medical Publishers, 1989:75–119.

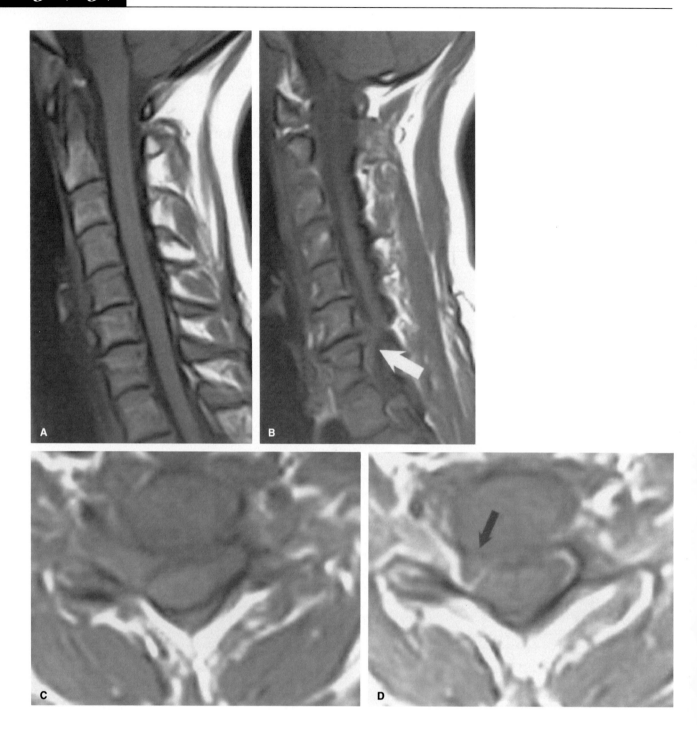

HISTORY

A 49-year-old patient with excruciating right arm pain

FINDINGS

(A) A midline T1-weighted sagittal image demonstrates small spurs and end plate degenerative changes at the C5–6 and C6–7 levels. (B) A T1-weighted sagittal image to the right of midline demonstrates abnormal soft tissue (*arrow*) extending posterior to the vertebral bodies at the C6–7 level. This abnormality was isointense to disk material and contiguous with the C6–7 disk on both this image and the corresponding T2-weighted scans (*images not shown*). (C) An axial T1-weighted image at the C6–7 level does not clearly demonstrate the abnormality. However, the spinal cord does appear mildly shifted to the left. (D) Following contrast administration, the soft tissue abnormality (*arrow*) is highlighted by the enhancement of the epidural venous plexus within the neural foramen. The abnormality fills the right neural foramen at C6–7.

DIAGNOSIS

Right foraminal disk herniation at C6–7

DISCUSSION

Central disk herniations in the cervical spine often result in myelopathy, with resultant vague symptoms that make determination of the exact level of disease difficult. In contrast, posterolateral or foraminal disk herniations frequently cause dramatic radiculopathies referable to a particular level. The symptoms are a result of the herniated disk compressing a single nerve root as it courses through the neural foramen.

Detection of lateral herniations using sagittal scans is often difficult. It is particularly important to carefully scrutinize the lateral sagittal images. Of course, to achieve high sensitivity, sagittal images must be correlated with axial scans. Many radiologists prefer gradient echo techniques for acquisition of axial images. Such studies are commonly designed to provide high-signal-intensity cerebrospinal fluid, thus achieving a myelographic effect. An alternative approach is to obtain T1-weighted axial images following administration of paramagnetic contrast. This technique often dramatically improves lesion conspicuity, as illustrated in the current case.[1] One reason for the increased conspicuity is the enhancement of reactive granulation tissue that forms as a result of disk disruption. This effect can be quite prominent even in virgin disk herniations. A second factor is the enhancement of the epidural venous plexus and foraminal veins, which highlight the low-signal-intensity disk herniation. Such enhancement is particularly important in cases of foraminal disk herniation, as foraminal contents are relatively isointense to disk material on noncontrast T1-weighted images.

MR Technique

A recent study has demonstrated the utility of postinfusion T1-weighted gradient echo volume techniques in the evaluation of cervical disk disease.[2] These techniques allow rapid acquisition of a data set that can then be reformatted into any desired imaging plane. This method has been found to be equivalent in sensitivity for extradural disease to a combination of routine spin echo images and gradient echo scans.

Pitfalls in Image Interpretation

Although T1-weighted and gradient echo scans provide high sensitivity for disk herniations, these techniques lack sensitivity for intrinsic cord abnormalities. A multiple sclerosis plaque, for example, may mimic symptoms of disk herniation, but will frequently be inapparent without the use of T2-weighted images.

Clinical References

1. Modic MT. Degenerative disorders of the spine. In: Modic MT, Masaryk TJ, Ross JS, eds. MRI of the spine. Chicago, Year Book Medical Publishers, 1989:75–119.
2. Ross JS, Ruggieri PM, Tkach JA. Gd-DTPA-enhanced 3D MR imaging of cervical degenerative disk disease: initial experience. AJNR 1992;13:127–136.

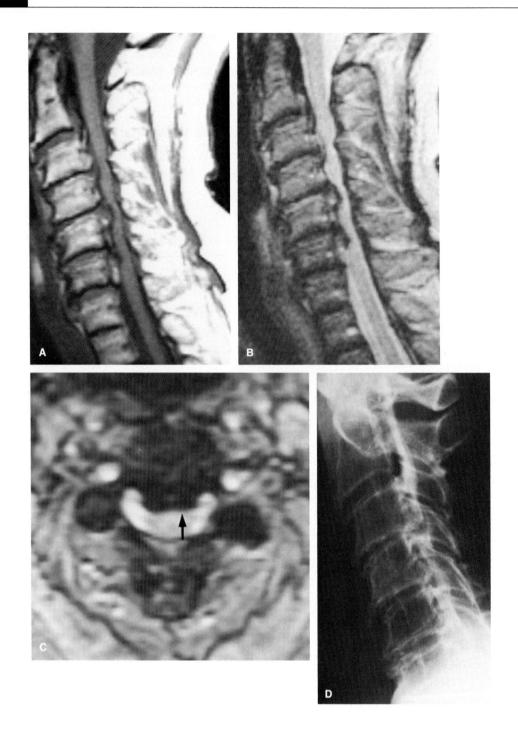

HISTORY

An 81-year-old woman with left arm numbness in a C5 to C7 distribution

FINDINGS

Sagittal T1-weighted (*A*) and T2-weighted (*B*) images of the cervical spine demonstrate a thin, low-signal-intensity extra-axial mass immediately anterior to the dural sac, extending from C2 to C6. This mass, which is chronic in nature, has led to spinal stenosis. There is effacement of the dural sac and compression of the cord (*arrow*), which is well demonstrated on the gradient echo axial image (*C*). The lateral plain film of the cervical spine demonstrates ossification of the spinous ligament (*D*).

DIAGNOSIS

Ossification of the posterior longitudinal ligament

DISCUSSION

Acquired spinal stenosis may result from a number of neoplastic and nonneoplastic causes. Of the nonneoplastic causes, ligamentous and facet joint hypertrophy are common etiologies.[1] In rare cases, the posterior longitudinal ligament will actually ossify with membranous bone containing bone marrow elements. This condition, known as ossification of the posterior longitudinal ligament (OPLL), is common in Asians. In the United States about half of patients with diffuse idiopathic skeletal hyperostosis will demonstrate OPLL. Patients with OPLL are at increased risk for traumatic spinal cord injury as compared to patients with hypertrophy alone.

Ossification of the posterior longitudinal ligament can be classified into three types: continuous, discontinuous, and segmental. Segmental is defined as that confined to the posterior edge of the vertebral column.[2] Cord compression is more commonly associated with the continuous type. Ossification of other spinal ligaments is also more common with continuous OPLL.

OPLL is visualized on MR as very low signal intensity on both T1- and T2-weighted images and may be difficult to distinguish from bony spurs on axial images. Intermediate or high signal intensity representing bone marrow may be seen centrally within the ligament.

MR Technique

OPLL is best demonstrated on sagittal T2-weighted images.

Pitfalls in Image Interpretation

The differential diagnosis of a lesion anterior to the spinal cord that is low signal intensity on both T1- and T2-weighted images includes calcified meningioma, arteriovenous malformation, hemosiderin/ferritin, and ligament hypertrophy.

Clinical References

1. Grenier A, Kressel H, Schiebler M, et al. Normal and degenerative posterior spinal structures: MR imaging. Radiology 1987;165:517–525.
2. Yamashita Y, Takahashi M, Matsuno Y, et al. Spinal cord compression due to ossification of ligaments: MR imaging. Radiology 1990;175:843–848.

(Images courtesy of Mark Osborne, MD)

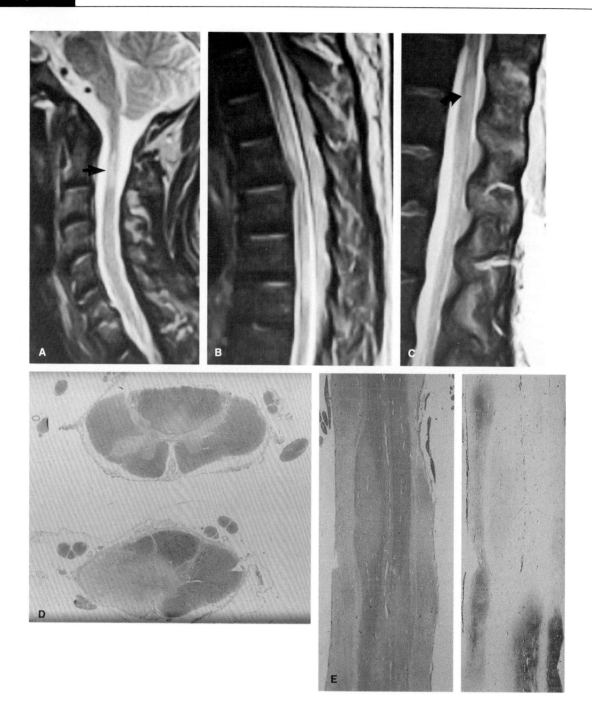

HISTORY

A 52-year-old white man with a long-standing neurologic disorder. Ambulation is with a cane; bowel function is intact but there is bladder incontinence.

FINDINGS

Heavily T2-weighted (TE = 90) sagittal images of the (*A*) cervical, (*B*) thoracic, and (*C*) lumbar spine are presented. A single hyperintense intrinsic cord abnormality (*arrow in A*) is noted in the cervical spine at the C2 level, with a suggestion of cord atrophy. Two thoracic cord lesions are also seen, both somewhat elongated in appearance. Incidental note is made of an osteophyte situated between the two thoracic cord lesions, causing anterior compression of the thecal sac. A subtle hyperintense conus lesion (*curved arrow in C*) is noted on the lumbar exam. There was no abnormal contrast enhancement (*images not shown*).

DIAGNOSIS

Multiple sclerosis (chronic disease)

DISCUSSION

On MR, spinal cord involvement in multiple sclerosis (MS) can appear as (1) abnormal T2 signal without cord enlargement, (2) abnormal T2 signal with cord enlargement, or (3) cord atrophy.[1] Cord swelling is seen with acute disease exacerbation, whereas cord atrophy correlates with longer-standing disease and greater disability. Up to one fifth of MS patients with spinal cord lesions on MR will not have cranial evidence of disease on MR. In rare cases, there is accompanying noncommunicating syringomyelia.[2]

Multiple sclerosis (MS) is primarily a disease of oli-godendroglial cells and myelin, in which multifocal areas of sharply marginated demyelination are noted with little axonal degeneration.[3] Demyelination, lipid-laden macrophages, reactive astrocytes, and perivascular inflammation are seen histologically in active lesions. Fibrillary gliosis, with little or no perivascular inflammation, is seen in inactive lesions.

MS typically presents in early adult life with recurrent focal neurologic attacks. These tend to remit and recur, often with progressive deterioration over years leading to permanent neurologic dysfunction. Classic features include decreased vibration and position sense, weakness of one or more extremities, impaired vision, and bladder problems. Dissemination of lesions in space and time is part of the clinical diagnostic criteria.

Pathologic Correlate

On pathologic exam, spinal cord lesions in MS are haphazard in distribution, both in cross section (*D*) and longitudinally (*E*). Spinal cord lesions disregard anatomic and functional boundaries. Spinal cord involvement can be found in most cases of MS, with such lesions dominating in the so-called spinal form of the disease.

Clinical References

1. Honig LS, Sheremata WA. MRI of spinal cord lesions in multiple sclerosis. J Neurol Neurosurg Psychiatry 1989;52:459–466.
2. Ransohoff RM, Whitman GJ, Weinstein MA. Noncommunicating syringomyelia in multiple sclerosis: detection by MRI. Neurology 1990;40:718–721.
3. Nesbit GM, Forbes GS, Scheithauer BW, et al. Multiple sclerosis: histopathologic and MR and/or CT correlation in 37 cases at biopsy and 3 cases at autopsy. Radiology 1991; 180:467–474.

(D and E *from Okazaki H, Scheithauer B. Atlas of neuropathology. New York, Gower Medical Publishing, 1988, p. 236. By permission of Mayo Foundation.*)

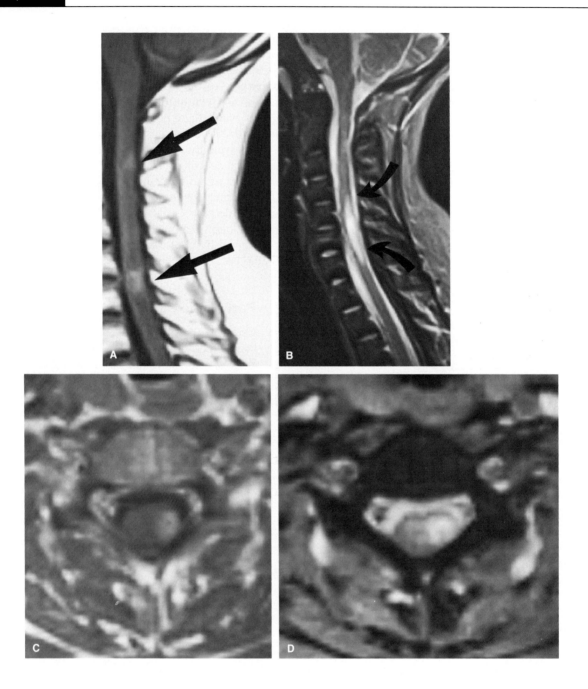

HISTORY

Two patients. The first is a 28-year-old white woman with new onset (2 months ago) of numbness below the waist, now also involving the left arm. Several episodes of blurred vision in one eye have occurred during the past 2 years. The second patient is a 40-year-old white woman with new onset of right arm weakness. In both patients the cerebrospinal fluid was positive for oligoclonal bands.

FINDINGS

(*A*) On the sagittal postcontrast T1-weighted scan from the first patient, two areas of abnormal enhancement (*arrows*) are noted in the cord. Subtle low signal intensity extends in a flamelike distribution above and below the lesion at C5–6. (*B*) The sagittal postcontrast T2-weighted scan confirms the lower lesion, with the higher one poorly seen. On the T2-weighted scan, the edema (with high signal intensity, *curved arrows*), which extends

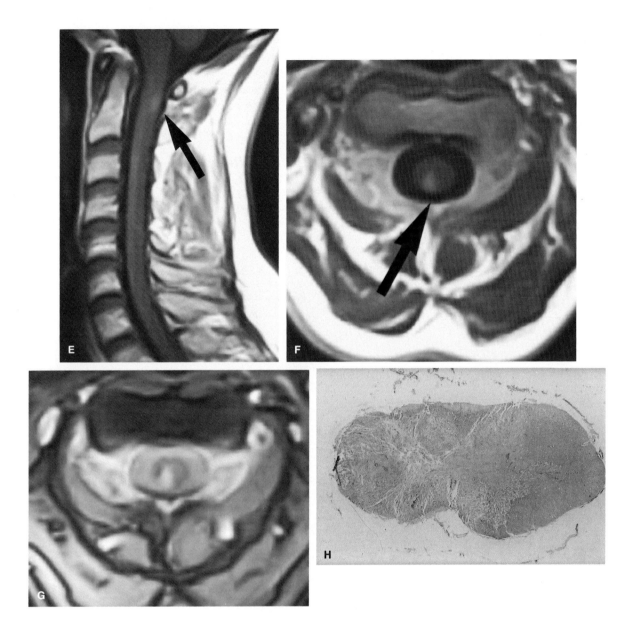

above and below the enhancing lesion at C5–6, is well depicted. The axial postcontrast T1-weighted spin echo (*C*) and T2-weighted gradient echo (*D*; FISP with TR/TE/tip angle = 250/12/20°) scans confirm the lower lesion, which is eccentrically located (on the left) and causes focal cord enlargement.

In the second patient, faint enhancement (*arrow*) is noted within the cord at the level of the dens on the sagittal postcontrast T1-weighted scan (*E*). On the axial postcontrast T1-weighted scan (*F*), lesion enhancement (*arrow*) is well seen. The T2-weighted gradient echo scan (*G*; FISP with TR/TE/tip angle = 250/12/20°) demonstrates a well-demarcated high-intensity lesion (located just to the right of midline) without surrounding edema or cord deformity.

DIAGNOSIS

Multiple sclerosis (active disease)

DISCUSSION

Symptomatic multiple sclerosis (MS) plaques in the cord may or may not demonstrate substantial surrounding edema and mass effect. Although in each case the lesions correlated with symptomatology, plaques in either the brain or the cord can be responsible for patient presentation.

MR Technique

MS lesions in the cord tend to be elliptical, with the greatest dimension in the craniocaudal direction. Thus, axial imaging may more clearly demonstrate a lesion, or enhancement of such (as in the second patient), due to smaller partial volume effects.

Positive lesion enhancement can also be visualized on postcontrast T2-weighted images (whether using gradient echo or spin echo technique), with clinical utility in certain instances. This occurs due to the large change in TI combined with a small but definite sensitivity to TI.

Pitfalls in Image Interpretation

Mass effect with central lesion enhancement occurs not uncommonly with active MS and should not be mistaken for neoplastic disease.[1]

Pathologic Correlate

Active lesions in MS are not often seen at autopsy because they are rarely fatal. Biopsy specimens can be misleading and may be misinterpreted as infarction or astrocytoma unless special stains are prepared and the sections are read by an experienced pathologist. Note the focal enlargement of the cord due to an MS plaque in this histologic cross section (*H*).

Clinical Reference

1. Larsson EM, Holtas S, Nilsson O. Gd-DTPA-enhanced MR of suspected spinal multiple sclerosis. AJNR 1989;10:1071–1076.

(H from Okazaki H, Scheithauer B. Atlas of neuropathology. New York, Gower Medical Publishing, 1988, p. 239. By permission of Mayo Foundation.)

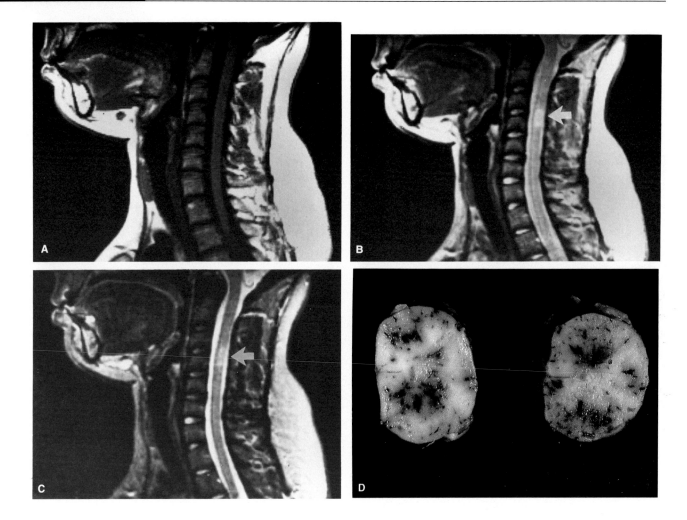

HISTORY

A 30-year-old patient with tingling and weakness in both arms, Lhermitte's sign (an electric-like shock down the spine on head flexion), and a normal cranial MR

FINDINGS

(A) The sagittal T1-weighted scan is normal. The (B) first (TE = 45) and (C) second (TE = 90) echoes of the T2-weighted exam reveal a focus of abnormal high signal intensity (arrows) within the cord at the C3–4 level.

DIAGNOSIS

Acute transverse myelitis

DISCUSSION

In acute transverse myelitis, there is a sudden loss of both sensory and motor function, with a segmental distribution, in the absence of other known neurologic disease. The pathogenesis remains unknown, with various etiologies including viral myelitis, vascular insults, and auto-immune reactions postulated.

In acute transverse myelitis, there is abnormal cord hyperintensity on T2-weighted sequences that commonly extends over multiple spinal segments.[1] There may be mild associated cord expansion and moderate enhancement postcontrast. MR is useful not only in diagnosis but also for exclusion of cord compression by an extramedullary lesion, which can mimic acute transverse myelitis clinically.

Subacute necrotizing myelopathy can mimic acute transverse myelitis on MR, with fusiform enlargement of the spinal cord and abnormal T2 hyperintensity over multiple segments.[2] A prolonged clinical course, however, distinguishes this disease from acute transverse myelitis. In most cases the underlying abnormality is a spinal dural arteriovenous fistula, but this need not be present.

Pitfalls in Image Interpretation

Pathologic processes that can cause abnormal high signal intensity in the cord on T2-weighted scans, in addition to transverse myelitis, include multiple sclerosis, vascular malformations (ischemia), infection, neoplastic disease, and acute spinal cord injury. Associated cord expansion will typically be detectable in the latter three instances.

Pathologic Correlate

(D) A cross section of the thoracic cord is illustrated in a case of subacute necrotic myelopathy. There is somewhat symmetric axonal necrosis, accompanied by a mild inflammatory reaction. There may also be limited accompanying hemorrhage. This syndrome is known to occur in patients with visceral carcinoma, perhaps related to viral invasion or antibody-mediated injury. It is also seen, as noted in the discussion, in the absence of carcinoma.

Clinical References

1. Barakos JA, Mark AS, Dillon WP, Norman D. MR imaging of acute transverse myelitis and AIDS myelopathy. J Comput Assist Tomog 1990;14:45–50.
2. Mirich DR, Kucharczyk W, Keller MA, Deck J. Subacute necrotizing myelopathy: MR imaging in four pathologically proved cases. AJNR 1991;12:1077–1083.

(A through C from Runge VM. Clinical magnetic resonance imaging. Philadelphia, JB Lippincott, 1990, p. 567. D from Okazaki H, Scheithauer B. Atlas of neuropathology. New York, Gower Medical Publishing, 1988, p. 259. By permission of Mayo Foundation.)

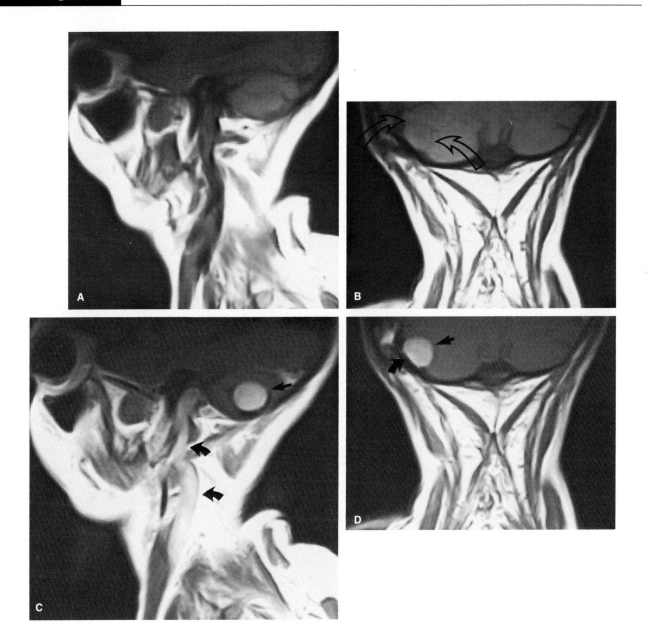

HISTORY

An 86-year-old woman with neck pain

FINDINGS

(A) The precontrast sagittal T1-weighted exam to the far right of midline is unremarkable. (B) A coronal precontrast T1-weighted exam was also obtained, although not part of standard protocol, due to a question of possible soft tissue disease. At first glance, this image is also normal. Postcontrast, on both (C) sagittal and (D) coronal images, a 1-cm round mass with intense uniform en-

hancement (*arrows in C and D*) is readily apparent within the posterior fossa. In retrospect, the lesion can be seen on the precontrast coronal exam. The broad base laterally (*curved arrow in D*) and the subtle low-signal-intensity cleft seen between the mass and normal brain precontrast (*open arrows in B*) suggest that the lesion is extra-axial in location. The internal jugular vein (*curved arrows in C*) is also well seen postcontrast and should not be mistaken for a lesion.

DIAGNOSIS

Posterior fossa meningioma

DISCUSSION

A consistent, thorough approach to the interpretation of cervical spine MRI exams will lead to a smaller percentage of missed lesions. Knowledge of common variants and the appearance of normal anatomy on multiplanar imaging is also important so that these and normal structures are not mistaken for significant pathology.

Attention should be directed in particular to the pituitary, paranasal sinuses, cerebellum, tonsils, thyroid, facet joints, and soft tissues.[1] Unsuspected disease that does not involve the central spinal structures can be commonly observed on cervical spine MRI exams—such lesions include pituitary macroadenoma, empty sella, retention cysts, cerebellar metastases, cerebellar infarction, Chiari I malformation, goiter, perched facets, and lymphadenopathy. In the thoracic and lumbar spine a similar situation exists, with abdominal aneurysms, renal disease, and pelvic abnormalities not uncommon.

MR Technique

IV contrast administration can be particularly valuable for detection and assessment of unsuspected pathology, in particular central nervous system neoplastic disease.

Pitfalls in Image Interpretation

In cervical MRI, significant pathology can be overlooked due to the physician's focus on the vertebral column and cord, the two anatomic areas most commonly involved by disease processes. Attention should always be paid in image interpretation to the extremes of the film, keeping in mind other, less common disease processes that might be present.

Clinical Reference

1. Mihara F, Murayama S, Gupta KL, et al. Peripheral findings in MR using surface coil. Comput Med Imaging Graph 1991;15:451–454.

Magnetic Resonance Imaging of the Spine, by Val M. Runge,
Mark H. Awh, Donald F. Bittner, and John E. Kirsch.
J.B. Lippincott Company, Philadelphia © 1995.

CHAPTER
THREE

Thoracic Spine

Mark H. Awh
Val M. Runge
Donald F. Bittner

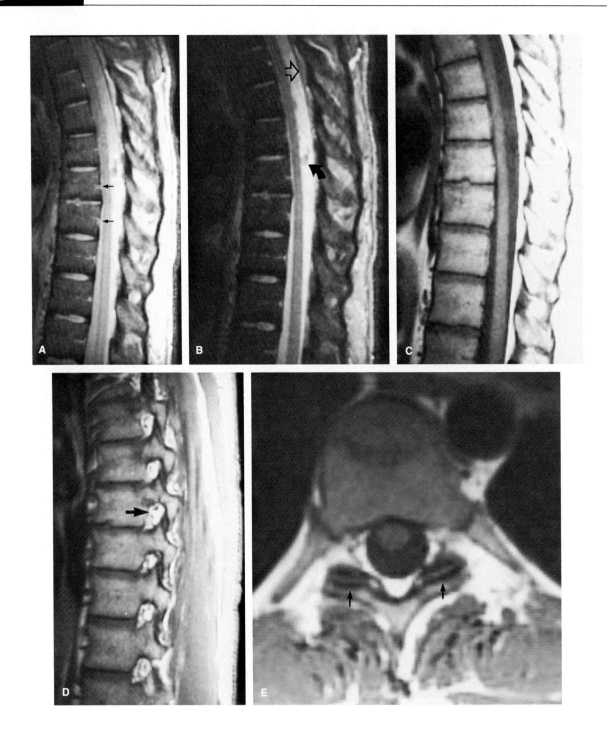

HISTORY

Normal volunteer

FINDINGS

On (*A*) intermediate (TE = 45) T2-weighted and (*B*) heavily (TE = 90) T2-weighted sagittal images of the thoracic spine, the vertebral bodies are low signal intensity, the spinal cord is intermediate signal intensity, and the intervertebral disks and cerebrospinal fluid (CSF) are high signal intensity. The exit foramina (*arrows in A*) for the basivertebral veins, seen posteriorly in the midbody, can be noted at multiple vertebral levels. Epidural fat (*open arrow in B*), prominent posterior to the thecal sac, has intermediate signal intensity on the heavily T2-weighted image. CSF motion accounts for the artifactual focal loss of signal intensity (*curved arrow in B*) posterior to the thoracic cord. On (*C*) midline and (*D*) off-midline (15

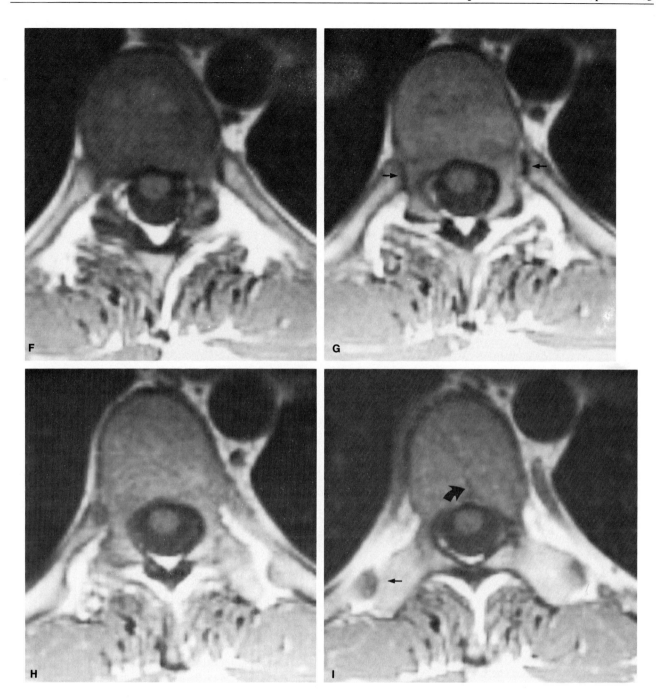

cm to the right) sagittal T1-weighted images (TR/TE = 500/10), vertebral bodies are high signal intensity, spinal cord and disks are intermediate signal intensity, and CSF is low signal intensity. The spinal nerves and accompanying blood vessels (both surrounded by fat) run within the intervertebral foramina (*arrow in D*) between the inferior and superior borders of the pedicles of adjacent vertebral bodies.

Six axial T1-weighted images (TR/TE = 750/10) are also shown (*E through J*). These are 3-mm-thick sections, adjacent in space from cranial to caudal, with a 30% (1.3 mm) interslice gap. Anatomic structures of note include

the facet joints (*arrows in E*), the intervertebral disk (*F*; note the lower signal intensity as compared to vertebral marrow on adjacent sections), the lateral costal facets (*arrows in G*), the articulation of the transverse processes with the costal heads (*arrow in I*), the basivertebral vein and branches (*curved arrow in I*), and the intervertebral foramina (*arrows in J*).

DIAGNOSIS

Normal thoracic spine anatomy

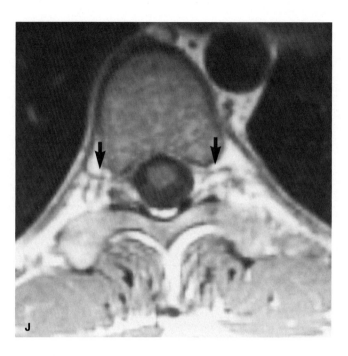

DISCUSSION

CSF and the normal hydrated nucleus pulposus have high signal intensity on T2-weighted images (long T2 values) and relatively low signal intensity on T1-weighted images (long T1 values) due to their free water content. Marrow appears low signal intensity on T2-weighted spin echo images mainly due to T2* (susceptibility) effects, caused by the presence of iron, and high signal intensity on T1-weighted spin echo images due to fat content.[1]

MR Technique

In the thoracic spine, the use of a coronal presaturation slab or pulse is important to eliminate motion artifacts from both the anterior chest wall and the heart. Both ECG gating and gradient moment nulling are necessary with T2-weighted spin echo techniques to reduce the effects of CSF pulsation, but adequate images can be obtained without gating using fast spin echo techniques. A maximum slice thickness of 3 mm is recommended (regardless of the plane of acquisition) due to the small size of the normal thoracic disk and the potential for missing a disk herniation or other significant pathology with thicker sections. These factors combine to make thoracic spine imaging relatively less efficacious than cervical spine imaging, where a dedicated wraparound coil can also be applied, and lumbar spine imaging, where slice thickness is also less critical. For sagittal T1-weighted scans, short TRs in the range of 500 are often used, as the scan is not limited by the number of sections required. For axial images the TR is often lengthened (750 in this example) to increase the number of sections that can be acquired in one scan sequence.

Pitfalls in Image Interpretation

Focal signal loss is commonly observed on T2-weighted scans within the thecal sac, particularly in the thoracic spine, secondary to pulsatile CSF motion.[2] Such an area of decreased signal intensity should not be mistaken for an intrathecal mass. Correlation with T1-weighted scans, which are less sensitive to this effect, is often of value.

Clinical References

1. Hackney DB. MRI of the spine. Normal anatomy. Top Mag Reson Imag 1992;4:1–6.
2. Hinks RS, Quencer RM. Motion artifacts in brain and spine MR. Radiol Clin North Am 1988;26:737–753.

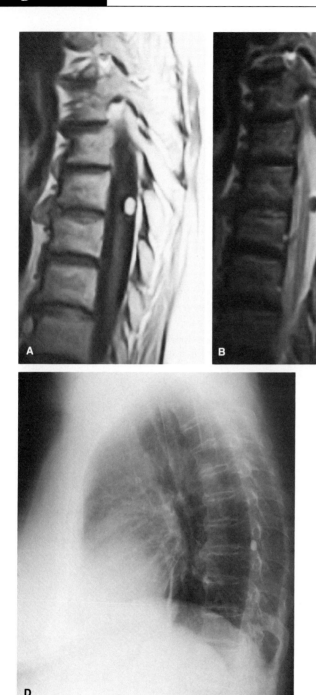

HISTORY

An 81-year-old patient with progressive left upper and lower extremity weakness

FINDINGS

Cervical MR (*images not shown*) revealed severe spinal stenosis at the C3–4 and C4–5 levels secondary to degenerative disease. The thoracic MR was obtained immediately after completion of the cervical exam. The sagittal T1-weighted exam (*A*), performed postcontrast, reveals a round, high-signal-intensity, 1-cm lesion just posterior to the cord at the T8–9 level. On the (*B*) first (TE = 45) and (*C*) second (TE = 90) echoes of the T2-weighted exam, the lesion appears markedly hypointense relative to CSF. On the lateral view from a chest x-ray (*D*), the lesion is noted to be radiopaque.

DIAGNOSIS

Pantopaque (iophendylate)

DISCUSSION

Pantopaque was used as a contrast agent for myelography before the introduction of safe water-soluble contrast media. After completion of a myelogram, it was not unusual to leave a small amount of contrast within the thecal sac. This material would then persist for years due to extremely slow resorption. Thus, Pantopaque can still be found in some patients referred today for spine MR.[1]

Residual Pantopaque may be free within the thecal sac or trapped within diverticula or root sleeves. When mobile, it is typically found within the posterior thecal sac in the thoracic region with the patient supine, as for an MR exam. Retained contrast may appear linear or more commonly globular.

Pantopaque is an oily contrast material with a short T1 and T2.[2] Thus, on T1-weighted spin echo images it appears hyperintense, similar to fat, and on T2-weighted spin echo and gradient echo images it appears markedly hypointense (relative to CSF).

MR Technique

When IV contrast is used, acquisition of both pre- and postcontrast T1-weighted images is strongly recommended. By comparing these scans, abnormal contrast enhancement can be identified with certainty. In the case illustrated, scans were obtained only postcontrast in the thoracic region, with the Pantopaque initially mistaken for an enhancing intradural lesion (a meningioma).

Pitfalls in Image Interpretation

Due to its very high signal intensity on T1-weighted images, Pantopaque can be mistaken for fat or blood (methemoglobin). On gradient echo images, retained Pantopaque may mimic a densely calcified mass, signal loss due to magnetic susceptibility effects, or flow-related phenomena.[3] Correlation with conventional radiographs of the spine is recommended.

Clinical References

1. Mamourian AC, Briggs RW. Appearance of Pantopaque on MR images. Radiology 1986;158:457–460.
2. Braun IF, Malko JA, Davis PC, et al. The behavior of Pantopaque on MR: in vivo and in vitro analyses. AJNR 1986;7:997–1001.
3. Jack CR Jr, Gehring DB, Ehman RL, Felmlee JP. CSF-iophendylate contrast on gradient echo MR images. Radiology 1988;169:561–563.

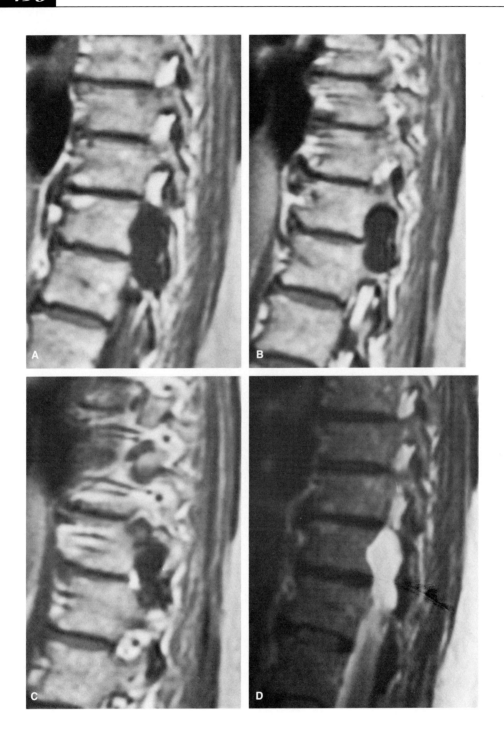

HISTORY

A 49-year-old woman referred for low back pain. On the lumbar MR exam a lesion was noted in the low thoracic spine; images of this region were subsequently obtained.

FINDINGS

Sagittal (*A through C*, T1-weighted; *D through F*, T2-weighted) and axial (*G*, T1-weighted) images of the thoracic spine are presented. A mass is noted within the right

neural foramen at T10–11, with low signal intensity on T1-weighted images and high signal intensity (slightly hyperintense to CSF) on T2-weighted images. There is enlargement of the neural foramen, with scalloping of the adjacent pedicles and the posterior margins of both T10 and T11.

DIAGNOSIS

Lateral meningocele

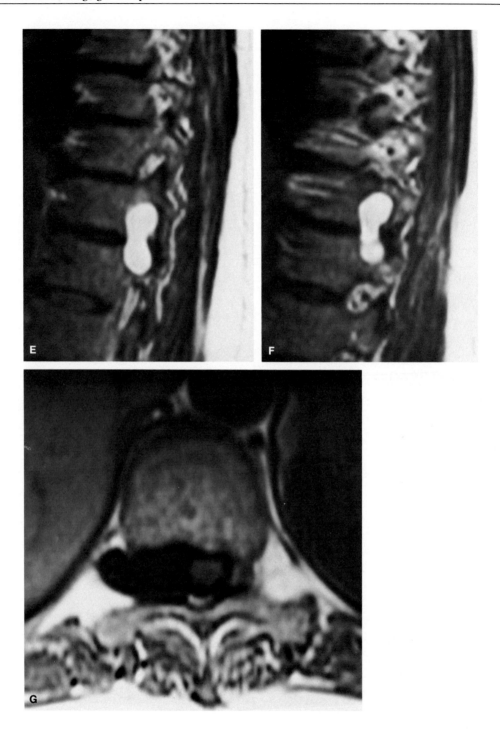

DISCUSSION

Lateral paravertebral meningoceles are an uncommon malformation of the meninges, with protrusion of the dura and arachnoid laterally through an enlarged intervertebral foramen.[1] Males and females are equally affected, with most lesions noted in patients between the ages of 30 and 50 years. Eighty-five percent occur in patients with neurofibromatosis. Indeed, thoracic paraspinal masses in neurofibromatosis are more likely to

be meningoceles, not neurofibromas. Other spinal and paraspinal abnormalities seen in neurofibromatosis include bony dysplasias, cord lesions, and dural ectasia.[2]

Most lateral meningoceles are right-sided, occupying a single foramen in the upper thoracic spine (T3 to T7). Lesions are rare in the cervical, lumbar, and sacral regions.[3] Their size varies widely. Cough or dyspnea may be present, but most are asymptomatic (with treatment conservative). Neurologic symptoms occur in a small number. Plain films often reveal a short focal scoliosis, convex toward the lesion. The neural foramen is often enlarged, with thinning of the adjacent pedicles and lamina, and scalloping along the dorsal surface of the adjacent vertebral bodies. The MR signal intensity on T2-weighted scans may be greater than that of CSF within the spinal canal, due to dampening of CSF pulsations. Lateral meningoceles can be demonstrated by myelography, CT, and MR.

MR Technique

MR is the ideal imaging modality for demonstration of a lateral meningocele, due to the ability to obtain multiplanar high-resolution images with excellent soft tissue contrast. Coronal images best display the lateral extension through the neural foramen. Axial images are important for examination of the paraspinal soft tissues. T1-weighted images are used for high-resolution anatomic information. T2-weighted images delineate well

the size and shape of these abnormal CSF spaces. T2-weighted images are also highly sensitive for detection of peripheral neurofibromas, which display markedly increased signal intensity, frequently with a central area of decreased signal intensity.

Clinical References

1. Gibbens DT, Argy N. Chest case of the day: lateral thoracic meningocele in a patient with neurofibromatosis. AJR 1991;156:1299–1300.
2. Burk DL, Brunberg JA, Kanal E, et al. Spinal and paraspinal neurofibromatosis: surface coil MR imaging at 1.5 T. Radiology 1987;162:797–801.
3. Nakasu Y, Minouchi K, Hatsuda N, et al. Thoracic meningocele in neurofibromatosis: CT and MR findings. J Comput Assist Tomogr 1991;15:1062–1064.

(Images courtesy of Kevin Nelson, MD)

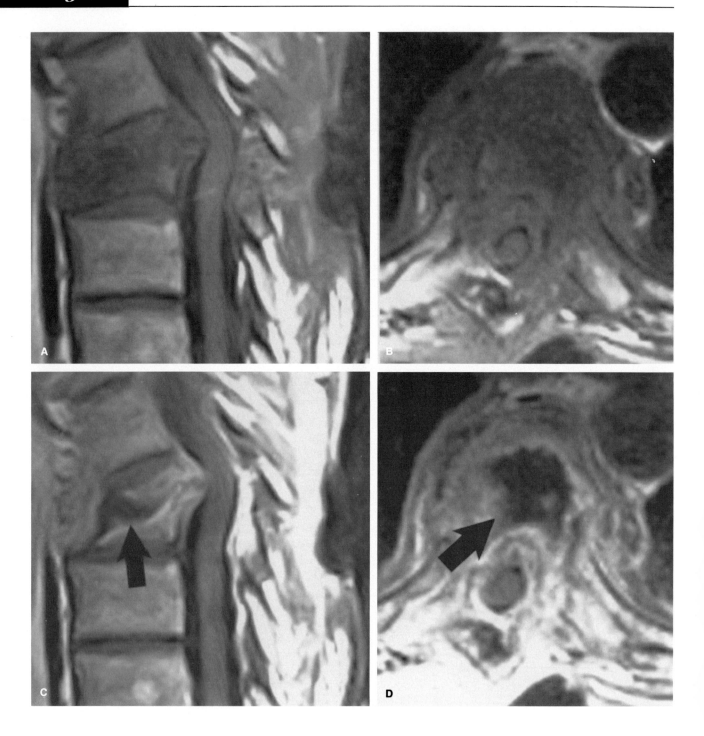

HISTORY

A 74-year-old patient with upper back pain for 2 months

FINDINGS

T2-weighted sagittal images (*images not shown*) demonstrated abnormally increased signal intensity within the T6 and T7 vertebral bodies. A particularly intense

area of abnormal high signal intensity was noted within the inferior T6 vertebral body. (*A*) The midline T1-weighted sagittal image reveals markedly decreased signal intensity throughout T6 and much of T7. It is difficult to separate the two affected vertebral bodies on this image. Loss of vertebral body height of both T6 and T7 is noted. There is marked deformity of the thecal sac and moderate cord compression. (*B*) The precontrast T1-weighted axial image reveals abnormal paraspinous and epidural soft tissue. (*C*) Following contrast administration, enhancement of T6, T7, and the epidural component of the lesion is identified. The portion of the T6 vertebral body that was of very high signal on the T2-weighted image does not enhance (*arrow*). The signal characteristics of this region are compatible with fluid. (*D*) A postcontrast axial image through the T6 vertebral body (corresponding in position to *B*) demonstrates enhancement of the abnormal paravertebral and epidural soft tissue. The central nonenhancing fluid collection (*arrow*) is again demonstrated. The compressed thoracic spinal cord is now well differentiated from the enhancing intraspinal soft tissue.

DIAGNOSIS

T6–7 osteomyelitis with epidural abscess

DISCUSSION

At surgery, the disk space contained yellowish, serous fluid. A large pocket of frank pus was present next to the disk. Although no organism was cultured from the surgical site (the patient was on broad-spectrum antibiotics at the time), the pathologic findings were compatible with a chronic bacterial infection.

Spinal osteomyelitis in the modern era is often an insidious process that can mimic a variety of other pathologic states. Delays in diagnosis and treatment result in a dramatic increase in morbidity and mortality. Plain film findings frequently remain unremarkable until late in the disease. MR allows noninvasive, multiplanar evaluation of vertebral osteomyelitis, with sensitivity and specificity that surpass radionuclide scintigraphy and plain radiography.[1] With MR, the intervertebral disk and spinal cord can be directly visualized. Spinal punctures, which may spread an infectious process, are avoided.

Osteomyelitis in children is usually the result of hematogenous spread of bacteria to the vascularized intervertebral disk. In adults, seeding to the relatively more vascular end plate occurs, and the disk is involved secondarily. The inflammatory process results in increased water content in affected areas, with resultant lower signal intensity on T1-weighted images and increased signal intensity on T2-weighted scans. Increased signal intensity within the disk on T2-weighted images is an early indicator of diskitis and osteomyelitis.[1,2] In such cases, the usual low-signal-intensity intranuclear cleft becomes inapparent. The involvement of the disk in osteomyelitis provides a classic means of distinguishing infection from metastatic disease.

MR Technique

With routine precontrast MR, an epidural abscess may be inapparent or difficult to distinguish from surrounding structures.[2] The use of intravenous contrast dramatically increases lesion conspicuity. Additional advantages of intravenous contrast include increased observer confidence in the diagnosis of diskitis and improved recognition of areas likely to yield positive biopsies. Varying patterns of contrast enhancement also aid in evaluating the response of lesions to antibiotic therapy.[3]

Pitfalls in Image Interpretation

In the postoperative state, enhancement of disk and scar tissue must be differentiated from an epidural abscess. Careful consideration of the clinical situation and attention to the extent of contrast enhancement are critical in such cases.

Clinical References

1. Modic MT, Feiglin DH, Piraino DW, et al. Vertebral osteomyelitis: assessment using MR. Radiology 1985;157:157–166.
2. Post MJD, Quencer RM, Montalvo BM, et al. Spinal infection: evaluation with MR imaging and intraoperative US. Radiology 1988;169:765–771.
3. Post MJD, Sze G, Quencer RM, et al. Gadolinium-enhanced MR in spinal infection. J Comput Assist Tomog 1990;14:721–729.

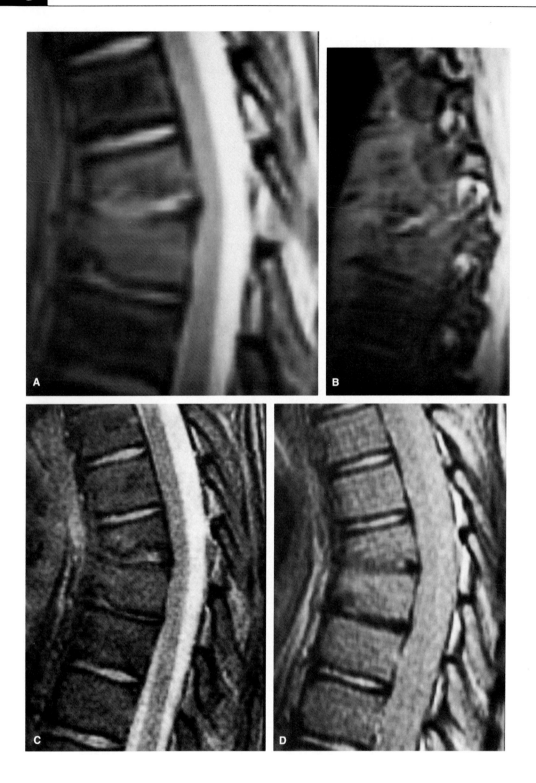

HISTORY

A 14-year-old patient from South America

FINDINGS

On the midline sagittal T2-weighted gradient echo scan (A), there is abnormal increased marrow signal intensity throughout T7 and T8, with irregularity and loss of definition of the T7–8 vertebral end plates and relative sparing of the intervening disk. Vertebral body destruction has led to an abnormal angulation at T7–8. Off midline (B), an anterior epidural soft tissue mass is noted that appears to extend over three or four vertebral body segments. On the follow-up exam (C), after initiation of medical therapy, the degree of marrow involvement is less. This finding is confirmed on sagittal (D) proton den-

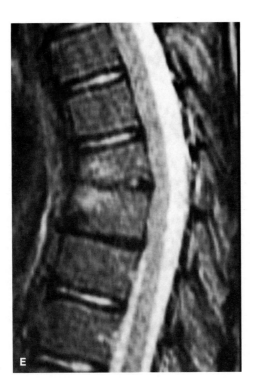

sity and (*E*) T2-weighted spin echo images. Abnormal high signal intensity is now confined to the more anterior portion of each vertebral body. The epidural disease component was also decreased in size (*images not shown*).

DIAGNOSIS

Tuberculous spondylitis

DISCUSSION

Disk space narrowing, abnormal marrow signal intensity (within two adjacent vertebral bodies), cortical bone destruction, and abnormal epidural soft tissue are characteristic findings on MR in pyogenic infectious spondylitis. Findings more suggestive of tuberculous spondylitis include relative sparing of the disk (given the extent of disease) and a large epidural mass.[1] This disease is relatively uncommon in the United States except in immigrants, particularly those from Southeast Asia and South America.

In tuberculous spondylitis, the disease often spreads along the anterior longitudinal ligament, involving multiple contiguous vertebral bodies. The epidural soft tissue component, although typically prevertebral in location, can also extend within the spinal canal. The clinical course is usually more indolent than with pyogenic in-

fection. In long-standing disease there may be extensive bony destruction, leading to a gibbus deformity. Cord compression can occur due to the abnormal angulation or the presence of a soft tissue mass.

Compared with more conventional imaging techniques, MR provides improved anatomic localization of both vertebral and paravertebral involvement.[2] MR can also be used to follow response to therapy. In spondylitis of all types, with healing there is restoration of the normal marrow signal intensity on T1-weighted images, decreased abnormal signal intensity on T2-weighted images, and reduction in the degree of abnormal contrast enhancement.

MR Technique

In tuberculous spondylitis, IV contrast enhancement is recommended for improved depiction and demarcation of epidural disease.

Clinical References

1. Thrush A, Enzmann D. MR imaging of infectious spondylitis. AJNR 1990;11:1171–1180.
2. Bell GR, Stearns KL, Bonutti PM, Boumphrey FR. MRI diagnosis of tuberculous vertebral osteomyelitis. Spine 1990; 15:462–465.

(Images courtesy of Clifford Wolf, MD)

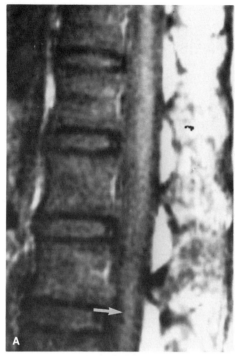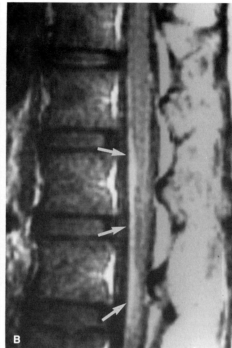

HISTORY

A 36-year-old homosexual man with AIDS who now presents with progressive lower extremity weakness, urinary retention, and bowel incontinence

FINDINGS

T2-weighted images were unremarkable (*images not shown*). The sagittal T1-weighted image (*A*) demonstrates a questionable focus (*arrow*) of slight hyperintensity within the lumbar thecal sac. The postcontrast exam (*B*) reveals diffuse leptomeningeal enhancement involving specifically the cauda equina (*arrows*). Cerebrospinal fluid (CSF) cultures were positive for cytomegalovirus (CMV).

DIAGNOSIS

CMV polyradiculopathy in AIDS

DISCUSSION

Polyradiculopathy is an uncommon complication of AIDS, with CMV implicated in multiple reports.[1] Treatment is with ganciclovir. Myelopathies also occur in AIDS, and may be the result of cord-compressing lesions (neoplasm) or viral infection.[2] Involvement of the cord in viral disease can be direct or indirect, the latter due to either postinfectious demyelination or parainfectious vasculitis. Direct involvement of the cord by CMV, herpes simplex virus type 2, varicella-zoster virus, and toxoplasmosis has been reported in AIDS.[3] Lymphoma and tuberculosis should also be considered in the differential diagnosis of a cord lesion in AIDS.

MR Technique

Patients with polyradiculopathy should receive intravenous contrast, as precontrast images alone may be normal.

Pitfalls in Image Interpretation

Infectious, neoplastic, and vascular etiologies should be considered when a cord lesion is present in an AIDS patient.[3]

Clinical References

1. Bazan C, Jackson C, Jinkins JR, Barohn RJ. Gadolinium-enhanced MRI in a case of CMV polyradiculopathy. Neurology 1991;41:1522.
2. Shabas D, Gerard G, Cunha B, et al. MR imaging of AIDS myelitis. AJNR 1989;10:S51–52.
3. Harris TM, Smith RR, Bognanno JR, Edwards MK. Toxoplasmic myelitis in AIDS: gadolinium-enhanced MR. J Comput Assist Tomog 1990;14:809–811.

(Images from reference #1, with permission)

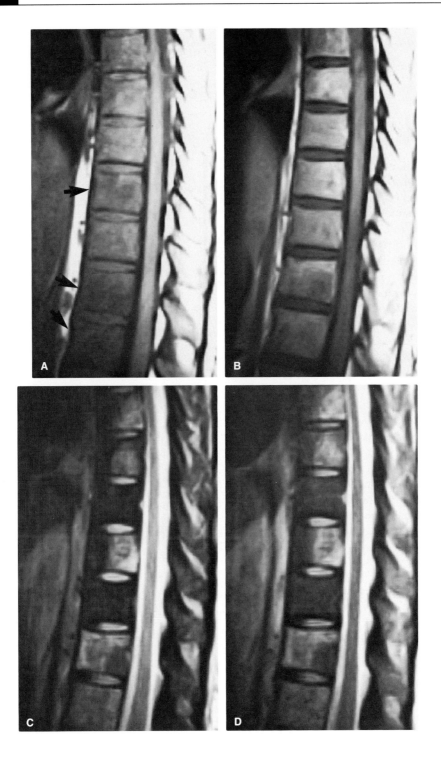

HISTORY

A 34-year-old woman with breast cancer and severe back pain

FINDINGS

(A) A T1-weighted midline sagittal image reveals irregularly decreased signal intensity within multiple thoracic vertebral bodies. The abnormally low signal intensity is most prominent at T9, T11, and T12 (*short arrows*). (B) Following contrast administration, enhancement of the abnormal regions results in decreased lesion conspicuity, although abnormally low signal intensity is still apparent within T11. (*C and D*) Conventional and fast spin echo T2-weighted sagittal images reveal increased signal intensity within the T6, T7, T9, T11, and T12 vertebral bodies. No vertebral body expansion or evidence for extension of lesions into the spinal canal is noted. The signal characteristics of the thoracic spinal cord are normal.

DIAGNOSIS

Vertebral metastases from breast carcinoma

DISCUSSION

Radionuclide bone scanning provides a useful whole-body screen for metastatic disease and is relatively inexpensive. However, when one is interested in evaluating spinal metastases, MR's superior sensitivity and anatomic detail make it the study of choice. MR may detect metastatic lesions despite a normal bone scan.[1] Additionally, degenerative changes, infection, healing fractures, and metabolic disorders may result in false-positive bone scans. The differing appearance of such abnormalities on MR allows a much higher level of discrimination between benign and malignant etiologies. Perhaps most importantly, MR allows simultaneous evaluation for possible paraspinal lesions, tumor within the spinal canal, and intrinsic cord abnormalities. Possible cord compression can be directly visualized.

In general, T1-weighted images provide the greatest sensitivity for vertebral metastases.[2] The increased cellularity of malignant lesions results in lower signal intensity than the normal marrow fat on T1-weighted images. Increased cellularity and edema account for the typical hyperintensity of malignant lesions on T2-weighted scans. However, the quantity of marrow fat increases with age. In young patients, normal high marrow cellularity will decrease the sensitivity of T1-weighted images for metastatic disease. This may account for the fact that the metastases are more apparent on the T2-weighted images in the current patient, a 34-year-old female. Similarly, metastases in elderly patients, who often have heterogeneous vertebral marrow, may be better seen on T2-weighted scans.

MR Technique

Paramagnetic contrast has shown promise in assessing the response to therapy of vertebral metastatic disease.[3] Posttreatment, responding lesions tend to enhance considerably less than nonresponding metastases.

Pitfalls in Image Interpretation

MR in patients who have had therapy for vertebral metastases must be interpreted with caution. Posttherapeutic changes such as osteosclerosis, fibrosis, and reactive bone marrow may result in abnormally low signal intensity on T1-weighted images.

Clinical References

1. Algra PR, Bloem JL, Tissing H, et al. Detection of vertebral metastases: comparison between MR imaging and bone scintigraphy. Radiographics 1991;11:219–232.
2. Jahre C, Sze G. MRI of spinal metastases. Top Magn Reson Imag 1988;1:63–70.
3. Sugimura K, Kajitani A, Okizuka H. Assessing response to therapy of spinal metastases with gadolinium-enhanced MR imaging. J Magn Reson Imag 1991;1:481–484.

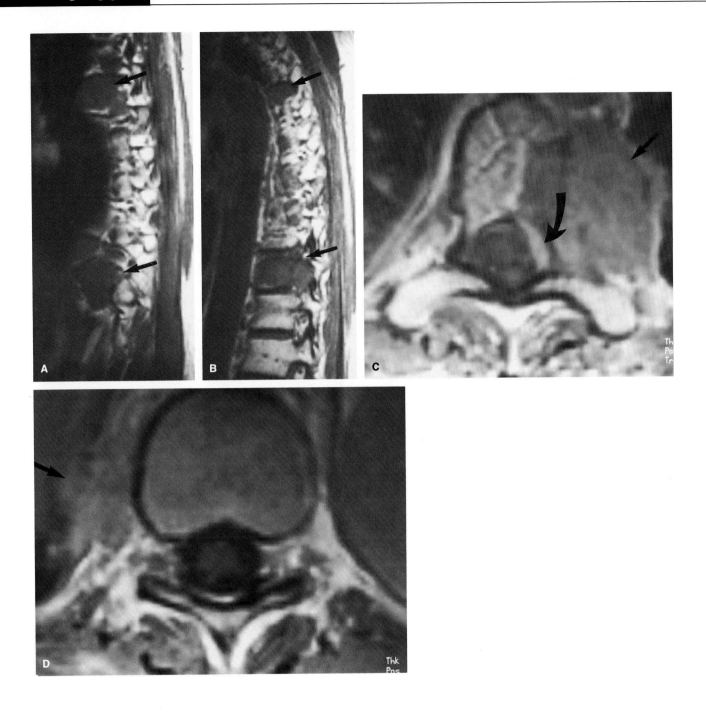

HISTORY

A 52-year-old patient with carcinoid tumor and severe back pain

FINDINGS

(A) A T1-weighted sagittal image in the right paraspinal region reveals prominent paraspinal soft tissue masses (*arrows*) at the T5 and T10 levels. (B) A sagittal T1-weighted image to the left of midline demonstrates an additional large lesion (*arrow*) that involves the body

and pedicle of the T9 vertebral body. A small paraspinal lesion (*arrow*) is also identified at T5. These abnormalities are of relatively low signal intensity on the T1-weighted images. On the T2-weighted images (*images not shown*), the lesions were of relatively high signal intensity. (C) A postinfusion T1-weighted axial image at the T9 level reveals enhancement of the left paraspinal lesion (*arrow*). Involvement of the left body and pedicle of T9 is apparent. A small amount of enhancing tissue has extended into the left side of the spinal canal (*curved arrow*), with resultant mild displacement of the thoracic cord to the right. (D) A postcontrast T1-weighted axial image at the T10 level demonstrates a separate enhancing paraspinal mass (*arrow*) to the right of the vertebral body. No evidence for vertebral destruction is seen at this level.

DIAGNOSIS

Nodal metastases from carcinoid tumor with vertebral body destruction and intraspinal extension at T9

DISCUSSION

Carcinoid tumors are one of the endocrine-secreting tumors of the gastrointestinal tract, which include pancreatic islet cell tumors, medullary thyroid carcinoma, small cell lung carcinoma, pituitary adenoma, and parathyroid adenoma. Because of a presumed common derivation associated with amine precursor uptake and decarboxylation, these neoplasms are sometimes referred to as APUDomas. The most common site of carcinoid tumor is the appendix, followed by the small intestine and rectosigmoid colon. The tumor metastasizes early to the liver and lymph nodes. Lung, bone, or brain metastases generally signify advanced disease.[1] A caveat to this appearance applies in carcinoid tumors that arise in foregut-related structures such as the bronchi and stomach. These carcinoids have a higher propensity for skeletal metastases, which are frequently blastic in nature.[2] In cases of metastatic carcinoid tumor, distant lesions may attain a large size while the primary tumor remains quite small.

In the current case, the marked destruction of the T9 vertebral body secondary to the adjacent nodal metastasis is readily apparent as abnormally low signal intensity on the T1-weighted images and increased signal intensity on T2-weighted scans. The smaller, additional areas of lymphadenopathy are less striking because the adjacent vertebral bodies are unaffected. When evaluating patients with malignancies that spread via lymphatics, it is essential to carefully scrutinize the lateral sagittal images for retroperitoneal lymphadenopathy. Axial images afford confirmatory views of the prevertebral region.

MR Technique

Many modern MR scanners allow the user to apply a saturation band to areas within the field of view that are not being evaluated. In the thoracolumbar spine, this technique is used to decrease the signal intensity and resultant motion artifact from the anterior abdominal fat and/or the aorta. Although this technique improves images of the vertebral bodies and spinal canal, if the saturation band extends far posteriorly, information in the prevertebral region will be lost. One must carefully weigh the advantage of limited aortic pulsation artifacts against decreased sensitivity for retroperitoneal disease.

Clinical References

1. Grage TB, Reed K, Wesen CA. Carcinoid tumors and the carcinoid syndrome. In: Moossa AR, Schimpff SC, Robson MC, eds. Comprehensive textbook of oncology, 2nd ed. Baltimore, Williams and Wilkins, 1991:1429–1436.
2. Silverman JM. Metastatic osteoblastic carcinoid tumor (primary in pancreas or gallbladder). Skeletal Radiol 1991; 20:149–151.

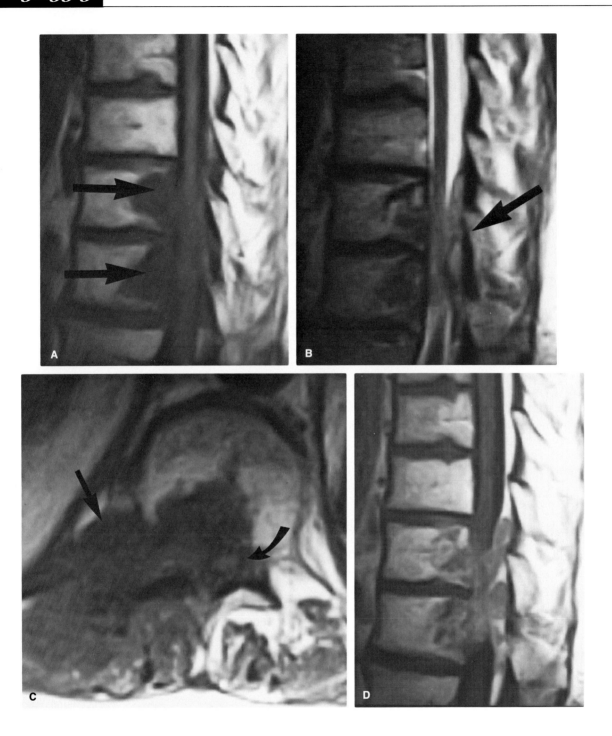

HISTORY

A 59-year-old patient with lung cancer and progressive paraplegia

FINDINGS

(A) The T1-weighted midline sagittal image reveals abnormally decreased signal intensity (*arrows*) within the posterior T10 and T11 vertebral bodies. Abnormal soft tissue is also present within the posterior spinal canal. On the fast spin echo T2-weighted sagittal view (*B*), the vertebral lesions demonstrate mixed low and high signal intensity. The intraspinal component (*arrow*) is of more homogeneously increased signal intensity. (*C*) A T1-weighted axial image at the T11 level confirms the markedly abnormal signal intensity within the posterior vertebral body. Paraspinal extension on the right (*arrow*) involves the adjacent rib and posterior musculature. The severely compressed spinal cord (*curved arrow*) lies to the left within the spinal canal. Both the vertebral and

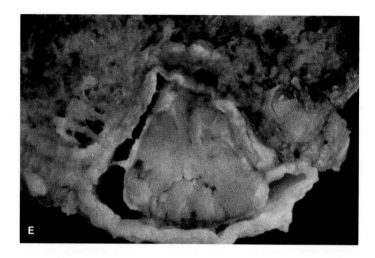

epidural lesions demonstrate irregular enhancement on the postinfusion T1-weighted sagittal image (*D*).

DIAGNOSIS

Lung carcinoma metastases with epidural extension resulting in severe cord compression

DISCUSSION

Lung cancer is the most common cause of metastatic disease to the vertebral column. Because of its high incidence, epidural extension of tumor with resultant cord compression is often seen with lung cancer. Myeloma, prostate, and renal cell carcinoma, however, appear to have a higher propensity for the development of epidural metastatic disease.[1]

A characteristic clinical picture is frequently seen in cases of epidural cord compression.[2] In the prodromal phase of disease, about 90% of patients will develop central back pain in the absence of radicular symptoms. The site of pain generally indicates the level of disease. Prodromal back pain may be present for a long duration before the development of the compressive phase, at which time neurologic deficits predominate. Neurologic deficits usually begin with motor impairment. Because of the prevalence of thoracic and lumbar metastatic lesions, lower body and lower extremity weakness are most common. In the early stages, breakthrough of tumor from the vertebral body leads to anterior cord compression, explaining the preponderance of motor signs rather than sensory deficits. Autonomic dysfunction tends to occur later in the disease, with the exception of conus lesions, in which autonomic dysfunction may occur in the absence of sensory or motor deficits.

MR Technique

MR and myelography have similar sensitivity for detection of epidural metastases with cord compression. MR, however, appears more sensitive for detection of epidural metastases in the absence of cord compression.[3] Detection of these early lesions provides valuable guidance for radiation therapy.

Pathologic Correlate

(*E*) A gross axial section of a thoracic metastatic lesion with metastatic dural involvement is shown. The dura is involved via contiguous spread from the posterior vertebral body.

Clinical References

1. Ratanatharathorn V, Powers WE. Epidural spinal cord compression from metastatic tumor: diagnosis and guidelines for management. Cancer Treat Rev 1991;18:55–71.
2. Bruckman JE, Bloomer WD. Management of spinal cord compression. Semin Oncol 1978;5:135–140.
3. Carmody RF, Yang PJ, Seeley GW, et al. Spinal cord compression due to metastatic disease: diagnosis with MR imaging versus myelography. Radiology 1989;173:225–229.

(E from Okazaki H, Scheithauer B. Atlas of neuropathology. New York, Gower Medical Publishing, 1988, p. 166. By permission of Mayo Foundation.)

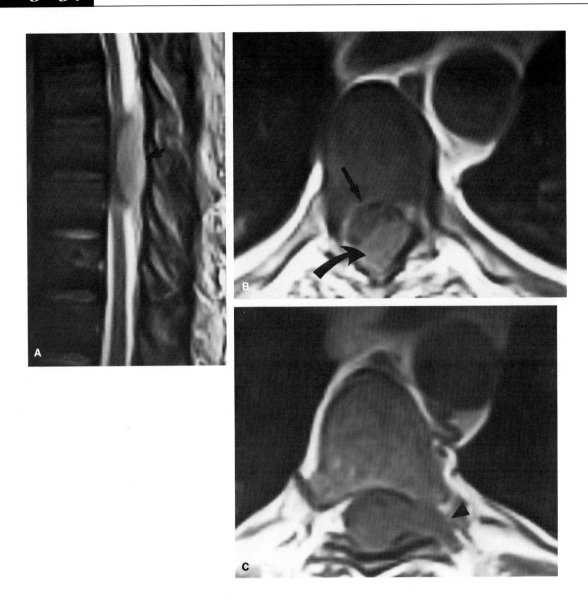

HISTORY

3-month history of progressive lower extremity numbness

FINDINGS

(A) A T2-weighted midline sagittal image reveals a large epidural mass (*arrow*) at the T8–T9 level. The lesion is slightly hyperintense relative to the spinal cord. There is severe spinal canal compromise and cord compression. The postcontrast T1-weighted sagittal image (*image not shown*) demonstrated moderate, homogeneous enhancement of the mass, which was isointense to the spinal cord on noninfused T1-weighted images. (*B and C*) T1-weighted axial images following contrast administration confirm the severe compression of the thoracic cord (*arrow*) by the enhancing mass (*curved arrow*). A por-

tion of the lesion (*arrowhead*) extends into the left T8–T9 neural foramen.

DIAGNOSIS

Epidural lymphoma with severe spinal cord compression

DISCUSSION

Spinal involvement is present in up to 15% of lymphoma patients. Several vertebral levels are often affected. Paravertebral, vertebral, or epidural lesions may exist separately or in any combination. Most commonly, spinal lymphoma is caused by local spread from retroperitoneal nodes. Isolated epidural lesions, however, may result from hematogenous spread of tumor or de novo tumor formation within epidural lymphatics.[1] Epidural tumor

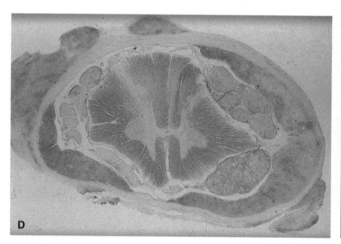

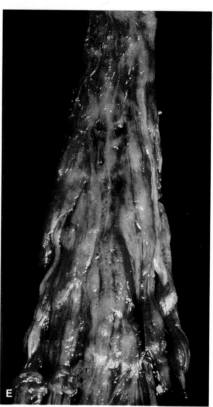

frequently results in clinically significant cord compression. Although overall spinal involvement is more common with non-Hodgkin's lymphoma, epidural lesions are more likely to be secondary to Hodgkin's disease.[2]

Magnetic resonance is well suited for imaging the varied sites of involvement in spinal lymphoma. MR is more sensitive for the infiltrative marrow lesions of lymphoma than either plain radiographs or CT. Detection of soft tissue masses, which is crucial to radiation therapy planning, is vastly improved with MR's multiplanar capability and superior soft tissue contrast. On T1-weighted images, epidural lymphoma is generally isointense or slightly hypointense to the spinal cord. The lesions are hyperintense to the spinal cord on T2-weighted images. Homogeneous enhancement is commonly seen following contrast administration. Vertebral disease generally manifests as inhomogeneously low signal intensity (relative to normal bone marrow) on T1-weighted images and iso- or hyperintense signal intensity on T2-weighted images.

MR Technique

Because epidural lymphoma is similar in signal intensity to the spinal cord on T1-weighted images, distinguishing the cord from the lesion may be difficult. On T2-weighted images, small hyperintense abnormalities may be obscured by the high signal intensity of cerebrospinal fluid (CSF). The use of postinfusion T1-weighted im-

ages allows clear delineation of enhancing tumor from the spinal cord and CSF.

Pitfalls in Image Interpretation

Because lymphoma patients are often immunocompromised, care must be taken in distinguishing epidural lymphoma from possible inflammatory processes. Coexistent coagulopathy may require that epidural hematoma also be considered.

Pathologic Correlate

Epidural and subdural involvement of the distal cord is evident on (D) an axial section through the lumbar spine in a patient with Hodgkin's disease. (E) The corresponding gross specimen reveals prominent thickening of the dura and lumbar nerve roots.

Clinical References

1. Li MH, Holtas S, Larsson EM. MR imaging of spinal lymphoma. Acta Radiologica 1992;33:338–342.
2. Greco A, Jelliffe AM, Maher EJ, Leung AWL. MR imaging of lymphomas: impact on therapy. J Comput Assist Tomogr 1988;12:782–785.

(D and E *from Okazaki H, Scheithauer B. Atlas of neuropathology. New York, Gower Medical Publishing, 1988, p. 177. By permission of Mayo Foundation.*)

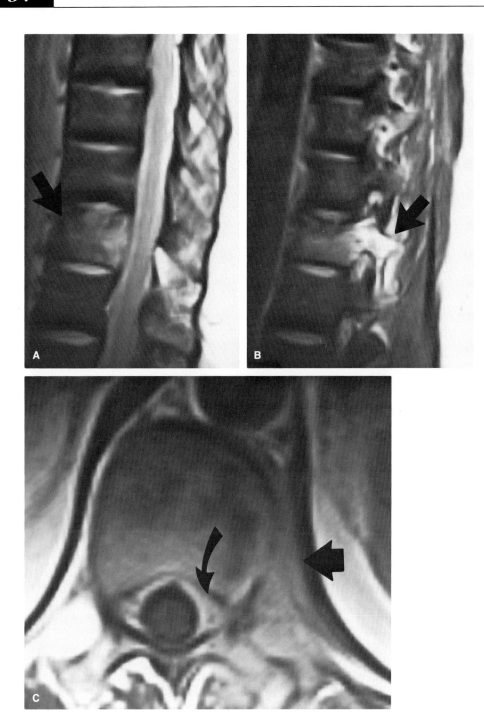

HISTORY

A 33-year-old patient, 12 months after bone marrow transplant for acute leukemia, who now presents with increasing back pain

FINDINGS

(*A*) A midline T2-weighted sagittal image demonstrates irregularly increased signal intensity (*arrow*) within T11.

The signal abnormality (*arrow*) extends into the posterior elements of T11 on (*B*) the T2-weighted left parasagittal view. (*C*) A postinfusion T1-weighted axial image at the inferior T11 level demonstrates uneven enhancement of the T11 vertebral body. A small paraspinal enhancing soft tissue mass (*arrow*) is present on the left. Both the T11 vertebral body and the left paraspinal mass were of homogeneously low signal intensity on noninfused T1-weighted images (*images not shown*). Abnormal enhancing tissue is also present around the spinal cord (*curved arrow*), with circumferential compression of the thecal sac. No significant cord compression is evident.

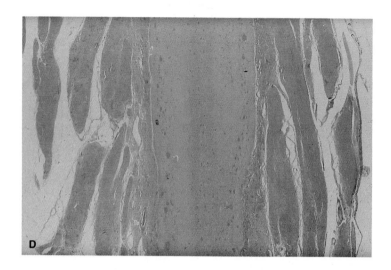

DIAGNOSIS

Vertebral relapse of acute lymphocytic leukemia

DISCUSSION

Leukemia is the most common malignancy of childhood and the ninth most common malignancy in the adult years. Leukemia is characterized by the malignant proliferation of hematopoietic cells. Leukemia arises in sites where hematopoietic cells normally reside, namely lymphoid tissue and bone marrow. Bone pain associated with leukemia is secondary to pressure caused by the rapidly proliferating leukemic cells. Bony involvement is most common at sites containing large amounts of blood-forming marrow, such as the spine, iliac crests, and proximal femurs. Bony involvement is most often diffuse. Focal bony involvement may be present in any leukemia but is most common in the acute myelogenous forms.

During chemotherapy the central nervous system (CNS) serves as a sanctuary for leukemic cells. The CNS is thus a frequent site of relapse for leukemia, particularly in cases of acute lymphocytic leukemia. Back pain in such patients should be considered a sign of relapse until proven otherwise.[1]

MR Technique

The composition of bone marrow, and particularly the amount of marrow fat, undergoes significant change during the treatment of acute leukemia. Quantitative chemical shift imaging has demonstrated great promise in monitoring the response to therapy in leukemia. Such techniques appear quite sensitive for detection of early leukemic relapse.[2]

Pitfalls in Image Interpretation

Marrow replacement in leukemia generally results in homogeneously decreased signal intensity on T1-weighted images. Normal young children often have little fat in their marrow, which makes detection of this relative decrease in signal intensity more difficult. Contrast administration is helpful in such cases, as leukemic infiltrates enhance while normal marrow does not.

Pathologic Correlate

A coronal section through the distal spinal cord (D) in a case of leukemia demonstrates severe leukemic infiltration of the meninges. This patient's leukemia was otherwise in remission, illustrating the propensity of the CNS to serve as a sanctuary for leukemic cells.

Clinical References

1. Williams MP, Olliff JFC, Rowley MR. CT and MR findings in parameningeal leukaemic masses. J Comput Assist Tomog 1990;14:736–742.
2. Gerard EL, Ferry JA, Amrein PC, et al. Compositional changes in vertebral bone marrow during treatment for acute leukemia: assessment with quantitative chemical shift imaging. Radiology 1992;183:39–46.

(D from Okazaki H, Scheithauer B. Atlas of neuropathology. New York, Gower Medical Publishing, 1988, p. 178. By permission of Mayo Foundation.)

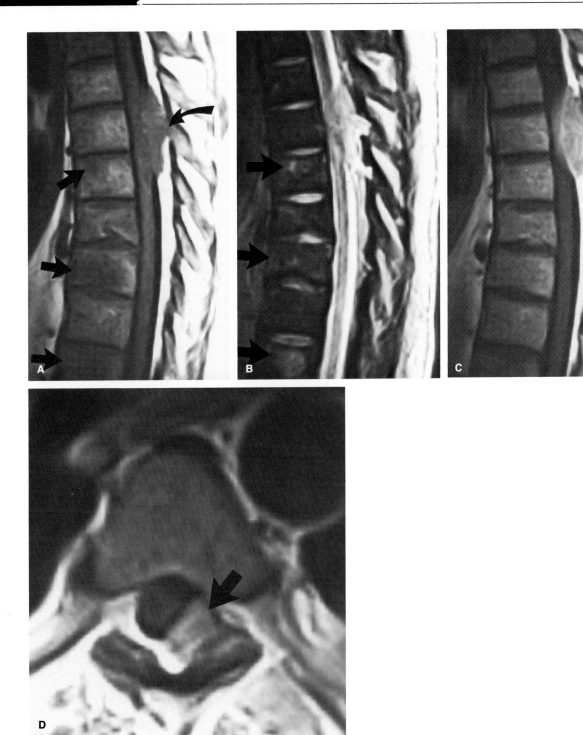

HISTORY

A 52-year-old patient with a pathologic fracture of the right femur and increasing back pain

FINDINGS

On the T1-weighted sagittal image (*A*), multiple areas of irregularly decreased signal intensity (*arrows*) are seen within the thoracic spine. A soft tissue mass (*curved arrow*) is apparent posterior to the spinal cord at the T6 level. The affected vertebral bodies demonstrate inhomogeneously increased signal intensity (*arrows*) on the T2-weighted sagittal view (*B*). Following contrast administration (*C*), the vertebral abnormalities enhance mildly and as a result become more isointense to normal marrow on T1-weighted images. The paraspinous mass (*arrow*), however, is more apparent postcontrast. The cord compression caused by the mass and the extradural location of the mass (*arrow*) are well depicted on the post-infusion T1-weighted axial image (*D*).

DIAGNOSIS

Multiple myeloma with an extradural soft tissue mass at T6

DISCUSSION

Multiple myeloma is characterized by a neoplastic overgrowth of plasma cells. Myeloma accounts for about one third of bone malignancies. It is found predominantly in older individuals, with a peak incidence between ages 50 and 70 years. Vertebral involvement is most common in the thoracic spine (about two thirds), followed by the lumbar and cervical regions.

Magnetic resonance is more sensitive than plain radiographs or radionuclide bone scans for the detection of myeloma. The appearance of myeloma on MR is variable.[1] Diffuse infiltration of the marrow by myeloma is most common, but nodular deposits of myeloma cells within normal marrow can also be seen. Areas of tumor demonstrate decreased signal intensity on T1-weighted images and increased signal intensity on T2-weighted images relative to normal marrow.

MR Technique

Diffuse marrow infiltration by myeloma is generally well seen on either T1- or T2-weighted images. T2-weighted images have greater sensitivity for nodular myeloma deposits.[1] Contrast administration is useful for increasing the conspicuity of myelomatous soft tissue masses and allows better delineation of the relationship of such masses to the spinal cord.

Pitfalls in Image Interpretation

MR is useful for distinguishing benign from malignant causes of vertebral compression fractures,[2] with differentiation based primarily on the degree and configuration of marrow replacement. Complete marrow replacement or incomplete but irregular marrow replacement suggests a pathologic fracture. However, in early cases of purely diffuse myeloma, signal changes within an affected vertebra can be subtle or imperceptible. As a result, patients with myelomatous compression fractures may have normal-appearing marrow in the affected vertebral body.[1] MR is thus of limited value in excluding multiple myeloma as a cause of vertebral compression fractures.

Clinical References

1. Libshitz HI, Malthouse SR, Cunningham D, et al. Multiple myeloma: appearance at MR imaging. Radiology 1992; 182:833–837.
2. Yuh WTC, Zachar CK, Barloon TJ, et al. Vertebral compression fractures: distinction between benign and malignant causes with MR imaging. Radiology 1989;172:215–218.

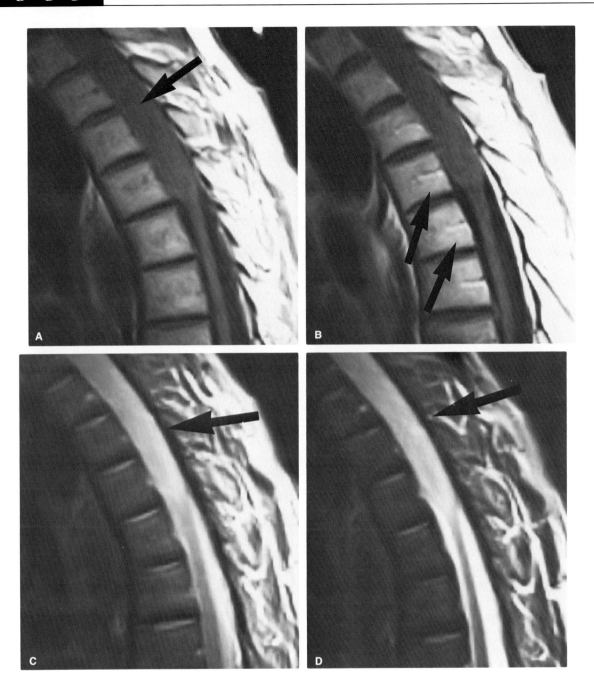

HISTORY

A 56-year-old patient with bilateral lower extremity paresthesias and weakness

FINDINGS

(A) The T1-weighted sagittal image demonstrates abnormal expansion (*arrow*) of the lower cervical and upper thoracic spinal cord. The expanded region is of slightly lower signal intensity than the normal spinal cord. (B) A postinfusion sagittal T1-weighted image reveals no significant enhancement of the abnormality. Normal en-

hancement of the basivertebral veins (*arrows*) is present. On (C) intermediate and (D) heavily T2-weighted sagittal images, the lesion is of homogeneously increased signal intensity (*arrows*), although it is not as intense as cerebrospinal fluid. (E) A T1-weighted axial image at the upper thoracic level obtained following contrast administration redemonstrates the marked expansion of the spinal cord by this nonenhancing intramedullary abnormality. The expanded cord fills the spinal canal.

DIAGNOSIS

Grade I astrocytoma

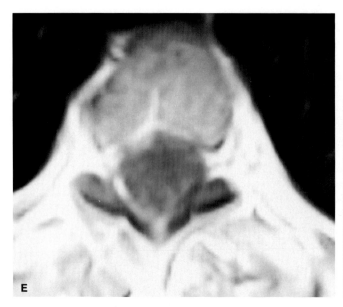

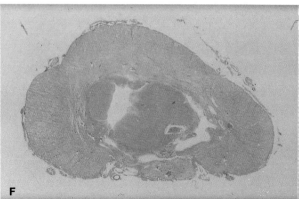

DISCUSSION

Astrocytomas and ependymomas account for the vast majority of intramedullary spinal cord neoplasms.[1] Ependymomas are somewhat more common in adults, whereas astrocytomas predominate in children. MR cannot reliably distinguish astrocytomas from ependymomas in all cases. However, certain patterns that aid in the differentiation of these lesions are known.[2] A tumor that involves the entire width of the cord and demonstrates homogeneously increased signal intensity on T2-weighted images is more likely to be an astrocytoma. The current case illustrates such an appearance. A small, nodular tumor with associated cysts is more likely to be an ependymoma.

Three fourths of astrocytomas are found in the cervical and thoracic regions. Patients commonly present in the fourth and fifth decades, with variable complaints that often include pain in the neck, back, or legs. The grade of the tumor is the primary determinant of prognosis.

MR Technique

Paramagnetic contrast administration provides valuable information in most cases of intramedullary spinal lesions.[3] Enhancing tumor can be differentiated from low-signal-intensity edema on postinfusion T1-weighted images. Better depiction of tumor nodules within cysts provides valuable guidance for the neurosurgical approach. Finally, recurrent tumor postoperatively is more easily recognized.

Pitfalls in Image Interpretation

The vast majority of intramedullary spinal tumors enhance following contrast administration.[3] Contrast en-

hancement, however, depends on breakdown of the blood–brain (blood–cord) barrier, which may not be present in low-grade neoplasms.[1] With nonenhancing lesions, it is often difficult to differentiate tumor from tumor-related edema. Edema, like the tumor itself, generally has decreased signal intensity on T1-weighted images and increased signal intensity on T2-weighted images. Signal changes secondary to edema may thus cause overestimation of the boundaries of an intraspinal tumor.[3]

Pathologic Correlate

(F) A thoracic astrocytoma is seen in cross section in a specimen with H & E (hematoxylin and eosin) staining. A small central cyst is noted within the tumor (which is also centrally located), with a syrinx evident at the tumor's periphery.

Clinical References

1. Enzmann DR, DeLaPaz RL. Tumor. In: Enzmann DR, ed. Magnetic resonance of the spine. St. Louis: CV Mosby Company, 1990:301–422.
2. Scotti G, Scialfa G, Colombo N, Landoni L. Magnetic resonance diagnosis of intramedullary tumors of the spinal cord. Neuroradiology 1987;29:130–135.
3. Parizel PM, Baleriaux D, Rodesch G, et al. Gd-DTPA-enhanced MR imaging of spinal tumors. AJNR 1989;10:249–258.

(F from Okazaki H, Scheithauer B. Atlas of neuropathology. New York, Gower Medical Publishing, 1988, p. 88. By permission of Mayo Foundation.)

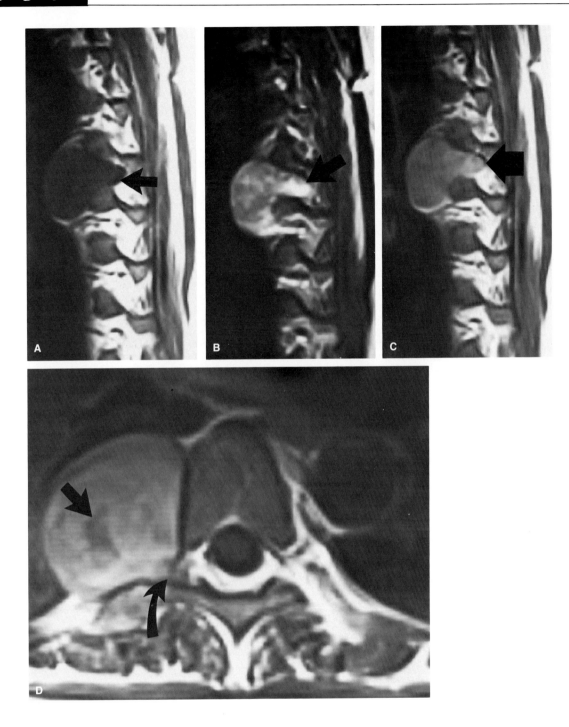

HISTORY

A 44-year-old patient with a paraspinal mass detected on routine chest x-ray

FINDINGS

(A) A T1-weighted right parasagittal image reveals a 3.5-cm paraspinal soft tissue mass (*arrow*) at the level of T7. This posterior mediastinal abnormality is heterogeneously hyperintense (*arrow*) on the corresponding T2-weighted sagittal view (B). Following contrast administra-

tion (C), intense enhancement of the lesion (*arrow*) is apparent. (D) The postinfusion axial image at the inferior T7 level confirms the enhancing paraspinal mass. Relatively less enhancement is seen within the central portion of the lesion (*arrow*). The mass appears to extend into the right T7–8 neural foramen (*curved arrow*). No spinal cord compression is identified.

DIAGNOSIS

Thoracic paraspinal schwannoma

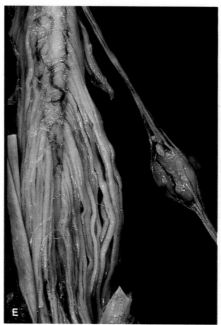 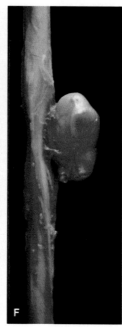

DISCUSSION

Neurogenic tumors account for the majority of thoracic paraspinal lesions. In adults, schwannomas and neurofibromas are the most prevalent of these tumors. Schwannomas are also referred to as neurinomas and neurilemmomas. These tumors arise from Schwann cells of the nerve root sheaths. Schwannomas thus arise extrinsic to the nerve root and do not typically envelop the nerve root. Schwannomas are usually unrelated to neurofibromatosis. Neurofibromas, in contrast, enlarge the nerve itself, and even when solitary are usually associated with neurofibromatosis.[1] The imaging characteristics of neurofibromas and schwannomas are quite similar.

In relation to the spinal cord, schwannomas are typically hypointense to isointense on T1-weighted images and hyperintense on T2-weighted scans. Signal intensity on T2-weighted images is often heterogeneous, with the more hyperintense regions corresponding pathologically to cystic areas within the tumor.[2] Contrast enhancement is also usually heterogeneous and often more intense peripherally. This pattern of peripheral enhancement may help distinguish schwannomas from neurofibromas and meningiomas, which typically demonstrate homogeneous enhancement.[3]

MR Technique

Sagittal images are important for assessing the size and level of involvement of a paraspinal lesion. The clinical impact of these abnormalities often depends on the extent of tumor within the spinal canal, which is generally best evaluated with postinfusion T1-weighted axial images.

Pitfalls in Image Interpretation

Spinal tumors usually show increased enhancement and more homogeneous enhancement with delayed scanning. If images are not obtained immediately after contrast administration, the typical peripheral enhancement of a schwannoma may be less conspicuous.[3]

Pathologic Correlate

(*E*) A gross example of a thoracic schwannoma that caused cord compression is depicted. Such lesions tend to arise along dorsal nerve roots. The cord appears atrophic at the site of prior compression. (*F*) A second example illustrates the typical eccentricity of these lesions to the nerves of origin.

Clinical References

1. Sze G, Twohig M. Neoplastic disease of the spine and spinal cord. In: Atlas SW, ed. MRI of the brain and spine. New York, Raven Press, 1991:921–965.
2. Demachi H, Takashima T, Kadoya M. MR imaging of spinal neuromas with pathological correlation. J Comput Assist Tomogr 1990;14:250–254.
3. Friedman DP, Tartaglino LM, Flanders AE. Intradural schwannomas of the spine: MR findings with emphasis on contrast-enhancement characteristics. AJR 1992;158:1347–1350.

(E and F from Okazaki H, Scheithauer B. Atlas of neuropathology. New York, Gower Medical Publishing, 1988, p. 185. By permission of Mayo Foundation.)

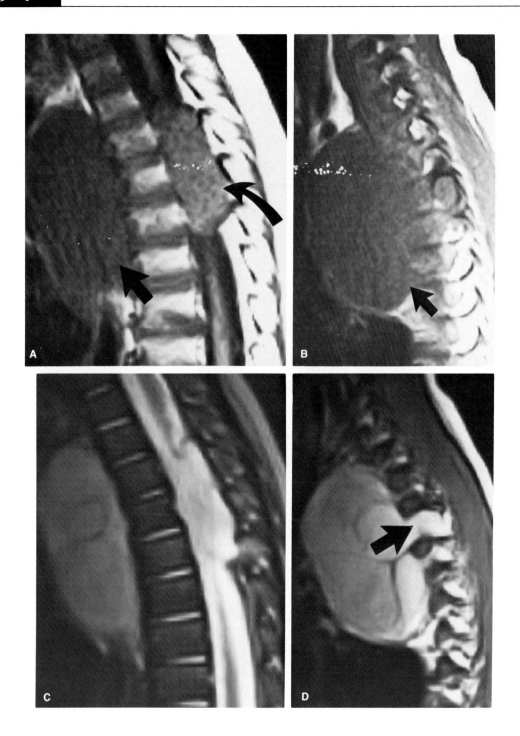

HISTORY

A 2-year-old child with respiratory distress

FINDINGS

Sagittal midline (*A*) and right parasagittal (*B*) T1-weighted images demonstrate a large paraspinal soft tissue mass (*arrows*) in the upper thoracic region. Exten-

sion of the mass (*curved arrow*) into the spinal canal is evident. On the midline sagittal T2-weighted image (*C*), both the paravertebral and intraspinal components are noted to be of increased signal intensity. On off-midline sagittal images with (*D*) intermediate and (*E*) heavy T2 weighting, extension of the mass into, and widening of, the T5–6 neural foramen (*arrow*) is noted. Moderate enhancement of the lesion is present on the postinfusion T1-weighted axial view, obtained at the T5–6 level (*F*). Extension of the mass through the right neural foramen

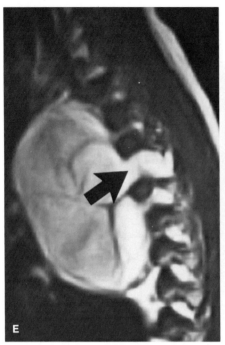

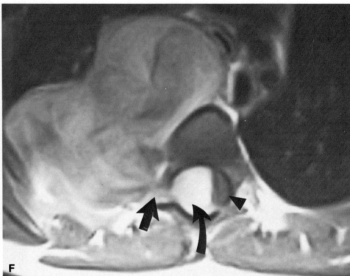

(*arrow*) is again noted. The portion of the mass within the spinal canal (*curved arrow*) enhances more intensely than the remainder of the lesion. The relationship of the mass to the severely compressed thoracic spinal cord (*arrowhead*) is well demonstrated postcontrast.

DIAGNOSIS

Thoracic ganglioneuroma

DISCUSSION

Neurogenic tumors are the most common cause of a posterior mediastinal mass. In young children, neuroblastoma is by far the most common of these neoplasms. Ganglioneuroblastoma and ganglioneuroma represent more differentiated forms of neuroblastoma. All of these tumors arise from primitive sympathetic neuroblasts of the embryonic neural crest; they are distinguished by varying degrees of cellular maturation. Both neuroblastoma and ganglioneuroblastoma are malignant neoplasms containing undifferentiated neuroblasts, with ganglioneuroblastomas containing mature ganglion cells as well. Ganglioneuromas are benign tumors of mature ganglion cells. The preoperative working diagnosis in this case was neuroblastoma. The pathologic finding of a ganglioneuroma was surprising, as this tumor is more common in adolescents and young adults.[1]

Most neuroblastomas arise from the adrenal glands. The remainder are found anywhere along the sympa-

thetic chain, with the most common extra-adrenal location being the thoracic paraspinal region. Prognosis is primarily based on the age of the patient, location of the tumor, and extent of disease. Overall survival decreases with increasing age at presentation. Patients with spinal neuroblastoma tend to fare better than those with abdominal or pelvic tumors. This difference is probably secondary to the early development of symptoms in patients with paraspinal lesions.[2]

MR Technique

Paravertebral neuroblastomas are notorious for extradural extension. MR allows noninvasive evaluation of the extent of tumor and the degree of intraspinal extension. The use of intravenous contrast allows excellent differentiation of intraspinal tumor from the spinal cord.

Pitfalls in Image Interpretation

The more mature forms of neuroblastoma are more likely to contain gross calcifications. These calcifications may be inapparent on MR.

Clinical References

1. Ng THK, Fung CF, Goh WG, Wong VCN. Ganglioneuroma of the spinal cord. Surg Neurol 1991;35:147–151.
2. Bousvaros A, Kirks DR, Grossman H. Imaging of neuroblastoma: an overview. Pediatr Radiol 1986;16:89–106.

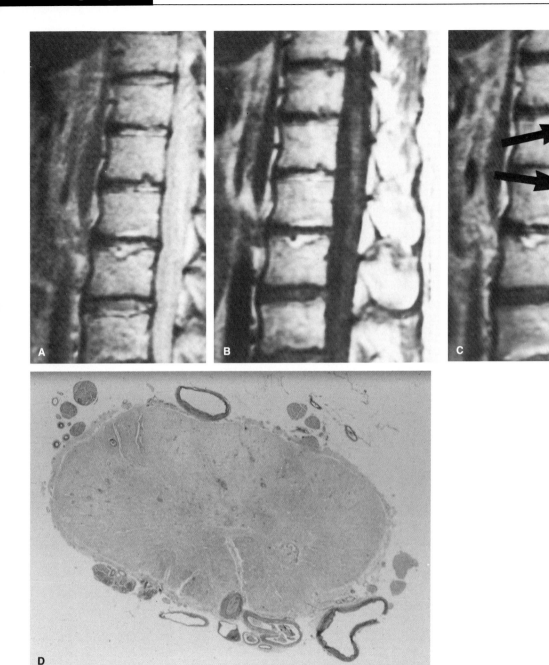

HISTORY

A 37-year-old patient with an 18-month history of progressive weakness and paresthesias below the waist, now with bladder and bowel dysfunction

FINDINGS

Precontrast T2-weighted (*A*) and T1-weighted (*B*) sagittal images are unremarkable, other than demonstrating moderate degenerative disease. Following IV contrast administration (*C*), abnormal enhancement (*arrows*) is

noted along the anterior surface of the cord. The lesion was confirmed by arteriography (*images not shown*) and subsequent surgery.

DIAGNOSIS

Arteriovenous malformation (AVM)

DISCUSSION

MR is an important noninvasive technique in the initial diagnosis of a spinal AVM.[1] Large abnormal vessels, in addition to associated hemorrhage (which may be spontaneous or due to treatment), are well depicted on unenhanced MR.[2] Vascular filling defects are best identified within the cord substance on T1-weighted sequences and within cerebrospinal fluid (CSF) on T2-weighted sequences. Other associated changes including myelomalacia, cord edema, and vascular thrombosis can be demonstrated.[3] Small lesions require contrast administration for detection, as in the current case.

Spinal AVMs are divided into two types, intramedullary and extramedullary. This differentiation can be made by MR. Intramedullary lesions are seen in young patients, present with acute hemorrhagic stroke, and have an anterior blood supply. Extramedullary lesions are seen in elderly men, present with progressive neurologic deficits, and have a posterior blood supply. In most extramedullary lesions, the nidus exists on or adjacent to the dura, with the intrathecal component being simply enlarged draining veins.

MR Technique

Flow-sensitive sequences can be of particular value in the study of AVMs for depiction of flow and differentiation of such from postsurgical changes and hemorrhage.

Pitfalls in Image Interpretation

Artifacts from CSF flow may mimic the appearance of a vascular flow void on T2-weighted scans, with caution advised in scan interpretation. It is important to give careful consideration to the choice of imaging technique and the implementation of motion artifact reduction schemes.

Pathologic Correlate

In (D) a spinal AVM, with the cord shown in cross section, abnormal vessels are seemingly confined to the surface of the cord. However, on close inspection, numerous small-caliber vessels are seen within the cord parenchyma. Focal faded histochemical staining reflects ischemic parenchymal damage.

Clinical References

1. Doppman JL, Di Chiro G, Dwyer AJ, et al. MRI of spinal arteriovenous malformations. J Neurosurg 1987;66:830–834.
2. Fahrendorf G, Sartor K, Gado MH. MRI of spinal cord hemangioblastomas and arteriovenous malformations. Acta Radiol Suppl 1986;369:730–733.
3. Minami S, Sagoh T, Nishimura K, et al. Spinal arteriovenous malformation: MR imaging. Radiology 1988;169:109–115.

(A, B, and C *reprinted with permission from Runge VM, Bradley WG, Brant-Zawadzki MN, et al. Clinical safety and efficacy of gadoteridol: a study of 411 patients with suspected intracranial and spinal disease. Radiology 1991;181:701–709; case provided courtesy of Steve Harms. D from Okazaki H, Scheithauer B. Atlas of neuropathology. New York, Gower Medical Publishing, 1988, p. 34. By permission of Mayo Foundation.)*

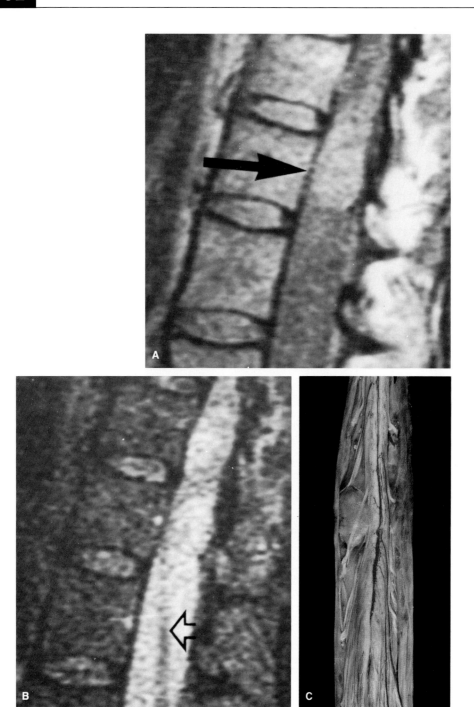

HISTORY

A 48-year-old woman

FINDINGS

(*A*) The sagittal proton density-weighted (TR/TE = 2000/25) spin echo scan reveals a soft tissue mass (*arrow*) within the bony spinal canal at T11. The lesion is isointense with CSF on the T2-weighted spin echo scan (*B*), which also reveals displacement of the spinal cord (*open arrow*) by the mass. The inferior capping of tumor by CSF marks the lesion as intradural and extramedullary in location. The lesion was subsequently surgically resected.

DIAGNOSIS

Meningioma

DISCUSSION

From surgical series,[1] one third of spinal meningiomas are in the cervical spine and two thirds in the thoracic spine, with a 3:1 female:male incidence. These tumors may be extra- or intradural, with the latter much more common. In elderly patients who present with a gait disorder, a spinal meningioma should be considered in the differential diagnosis. Complete tumor removal can be achieved in more than 95% of cases. The use of microsurgical technique is, however, important to minimize postoperative neurologic deficits. With complete removal, about 5% recur.[2]

MR Technique

IV contrast administration improves recognition of small tumors within the spinal canal and should be used routinely in this circumstance. This point is well illustrated by the present case, in which only precontrast scans were obtained, with resultant poor lesion conspicuity.

Pitfalls in Image Interpretation

In this case, an intradural extramedullary soft tissue mass is identified within the bony spinal canal. These findings are not specific for a meningioma, with the differential diagnosis including neurinoma and neurofibroma.

Pathologic Correlate

(C) This gross specimen shows a spinal meningioma, with typical lateral dural attachment adjacent to an exiting nerve root. The lesion causes mild mass effect on the cord and compresses the nerve root below. A tomogram revealed dense calcification, also common with spinal meningiomas.

Clinical References

1. Namer IJ, Pamir MN, Benli K, et al. Spinal meningiomas. Neurochirurgia 1987;30:11–15.
2. Solero CL, Fornari M, Giombini S, et al. Spinal meningiomas: review of 174 operated cases. Neurosurgery 1989; 25:153–160.

(A and B courtesy of Clifford Wolf, MD. C from Okazaki H, Scheithauer B. Atlas of neuropathology. New York, Gower Medical Publishing, 1988, p. 128. By permission of Mayo Foundation.)

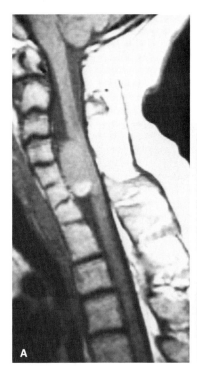
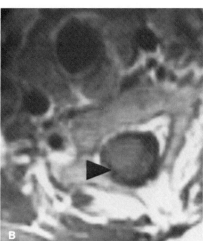
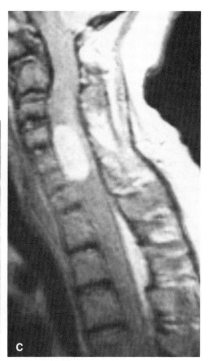

HISTORY

A 30-year-old woman with bilateral lower extremity weakness

FINDINGS

(*A*) The sagittal T1-weighted image of the cervical spine reveals an ovoid mass ventral to the spinal cord that is predominantly isointense with the spinal cord, with a high-signal-intensity layer inferiorly. The C5–7 and T1 vertebral bodies appear to be congenitally partially fused. (*B*) On the axial image, the mass is seen to compress the cord (*arrowhead*). The vertebral body anterior to the mass is intact. The lesion did not enhance on postcontrast images (*images not shown*). (*C*) The sagittal T2-weighted image reveals the mass to be of uniform high signal intensity, suggesting the diagnosis of a proteinaceous cyst.

DIAGNOSIS

Neuroenteric cyst

DISCUSSION

For a short time during early embryonic development, a communication exists between the amnion and primitive yolk sac. Usually this connection (canal of Kovalevsky) is obliterated, reestablishing the solid notochord. However, persistence of the canal establishes a fistula from the gut, through the vertebral bodies and spinal cord, to the dorsal skin surface. Mesenteric cysts, enteric diverticula, diastematomyelia, neuroenteric cysts, and spina bifida are all the result of persistence of various portions of the canal of Kovalevsky.[1] Neuroenteric cysts are enteric-lined cysts located within the spinal canal, and may have an extraspinal component. They are ventral to the cord, usually located at the cervicothoracic junction or conus medullaris, and are frequently associated with anomalies of the vertebral bodies.

MR imaging characteristics vary with protein content, viscosity, pulsatility, and presence of blood products.[2] High protein content and blood products will result in signal characteristics hyperintense to CSF. Pulsatile flow within the cyst can produce foci of decreased signal intensity, while high-viscosity contents may preclude such motion and associated signal dropout.

Arachnoid cysts, on the other hand, have a separate origin. They may be intradural or extradural, arising either as the result of alteration of arachnoid trabeculae or as a defect in the dura with herniation of the arachnoid membrane. They are isointense to CSF on all pulse sequences, unless complicated by hemorrhage, and have no associated vertebral anomalies.

Clinical References

1. Bentley JFR, Smith JR. Developmental posterior enteric remnants and spinal malformations: the split notochord syndrome. Arch Dis Child 1960;35:76–86.
2. Geremia GK, Russell EJ, Clasen RA. MR imaging characteristics of a neuroenteric cyst. AJNR 1988;9:978–980.

(A through C *courtesy of Mark Osborne, MD*)

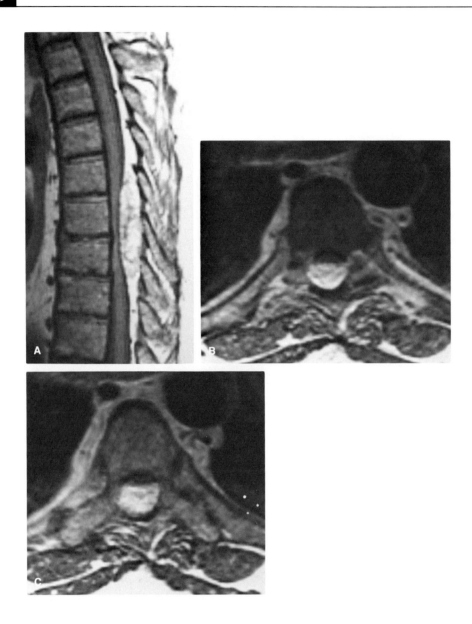

HISTORY

Paralysis

FINDINGS

A well-delineated, obtusely marginated epidural mass is noted that demonstrates hyperintense heterogeneous signal on (A) sagittal and (B and C) axial T1-weighted images. The lesion was isointense to CSF on the T2-weighted examination (*images not shown*).

DIAGNOSIS

Angiolipoma

DISCUSSION

The differential diagnosis of extradural masses in the thoracic spine includes benign tumor (neurinoma, meningioma, lipoma), hematoma, abscess, and metastatic lesions (including secondary foci of leukemia and lymphoma). A much less common entity is extradural lipomatosis, seen with chronic steroid use or in Cushing's disease.[1] The bright T1-weighted signal of the epidural lesion in this patient moves masses composed of fat and blood products to the top of our differential list.

The signal intensity of spinal hematomas is stage-dependent, similar to that described for brain lesions. Often it is difficult to separate epidural and subdural hematomas of the spine preoperatively. Spinal epidural and subdural hematomas may be associated with lumbar punctures, trauma (including disc herniation), bleeding diatheses, anticoagulants, vascular malformations, vasculitides, and pregnancy.[2]

The T2-weighted scans (*images not shown*) in this case revealed the mass to have a signal intensity approximately that of CSF; thus, it was not completely characteristic for fat, with lipomatous tissue being of lower signal intensity on T2-weighted images than on T1-weighted images. Spinal angiolipomas are rare benign neoplasms that are composed of mature lipocytes in combination with abnormal blood vessels.[3] The hyperintensity on T2-weighted images may be due to stagnant blood, which has a long T2 relaxation time. More than 90% of spinal angiolipomas are found in the epidural space.[4] Gadolinium chelate infusion can help evaluate the degree of vascularization in angiolipomas. Spinal angiolipomas are most often encountered in the midthoracic region, are most common in women, and can cause both erosive changes and pathologic fractures in bone. They produce signs and symptoms of spinal cord compression. Their symptomatology may be exacerbated by pregnancy and weight gain. Surgery is highly successful in relieving symptoms.

Clinical References

1. Mascalchi M, Arnetoli G, Dal Pozzo G, et al. Spinal epidural angiolipoma: MR findings. AJNR 1991;12:744–745.
2. Mark MS. Nondegenerative, nonneoplastic diseases of the spine and spinal cord. In: Atlas SW, ed. MRI of the brain and spine. New York, Raven Press, 1991.
3. Preul MC, Leblanc R, Tampieri D, et al. Spinal angiolipomas: report of three cases. J Neurosurg 1993;78:280–286.
4. Weill A, del Carpio-O'Donovan R, Tampieri D, et al. Spinal angiolipomas: CT and MR aspects. J Comput Assist Tomog 15:83–85.

(A through C courtesy of Mark Osborne, MD. Parts of this case, as well as 33.13-2, 33.1481-5, 33.33-5, and 33.417, were contributed by Joseph Kozlowski, MD.)

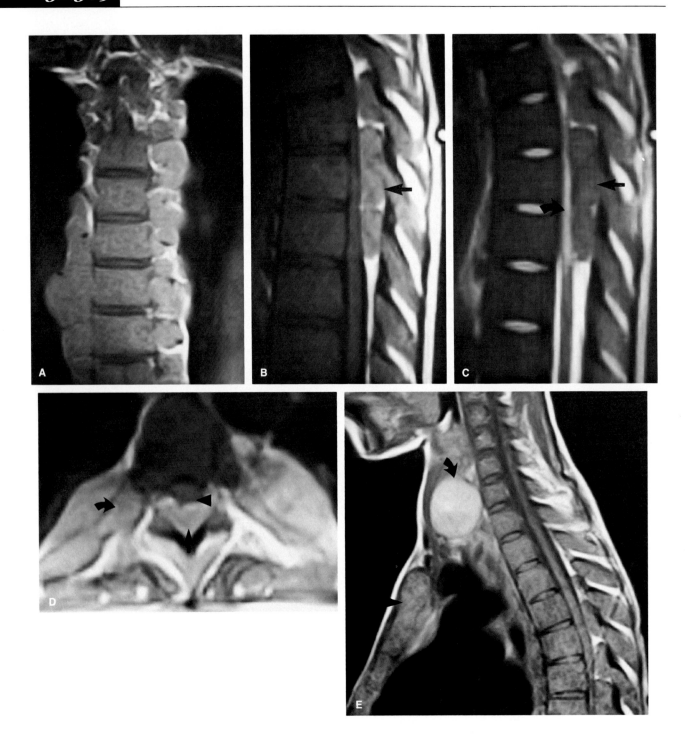

HISTORY

A 32-year-old patient with thalassemia and progressive paraplegia

FINDINGS

(A) A T1-weighted coronal image demonstrates large, bilateral lobulated paraspinal masses in the upper and mid-thoracic regions. On the T1-weighted midline sagittal view (B), large intraspinal masses (*arrow*) with resultant severe cord compression are identified at the T6 to T8 levels. The soft tissue masses lie within the same space as the thoracic epidural fat. Additional sagittal images (*images not shown*) revealed intraspinal lesions posterior to T3–5 as well. Also noted is a generalized decrease in signal intensity of the thoracic vertebral bodies. (C) A corresponding fast spin echo T2-weighted sagittal image confirms the abnormal intraspinal soft tissue masses (*arrow*). The lesions remain relatively low in signal intensity on the T2-weighted scan. Abnormally increased signal intensity compatible with edema and/or gliosis is identified within the compressed thoracic spinal cord (*curved arrow*). (*D*) A postinfusion T1-weighted axial image at the T4–5 level demonstrates mild, homogeneous enhancement of the paraspinal and the intraspinal (*arrow*) lesions. A thin, low-intensity line (*arrowhead*) between the intraspinal lesion and the compressed thoracic cord suggests the extradural location of the masses. The medial right T5 rib (*curved arrow*) is abnormally expanded. (*E*) A T1-weighted sagittal localizer image redemonstrates the severe cord compression in the upper thoracic region. Of note are moderate expansion of and generalized decreased signal intensity within the sternum (*arrow*). A thyroid goiter (*curved arrow*) is incidentally noted.

DIAGNOSIS

Extramedullary hematopoiesis (EH) with severe thoracic cord compression

DISCUSSION

EH is a compensatory response to insufficient bone marrow blood cell production. Thalassemia, hereditary spherocytosis, myelosclerosis, and metastatic bone marrow replacement are among the entities most commonly associated with this process. The favored sites of involvement are the spleen, liver, and lymph nodes. Thoracic cases of EH are relatively rare. Such cases are usually asymptomatic, although, as illustrated by the current case, intraspinal lesions may result in cord compression.

The origin of marrow-producing masses in thoracic EH is controversial.[1] The paraspinal lesions are probably the result of extrusion of proliferating marrow into a subperiosteal location. The intraspinal lesions may also form in this manner, or alternatively may be secondary to transformation of embryonic hematopoietic rests within the epidural space.

Intrathoracic EH usually presents with multiple, smoothly marginated paraspinal masses. No bony erosion should be present. The paraspinal lesions are most common in the mid- to lower thoracic region but may be present anywhere from T2 to T11.[2] MR of these lesions demonstrates relatively low signal intensity on both T1- and T2-weighted images, similar to the signal intensity characteristics of erythropoietic tissue.[3]

MR Technique

MR enhancement patterns in EH have not been described, but in light of the highly vascular nature of the lesions, the enhancement seen in this case is not unexpected. Following enhancement, the relationship of the compressed spinal cord to the intraspinal hematopoietic component is more clearly delineated.

Pitfalls in Image Interpretation

The diagnosis of EH can often be made confidently in light of patient history. However, patients with metastatic disease and lymphoma may present with imaging patterns very similar to those seen with EH. The key findings that distinguish EH are marrow expansion and abnormal signal intensity in locations apart from the spine. In the current case, the abnormalities in the posterior ribs and sternum clinch the diagnosis of EH. Another, although less reliable, difference is the signal intensity of the lesions on T2-weighted images. Hematopoietic tissue tends to have fairly low signal intensity on T2-weighted scans, while neoplastic cells generally demonstrate increased signal intensity.

Clinical References

1. Kalina P, Hillstrom MM. MR of extramedullary hematopoiesis causing cord compression in beta-thalassemia. AJNR 1992;13:1407–1409.
2. Korsten J, Grossman H, Winchester PH, Canale VC. Extramedullary hematopoieses in patients with thalassemia anemia. Radiology 1970;95:257–263.
3. Savader SJ, Otero RR, Savader BL. MR imaging of intrathoracic extramedullary hematopoiesis. J Comput Assist Tomog 1988;12:878–880.

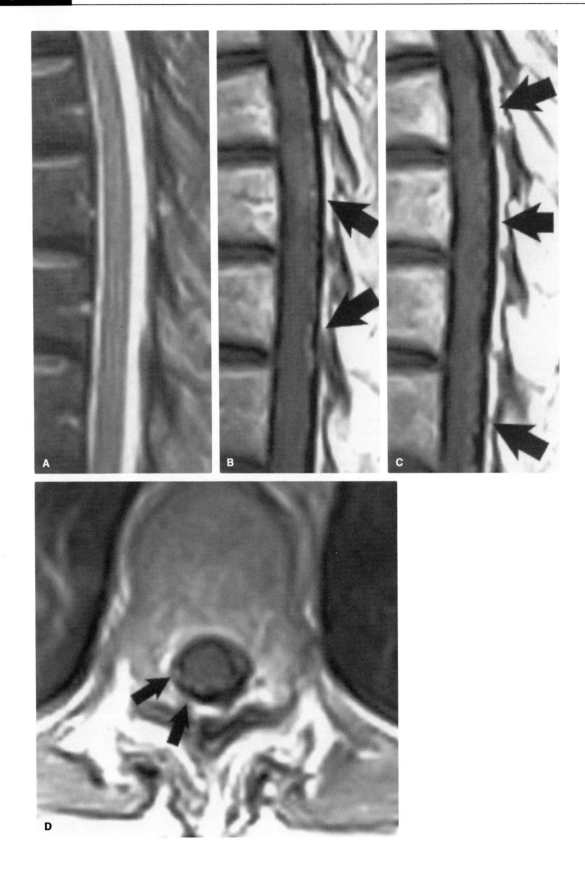

HISTORY

A 55-year-old patient with known lung cancer and increasing difficulty walking

FINDINGS

No abnormalities are noted on precontrast T1-weighted (*images not shown*) and T2-weighted (*A*) midline sagittal images. Following contrast administration (*B and C*), multiple tiny foci of abnormal enhancement (*arrows*) are identified along the dorsal aspect of the thoracic spinal cord. (*D*) An axial postinfusion image at the T10 level confirms the meningeal location of the enhancing abnormalities (*arrows*).

DIAGNOSIS

Thoracic leptomeningeal metastases

DISCUSSION

Leptomeningeal seeding of tumor can be seen from either primary central nervous system (CNS) or non-CNS tumors. Primary CNS neoplasms that cause leptomeningeal seeding include glioblastoma, ependymoma, medulloblastoma, and pineal tumors. Lung carcinoma, breast carcinoma, melanoma, and lymphoma are common non-CNS tumors that result in leptomeningeal metastatic disease.

Patients with leptomeningeal metastases may present with a variety of symptoms. Back pain, leg pain, headaches, cranial and spinal nerve deficits, and gait disturbances are common complaints.

Cerebral spinal fluid (CSF) cytology provides the gold standard for diagnosis of subarachnoid tumor spread but may be inaccurate unless multiple samples and large volumes of CSF are obtained. Nodular filling defects in the subarachnoid space or clumping of nerve roots suggest leptomeningeal metastases on computed tomography or nonenhanced MR, but these techniques are rather insensitive.[1] The use of paramagnetic contrast greatly increases the sensitivity of MR for spinal leptomeningeal metastases.[2]

MR Technique

Contrast administration is essential for sensitive detection of leptomeningeal tumor. On T2-weighted images, CSF and most leptomeningeal metastases demonstrate high signal intensity. As a result, small metastases are generally inapparent on T2-weighted scans. On postcontrast T1-weighted images, enhancing tumor is well differentiated from low-signal-intensity CSF.

Pitfalls in Image Interpretation

MR is more sensitive for leptomeningeal metastases in patients with non-CNS primaries than in those with primary CNS neoplasms. Sensitivity is further decreased in patients with hematologic malignancies such as lymphoma and leukemia, probably due to the lack of macroscopic meningeal invasion in these malignancies.[2]

Clinical References

1. Krol G, Sze G, Malkin M, Walker R. MR of cranial and spinal meningeal carcinomatosis: comparison with CT and myelography. AJNR 1988;9:709–714.
2. Yousem DM, Patrone PM, Grossman RI. Leptomeningeal metastases: MR evaluation. J Comput Assist Tomog 1990; 14:255–261.

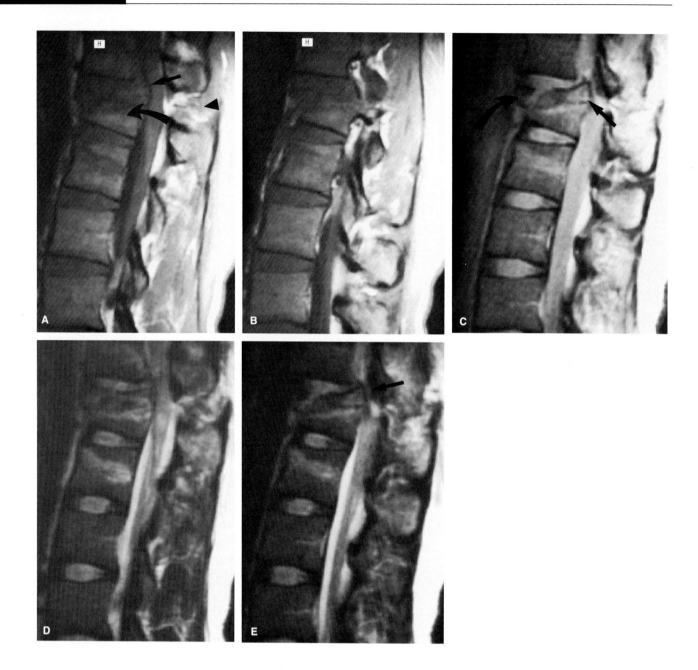

HISTORY

A 26-year-old patient who fell 15 feet while spelunking, with subsequent bilateral lower extremity weakness and numbness

FINDINGS

(A) The sagittal T1-weighted image shows increased anteroposterior dimension and mild anterior wedging of the T12 vertebral body (*curved arrow*). Low signal intensity fills the upper T12 body, which also demonstrates an indistinct margin with the adjacent T11–12 disk. The posterosuperior T12 fragment is retropulsed (*arrow*), par-

tially compromising the spinal canal. Anterior listhesis of T11 on T12 further compromises the canal, causing deformity and compression of the spinal cord. Posterior element abnormalities are present, with a widened distance between the T11 and T12 spinous processes (*arrowhead*) indicating ligamentous disruption. (B) A parasagittal image reveals facet joint distraction and facet malalignment on the left at T11–12. This was present bilaterally. (C) The parasagittal intermediate T2-weighted image (TE = 30) demonstrates the radial expansion of the upper T12 body with retropulsed (*arrow*) and anteriorly displaced (*curved arrow*) fragments. (D) The midline sagittal T2-weighted image demonstrates increased signal intensity in T12 as well as a horizontal band of high signal intensity in the adjacent T11 and L1 vertebral bodies due

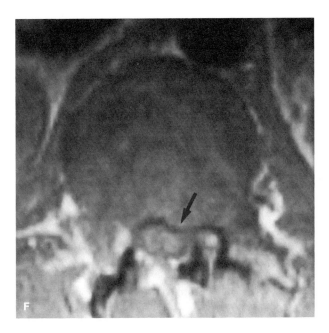

to marrow edema. Corresponding low-signal-intensity bands are seen on the T1-weighted images in the T11 and L1 vertebrae. These signal characteristics are consistent with microfractures. Severe canal narrowing is present with compression of the spinal cord. High signal intensity is present in the cord, indicating edema and contusion. (*E*) The parasagittal image, just to the left of midline, better depicts the retropulsed fragment (*arrow*). (*F*) The axial T1-weighted image demonstrates an expanded T12 vertebral body. The mottled marrow signal intensity is secondary to the complex fracture and edema. The spinal canal is narrowed, most prominently by the retropulsed fragment (*arrow*) projecting along the left posterior margin, producing cord compression. The abnormally aligned right T11 and T12 facets are identified.

DIAGNOSIS

Burst fracture of T12 with retropulsion and cord compression, combined with a fracture–dislocation injury at T11–12

DISCUSSION

A burst fracture is categorized as an axial loading injury. The vertical compression forces the nucleus pulposus into the vertebral body, resulting in a complex fracture with radial displacement of the fragments. This becomes particularly important when fragments are displaced posteriorly into the spinal canal, causing canal stenosis or cord injury. These fractures occur most commonly at the thoracolumbar junction from T9 to L5. A burst fracture is usually isolated to a single vertebral body, although multiple burst fractures can occur.[1] Traumatic injuries are frequently present at other levels.

In most cases, burst fractures have associated neurologic deficits, with the findings corresponding to the level of the fracture. Distraction or surgery can reduce the retropulsed fragment, but the neurologic deficit often persists. MR detects fractures extending into the pedicles so that adequate anchoring sites can be selected for surgical stabilization devices.

Computed tomography remains the study of choice for the initial evaluation of a burst fracture and the retropulsed fragment.[2] MR, however, has become a valuable imaging tool in the evaluation of the posttraumatic spine. This is especially true when spinal cord or paraspinal soft tissue abnormalities are suspected. MR allows direct visualization of cord abnormalities, including compression, edema, and hemorrhage. Previously unsuspected ligamentous injuries are often demonstrated.

MR Technique

Vertebral body fractures are often better visualized on sagittal images. Axial sections, however, usually show canal narrowing and other clinically relevant information with regard to the spinal cord to better advantage.

Clinical References

1. Atlas SW, Regenbogen V, Rogers LF, Kim KS. The radiographic characterization of burst fractures of the spine. AJR 1986;147:575–582.
2. Beale SM, Pathria MN, Masaryk TJ. MRI of spine trauma. Top Magn Reson Imag 1988;1:53–62.

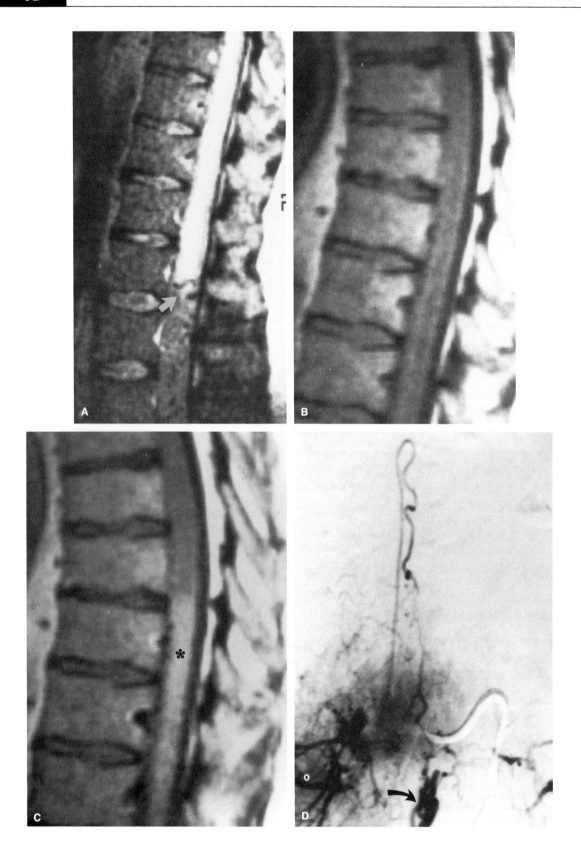

HISTORY

A 48-year-old patient with multiple episodes of transient lower extremity weakness

FINDINGS

(A) The midline T2-weighted (TR/TE = 2500/80) sagittal image at the level of the thoracolumbar junction demonstrates an expanded cord with abnormal hyperintensity. Enlarged serpentine vascular flow voids (*arrow*) are noted in the thecal space below the conus. Precontrast (B) and postcontrast (C) T1-weighted sagittal images in the thoracic region reveal abnormal cord enhancement (*asterisk*) that extends over several contiguous segments. Digital subtraction arteriography (D) demonstrates an enlarged feeding artery (artery of Adamkiewicz) and a caudally draining vein, the latter originating at the site of an arteriovenous fistula (*curved arrow*).

DIAGNOSIS

Spinal cord infarction, secondary to an intradural arteriovenous fistula

DISCUSSION

MR is the imaging modality of choice when spinal cord ischemia or infarction is suspected, both for diagnosis and to exclude other causes of thoracic myelopathy.[1] This disease involves primarily the lower thoracic cord and conus, and affects predominantly central gray matter. The extent of abnormality seen on MR correlates well with the clinical findings and prognosis. Signal abnormalities are first seen in the anterior horns of the gray matter, with more extensive disease involving the posterior horns, the adjacent central white matter, and in severe disease the entire cord cross section. The thoracolumbar cord is supplied by the artery of Adamkiewicz, which arises in 75% of cases from the 9th, 10th, 11th, or 12th intercostal artery. Blood flow is highest to the thoracolumbar segment of the spinal cord due to the abundance of gray matter (which has a higher metabolic need than white matter). Thus, this portion of the cord is most vulnerable to hypoperfusion. Ischemia leads to vasogenic edema and cord enlargement, with hyperintensity on T2-weighted scans. Contrast enhancement can occur due to disruption of the blood–cord barrier associated with cord ischemia.[2] Causes of spinal cord infarction include atherosclerosis, vasculitis, embolic events, infection, surgery (abdominal aortic aneurysm resection), radiation, and trauma.

Spinal arteriovenous malformations (AVMs) are classified into three types: intradural AVMs supplied by medullary arteries and drained by perimedullary veins, dural arteriovenous fistulas supplied by radiculomeningeal arteries and drained by perimedullary veins, and extradural AVMs supplied and drained by extradural vessels. The changes observed in the spinal cord on MR with AVMs are secondary to ischemia, edema, and venous infarction, with the latter due to venous stasis.

MR Technique

Axial T2-weighted and postcontrast T1-weighted images permit assessment of the geographic distribution of disease in spinal cord ischemia. Axial sections should be acquired in addition to sagittal sections.

Pitfalls in Image Interpretation

Entities similar in appearance on MR to spinal cord infarction include multiple sclerosis, transverse myelitis, and neoplasia. Recognition of a vascular distribution of disease involvement (in cord cross section and craniocaudal extent) facilitates diagnosis.

Bone marrow changes in patients with spinal cord infarction can represent associated disease (marrow ischemia), with recognition of such assisting diagnosis.[3]

Clinical References

1. Mawad ME, Rivera V, Crawford S, et al. Spinal cord ischemia after resection of thoracoabdominal aortic aneurysms: MR findings in 24 patients. AJR 1990;155:1303–1307.
2. Larsson EM, Desai P, Hardin CW, et al. Venous infarction of the spinal cord resulting from dural arteriovenous fistula: MR imaging findings. AJNR 1991;12:739–743.
3. Yuh WTC, Marsh EE, Wang AK, et al. MR imaging of spinal cord and vertebral body infarction. AJNR 1992;13:145–154.

(A through D from Sener RN, Larsson EM, Backer R, Jinkins JR. MRI of intradural spinal arteriovenous fistula associated with ischemia and infarction of the cord. Clinical Imaging 1993;17:73–76, courtesy of J.R. Jinkins, MD.)

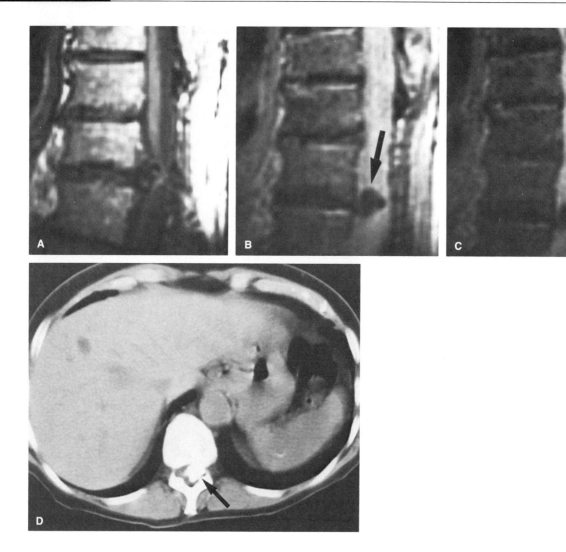

HISTORY

An elderly woman with persistent back pain

FINDINGS

(A) The sagittal T1-weighted exam reveals displacement of the lower thoracic cord at the T11–12 level by an apparent, but not well visualized, low-signal-intensity mass. This mass (*arrow in B*) is markedly hypointense on (B) proton density and (C) T2-weighted images. Contiguity with the native disk is best demonstrated on the T1-weighted exam. On (D) CT, the mass (*arrow*) and native disk are densely calcified. The diagnosis was confirmed at surgery.

DIAGNOSIS

Calcified thoracic disk herniation

DISCUSSION

Thoracic disk herniation can occur at any level but is most common at the lower four interspaces. A clear-cut clinical syndrome is often not present, with common symptoms including pain, paresthesias, and motor weakness.

Calcification of a herniated disk is rare, but can occur. In the pre-CT era, in a series of 61 thoracic disk herniations, five were calcified.[1] Two patterns of calcification can be seen, with calcification either within both the disk space and contiguous herniation or within only the herniation itself. Diagnosis is possible in these cases from plain film alone. In adults, disk calcification by itself, when restricted to one or two levels, is typically degenerative in nature and not necessarily of clinical significance.

The most common appearance of dense calcification on MR is that of a signal void, due to local variations in magnetic susceptibility. However, calcification can also be of high signal intensity on T1-weighted images, due to T1 shortening in hydrated regions.

MR Technique

Gradient echo images demonstrate to better advantage magnetic susceptibility effects, which result in a loss of signal intensity. These effects are accentuated at the interface between substances with a large difference in susceptibility—for example, between soft tissue and air or bone. Although not illustrated in this case, gradient echo images can thus provide improved depiction, relative to spin echo images, of vacuum disks, calcified disks, and bony hypertrophic change.[2]

Pitfalls in Image Interpretation

The presence of dense calcification could lead to misdiagnosis of the lesion as a meningioma. Although one would expect to be able to distinguish with certainty an extradural from an intradural extramedullary lesion, this distinction is not always possible.

Clinical References

1. Baker HL, Love JG, Uihlein A. Roentgenologic features of protruded thoracic intervertebral disks. Radiology 1965; 84:1059–1065.
2. Murayama S, Numaguchi Y, Robinson AE. Degenerative lumbar spine disorders in gradient refocused echo axial magnetic resonance images. Clin Imaging 1990;14:198–203.

(Images courtesy of Clifford Wolf, MD)

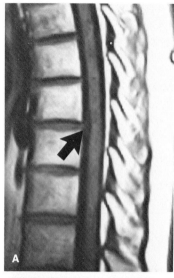

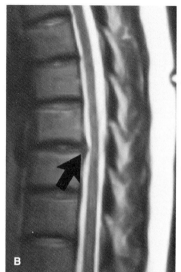

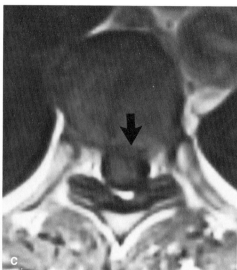

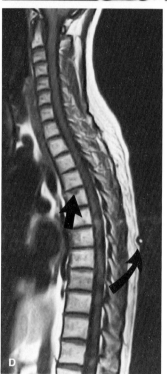

HISTORY

A 45-year-old patient with midthoracic back pain

FINDINGS

(*A*) The T1-weighted midline sagittal image demonstrates a small anterior extradural soft tissue abnormality (*arrow*) at the T8–T9 level. (*B*) A fast spin echo T2-weighted sagittal image redemonstrates the T8–T9 abnormality (*arrow*). The lesion appears similar in signal intensity to the intervertebral disk and contiguous with the disk on both T1- and T2-weighted images. The abnormality (*arrow*) is confirmed on the postinfusion T1-weighted axial view (*C*) and appears centered to the left of midline. Mild deformity of the left side of the spinal cord is well demonstrated.

DIAGNOSIS

Left paracentral disk herniation at T8–T9

DISCUSSION

Thoracic disk herniations are generally thought to be uncommon. Much of this impression may be secondary to the difficulty involved in imaging the thoracic spine with conventional myelography or computed tomography (CT).[1] Nevertheless, it is generally accepted that thoracic disk herniations are less common than those in the cervical or lumbar spine. Thoracic disk herniations are most prevalent in the lower thoracic spine, where the spine is more mobile. T10–11 and T11–12 are particularly vulnerable. Radiculopathies in association with thoracic disk disease are unusual. Symptoms are varied and often quite vague, with the most common complaint being back pain. The lack of a distinct symptom complex makes the clinical diagnosis of thoracic disk herniation difficult.

Although myelography and CT provide excellent visualization of bony structures, soft tissue details are notably lacking. Additionally, extensive scans are required to cover the entire thoracic spine with CT. MR provides direct multiplanar visualization of the entire thoracic spine, and iodinated contrast is of course unnecessary. Importantly, the mass effect of disk herniations on the cord and the contour of the cord itself are well demonstrated. The superior soft tissue contrast of MR also allows evaluation for the presence of intrinsic spinal cord pathology.

MR Technique

A common problem with MR is the inability to define accurately the exact level of a thoracic disk herniation.[2]

We commonly use a body coil total spine image (*D*) as a localizer, which on our system can be obtained with a dedicated spine coil already in position. Although this image has poor sensitivity for subtle abnormalities, landmarks within or near the spine such as the Schmorl's node at T5 (*arrow*) are almost always identified. A vitamin E capsule (or, alternatively, a piece of IV tubing filled with Johnson's Baby Oil) taped to the patient's back (*curved arrow*) serves as an additional reference. Correlation with the higher-resolution spine coil images allows precise localization of the level of abnormality.

Pitfalls in Image Interpretation

The use of paramagnetic contrast improves visualization of disk herniations due to enhancement of surrounding epidural structures. Nodular areas of enhancement are often seen above and below the herniated disk. At surgery, these enhancing regions have been found to represent dilated, congested epidural veins.[3] Without contrast, the presence of engorged epidural plexus may result in overestimation of the size of a disk herniation.

Clinical References

1. Williams MP, Cherryman GR, Husband JE. Significance of thoracic disc herniation demonstrated by MR imaging. J Comput Assist Tomog 1989;13:211–214.
2. Ross JS, Perez-Reyes N, Masaryk TJ, et al. Thoracic disk herniation: MR imaging. Radiology 1987;165:511–515.
3. Parizel PM, Rodesch G, Baleriaux D. Gd-DTPA-enhanced MR in thoracic disk herniations. Neuroradiology 1989; 31:75–79.

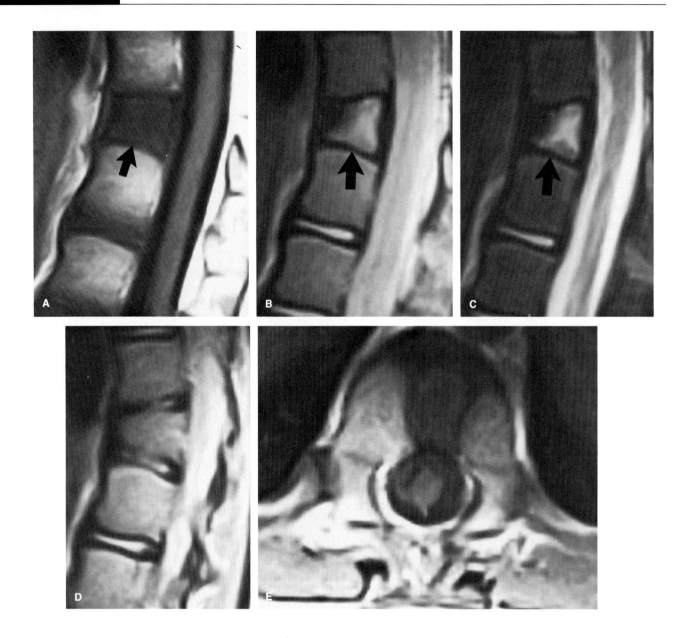

HISTORY

A 10-year-old patient with lower extremity weakness

FINDINGS

(*A*) A midline postinfusion T1-weighted sagittal image demonstrates abnormally decreased signal intensity within the T11 vertebral body (*arrow*). No areas of abnormal enhancement are identified. This abnormality (*arrows*) is of increased signal intensity on (*B*) the intermediate and (*C*) the heavily T2-weighted midline sagittal views. Mild anterior wedging of the T11 vertebral body is also present. The signal characteristics of the abnormal segment are identical to disk material on all sequences. (*D*) An intermediate T2-weighted sagittal image to the right of midline reveals normal-appearing signal characteristics within T11, although wedging of the vertebral body is still noted. The adjacent vertebral bodies are seen to conform to the wedge-shaped T11. (*E*) The postinfusion T1-weighted axial view of T11 reveals a low-signal-intensity cleft extending through the anterior vertebral body. (*F*) A T1-weighted axial view at the midthoracic level demonstrates splitting (*arrow*) of the thoracic cord, compatible with diastematomyelia. (*G*) A frontal radiograph of the thoracic spine confirms the defect (*arrow*) in the T11 vertebral body.

DIAGNOSIS

Butterfly vertebra at T11 and diastematomyelia

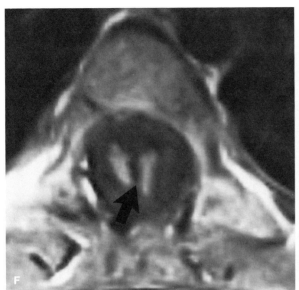

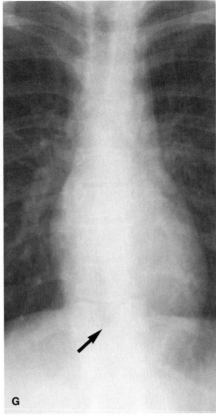

DISCUSSION

Butterfly vertebral body, sometimes referred to as anterior spina bifida, is so named because of its characteristic appearance on plain film. Concave superior and inferior end plates and the central osseous defect combine to produce the butterfly appearance. The appearance on MR is also characteristic.[1] On sagittal images, a defect is present through the central portion of the vertebral body. This defect is contiguous with the intervertebral disk above and below the affected level. Importantly, the defect should remain isointense to normal intervertebral disk material on all imaging sequences. Axial or lateral sagittal views demonstrate the normal-appearing marrow on either side of the midline cleft. On the lateral sagittal views, as on plain films, the adjacent vertebral bodies can be seen conforming to the abnormal shape of the butterfly vertebral body.

A butterfly vertebral body is often an incidental finding of no clinical significance. In the proper clinical context, however, one should keep in mind the association of butterfly vertebral body with intraspinal abnormalities such as diastematomyelia.

Pitfalls in Image Interpretation

A butterfly vertebral body should not be mistaken for an infiltrative vertebral lesion. The lack of enhancement, isointensity of the cleft to disk material, and adjacent bony changes should allay any such suspicions.

Clinical Reference

1. Duffrin D, Auer R, Moolsintong P, et al. MRI, CT, and plain film appearance of anterior spina bifida. Magn Reson Imag 1987;5:499–503.

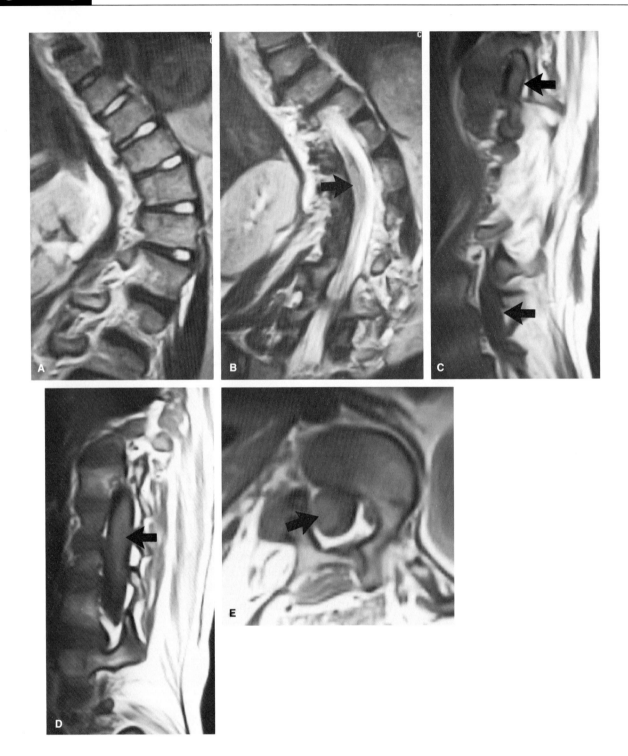

HISTORY

An 8-year-old boy with measured lumbar scoliosis of 77° and a minor thoracic curve. Three previous surgeries have been performed to remove a hemangioma from his lower back.

FINDINGS

(*A*) The coronal fast spin echo T2-weighted image shows marked lumbosacral scoliosis with the convexity to the left and the apex at L2. A compensatory thoracic scoliosis is present with curvature to the right in the thoracic region. (*B*) A more posterior coronal section through the spinal canal demonstrates the low signal intensity of the spinal cord surrounded by high-signal-intensity CSF. The conus (*arrow*) ends in a normal location, at the level of the lower L2 vertebral body. The nerve roots and cauda equina are well seen below the conus. The cord is positioned along the concave, right side of the lumbar curvature with high-signal CSF on the left side of the thecal sac. (*C*) The midline sagittal T1-weighted image reveals portions of the vertebrae in the lumbosacral and thoracolumbar junctions and only short segments of the spinal canal and cord (*arrows*). The vertebral bodies appear distorted in this projection. This is further complicated by rotation of the spine. (*D*) A sagittal image toward the convexity of the curvature demonstrates the L1 through L3 vertebral bodies and the intermediate-signal-intensity conus medullaris (*arrow*) terminating at the inferior L2 level. (*E*) The axial T1-weighted image at the upper L1 level demonstrates the round, intermediate-signal-intensity cord (*arrow*) positioned along the right side of the spinal canal. This is along the concave side of the curvature. The signal intensity of the vertebral body is lower on the right due to the oblique imaging plane and volume averaging of the intervertebral disk and the vertebral marrow. Obvious rotation of the spinal column is present.

DIAGNOSIS

Scoliosis

DISCUSSION

Scoliosis is a lateral curvature of the spine. Between 80% and 90% of patients with scoliosis have the idiopathic form with no detectable underlying cause for the abnormal curvature. This type is much more common in females, accounting for 80% to 90% of cases. In idiopathic

scoliosis, the thoracic or thoracolumbar curvature is usually convex to the right. Atypical features of scoliosis include a leftward curvature, associated pain or neuromuscular dysfunction, or rapid progression.[2] A curve that progresses or one that measures more than 50° usually requires surgical treatment.

In the remaining 10% to 20% of patients, scoliosis is due to a variety of causes, including congenital, neuromuscular, and posttraumatic causes. Congenital scoliosis may occur due to vertebral anomalies, including a butterfly vertebral body and hemivertebra. Intraspinal causes include Arnold-Chiari I and II malformations, syringohydromyelia, diastematomyelia, and spinal cord neoplasms. Neuromuscular scoliosis, such as that due to cerebral palsy, classically demonstrates a curve in the shape of a C, rather than the S shape of idiopathic scoliosis. Posttraumatic causes include fracture or previous insult such as prior osteomyelitis, surgery, or radiation therapy.

MR is the study of choice in the workup of atypical or progressive scoliosis.[2] MR is noninvasive and does not use ionizing radiation and is therefore ideal for evaluation of pediatric patients. MR provides accurate detection of lesions associated with scoliosis. Plain films remain necessary for quantitating the degree of curvature and monitoring progression. Plain films may also diagnose or suggest the underlying etiology for the spinal curvature.

MR Technique

Images in the coronal plane are frequently helpful to evaluate the spinal canal and contents in patients with scoliosis because sagittal images may demonstrate only a limited segment of the canal. This is particularly true when minimal kyphosis is present. A combination of sagittal and coronal images allows evaluation of the entire spine and cord from the craniocervical junction to the coccyx.

Pitfalls in Image Interpretation

Diastematomyelia is a cause of scoliosis that may be missed on sagittal images. Axial or coronal images frequently identify the split cord and may detect a fibrous or bony septum.

Clinical References

1. Nokes SR, Murtagh FR, Jones JD, et al. Childhood scoliosis: MR imaging. Radiology 1987;164:791–797.
2. Barnes PD, Brody JD, Jaramillo D, et al. Atypical idiopathic scoliosis: MR imaging evaluation. Radiology 1993;186:247–253.

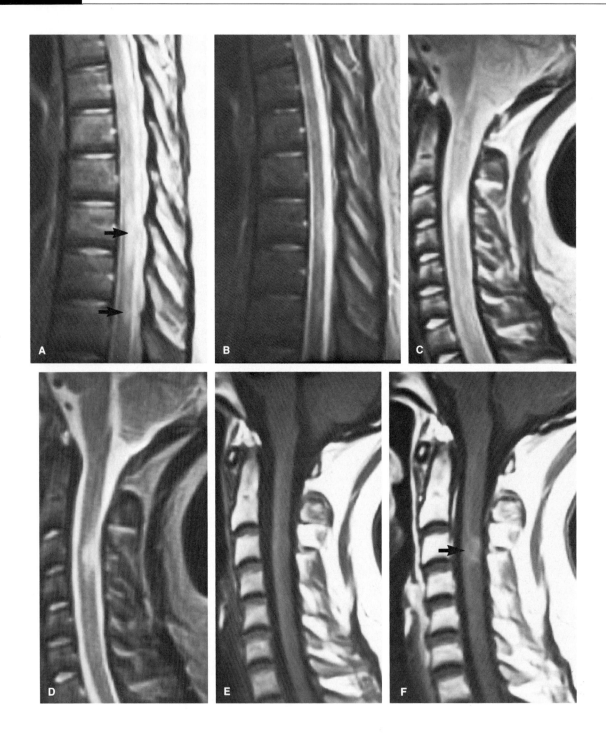

HISTORY

A 40-year-old white woman with recent onset of weakness and loss of sensation in her hands and lower extremities. Posterior tibial and median nerve somatosensory evoked potentials were abnormal (consistent with disruption of the somatosensory pathways between the spinal cord and cortex), suggesting a cervical lesion. The cerebrospinal fluid (CSF) was positive for oligoclonal bands.

FINDINGS

Sagittal T2-weighted images (*A*, TE = 45; *B*, TE = 90) reveal two intrinsic thoracic cord abnormalities (*arrows*), both hyperintense relative to the normal cord. These lesions are less apparent on the second echo (TE = 90) than on the first echo (TE = 45). The thoracic cord is normal in width. A single lesion is identified at the C3 level on the (*C*) first (TE = 45) and (*D*) second (TE = 90) echoes of the T2-weighted se-

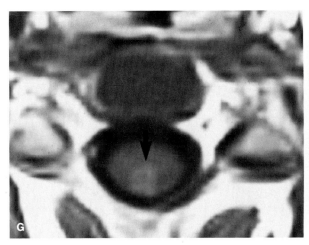

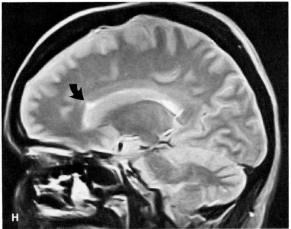

quence from the subsequent cervical MR scan. There is minimal cord expansion, best noted on the precontrast T1-weighted exam (*E*), with faint enhancement (*arrow*) postcontrast (*F and G*). On the T2-weighted head MR exam (*H*), only a single hyperintense periventricular abnormality (*curved arrow*) was noted.

DIAGNOSIS

Multiple sclerosis (chronic thoracic and active cervical cord disease)

DISCUSSION

Spinal cord plaques tend to be best detected on MR scans with intermediate T2 weighting (TE = 40 to 50). The contrast between the lesion and surrounding normal cord not uncommonly diminishes with heavier T2 weighting (TE ≥ 80). In patients with symptoms referable to the spinal cord, and a lesion demonstrated by MR, imaging of the brain is often used to support the diagnosis of multiple sclerosis.[1] However, not all patients with evidence by MR of spinal cord disease will demonstrate characteristic brain involvement.

MR Technique

Because inactive lesions are not well demonstrated on postcontrast T1-weighted scans, these should always be preceded by precontrast T2-weighted scans, which will detect both active and inactive disease.

Pitfalls in Image Interpretation

Multiple sclerosis can present with symptoms suggestive of a cord tumor, particularly in the cervical spine. Findings on MR can also mimic neoplasia, with focal cord enlargement and abnormal contrast enhancement not unusual in active disease.[2] Careful consideration of all test results, combined with imaging of the entire spine and head, can prevent misdiagnosis.

Clinical References

1. Edwards MK, Farlow MR, Stevens JC. Cranial MR in spinal cord MS: diagnosing patients with isolated spinal cord symptoms. AJNR 1986;7:1003–1005.
2. Lammoglia FJ, Short SR, Sweet DE, et al. Multiple sclerosis presenting as an intramedullary cervical cord tumor. Kans Med 1989;90(7):219–221.

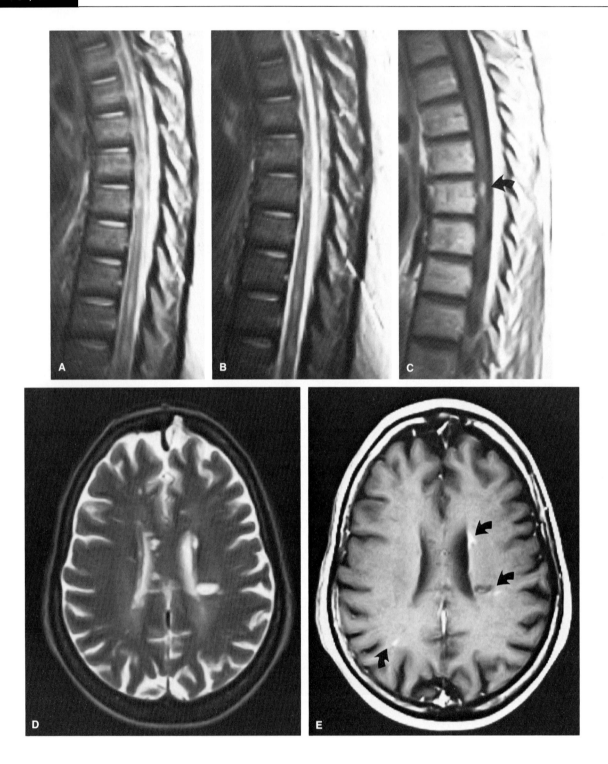

HISTORY

A 50-year-old white woman presenting 1 month before hospital admission with tingling and numbness of the right foot. This subsequently spread to include the right leg, and later the left. Although the patient became unable to walk, symptoms have recently regressed, with decreased burning sensation, and the patient can now walk with support. The cerebrospinal fluid (CSF) was positive for oligoclonal bands.

FINDINGS

Multiple intramedullary lesions with high signal intensity on T2-weighted images (*A*, TE = 45; *B*, TE = 90) are identified throughout the thoracic spinal cord. No cord expansion is evident. Enhancement of one of these lesions (*curved arrow*) is observed on the T1-weighted image postcontrast (*C*). On brain MR, multiple punctate white matter abnormalities are noted, located predominantly within the corpus callosum and immediate periventricular white matter (*D*, TE = 90). Postcontrast (*E*), there is enhancement of three brain lesions (*curved arrows*).

DIAGNOSIS

Multiple sclerosis (active thoracic cord disease)

DISCUSSION

Contrast enhancement is presumed to correlate with histologic lesion activity, a finding confirmed in a recent study of multiple sclerosis lesions of the brain.[1] The degree of enhancement tends to parallel the extent of macrophage infiltration. In cervical spinal disease, enhancement has been shown to correlate with clinical symptoms.[2] On brain MR, characteristic findings in multiple sclerosis include multiple punctate white matter lesions, asymmetrically distributed with regard to the right and left hemispheres, with a preference for the immediate periventricular white matter.

MR Technique

In multiple sclerosis, contrast enhancement provides information about disease activity not otherwise available. Enhancement, however, may be delayed following contrast administration.

Pitfalls in Image Interpretation

Although previously considered a monophasic disorder, relapse of acute transverse myelitis has been recently documented.[3] This disease, which demonstrates findings on spinal MR consistent with inflammation and/or demyelination not unlike multiple sclerosis, must be considered in the differential diagnosis. The presence of multiple cord lesions, combined with characteristic brain abnormalities, permits confident diagnosis of multiple sclerosis in the case presented here.

Clinical References

1. Nesbit GM, Forbes GS, Scheithauer BW, et al. Multiple sclerosis: histopathologic and MR and/or CT correlation in 37 cases at biopsy and three cases at autopsy. Radiology 1991;180:467–474.
2. Larsson EM, Holtas S, Nilsson O. Gd-DTPA-enhanced MR of suspected spinal multiple sclerosis. AJNR 1989;10:1071–1076.
3. Tippett DS, Fishman PS, Panitch HS. Relapsing transverse myelitis. Neurology 1991;41:703–706.

CHAPTER FOUR

Magnetic Resonance Imaging of the Spine, by Val M. Runge, Mark H. Awh, Donald F. Bittner, and John E. Kirsch. J.B. Lippincott Company, Philadelphia © 1995.

Lumbar Spine

Val M. Runge

Mark H. Awh

Donald F. Bittner

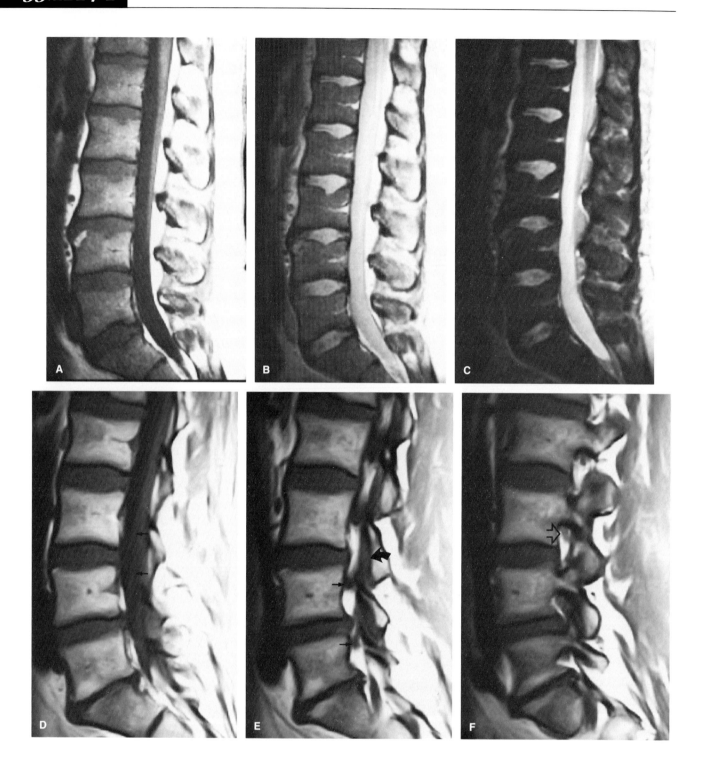

HISTORY

Normal volunteer

FINDINGS

Midline sagittal (*A*) T1-weighted (TR/TE = 450/10), (*B*) proton density (TR/TE = 3000/30), and (*C*) T2-weighted (TR/TE = 3000/80) spin echo images well demonstrate the conus medullaris, cauda equina, lumbar vertebral bodies, and intervertebral disks. The normally hydrated (nondegenerated) intervertebral disks are slightly hypointense relative to the vertebral bodies on the T1-weighted exam and markedly hyperintense on the T2-weighted exam.

In a second asymptomatic volunteer, parasagittal T1-weighted images (*D through G*) are displayed from just off the midline to the neural foramen laterally. In *D*, individual nerve roots (*arrows*) are noted coursing

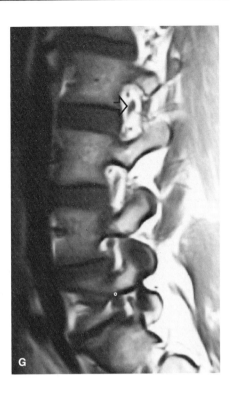

G

through CSF toward their exit points from the thecal sac. On *E*, the adjacent image laterally, the nerve root sleeves (*arrows*) are visualized. The normal ligamentum flavum (*curved arrow in E*) can be seen at the level of the disk spaces. On *F and G*, the two most lateral images, the nerve roots and dorsal root ganglia (*open arrows*) are seen within the neural foramina just beneath the pedicles. Incidentally noted are loss of height of the L5–S1 disk with type 2 end plate degenerative changes and narrowing of the L4–5 neural foramen.

DIAGNOSIS

Normal sagittal lumbar spine anatomy

DISCUSSION

Midline, within the thecal sac, the conus normally terminates between L1 and L2, continuing as a collection of nerve roots referred to as the cauda equina.[1] The posterior longitudinal ligament lies immediately posterior to the vertebral bodies and anterior to the thecal sac. This structure is only 1 mm thick in AP dimension, although 5 mm wide. The posterior longitudinal ligament is seen on sagittal images only near the midline. Laterally, the appearance of the facet joints varies depending on their location. The facet joints of the upper lumbar spine are oriented more in the sagittal plane, while those of the lower lumbar spine are oriented more in the coronal plane.

In parasagittal images of the lumbar spine, the dorsal root ganglion and smaller ventral root lie in the superior portion of the neural foramen.[2] Lateral to the dorsal root ganglion, the proximal spinal nerve is not a single structure, but is composed of seven to 15 fascicles. These lie centrally in the neural foramen, with intervening connective tissue containing fat and small blood vessels. Thus, a distinct spinal nerve is not visualized on conventional sagittal MR images lateral to the dorsal root ganglion. These fascicles, which comprise the proximal common spinal nerve, lie closer anatomically to the ligamentum flavum and intervertebral disk than the nerve root itself.

Sagittal images are particularly useful for grading the degree of foraminal stenosis and for demonstrating hypertrophy of the ligamentum flavum and facet joints.[3]

MR Technique

The normal sagittal exam of the lumbar spine includes both T1- and T2-weighted spin echo images. The slice thickness is typically 4 mm or less, with an interslice gap of 10% to 30%. Sections are obtained from pedicle to pedicle. For T1-weighted scans, TEs are typically in the range of 10 to 15 msec, with TRs from 400 to 500 msec. For T2-weighted scans, two echoes are typically acquired, the first at 20 to 30 msec and the second at 70 to 90 msec. Fields of view from 250 to 280 mm provide adequate in-plane spatial resolution. Application of a saturation pulse anterior to the spine is important to decrease motion artifacts that might otherwise degrade the image. Single or dual echo fast spin echo scans will probably replace conventional T2-weighted spin echo scans in the immediate future due to shorter scan times and reduced sensitivity to motion artifacts. Three-dimensional T1-weighted scans, with a voxel size of 1 × 1 × 1 mm, are currently feasible with techniques such as MP-RAGE and offer the possibility of high-resolution image reconstruction of arbitrary planes. However, three-dimensional techniques have not yet gained widespread acceptance in clinical practice.

Clinical References

1. Yu S, Haughton VM, Rosenbaum AE. MRI and anatomy of the spine. Radiol Clin North Am 1991;29:691–710.
2. Kostelic JK, Haughton VM, Sether LA. Lumbar spinal nerves in the neural foramen: MR appearance. Radiology 1991; 178:837–839.
3. Grenier N, Kressel HY, Schiebler ML, et al. Normal and degenerative posterior spinal structures: MR imaging. Radiology 1987;165:517–525.

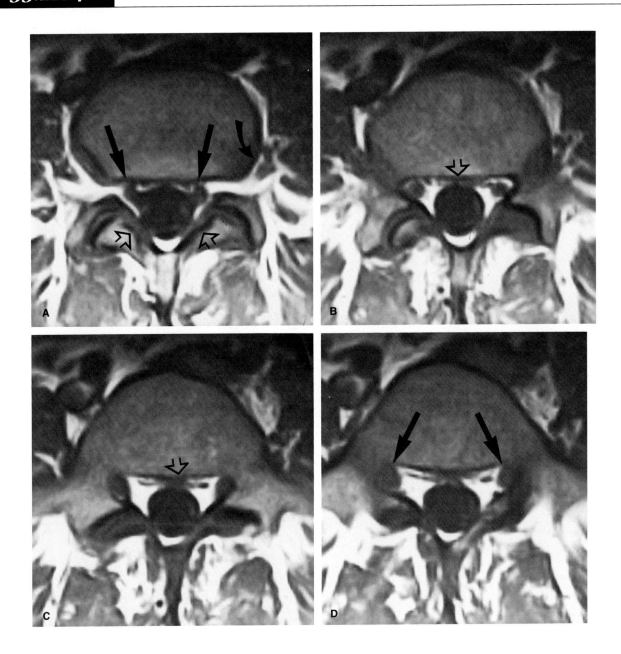

HISTORY

Normal volunteer

FINDINGS

Three-mm axial T1-weighted spin echo images (TR/TE = 650/10), with a 1.3-mm interslice gap, are shown from just inferior to the L4–5 disk to the level of the L5–S1 disk. On *A*, at the level of the L4–5 facet joints, the L5 nerve root sleeves (*arrows*) are noted emerging anterolaterally from the thecal sac. Just lateral to the vertebral body, a cluster of intermediate-signal-intensity foci

(*curved arrow*) corresponds to the L4 spinal nerve fascicles. The normal ligamentum flavum (*open arrows*) is well seen posterior to the thecal sac. On *B and C*, the next two sections caudally, the nerve root sleeves separate laterally from the thecal sac and become positioned immediately medial to the pedicle. Anterior to the thecal sac, the epidural venous plexus (*open arrows*) can be noted with intermediate signal intensity. On *D and E*, the next two sections, the L5 nerve roots (*arrows*) appear more bulbous, corresponding to the normal dorsal root ganglion. The next two sections (*F and G*) are through the L5–S1 foramina. Laterally the L5 spinal nerves now consist of multiple elements (fascicles), rather than a single root, as was the case proximally. The S1 nerve roots

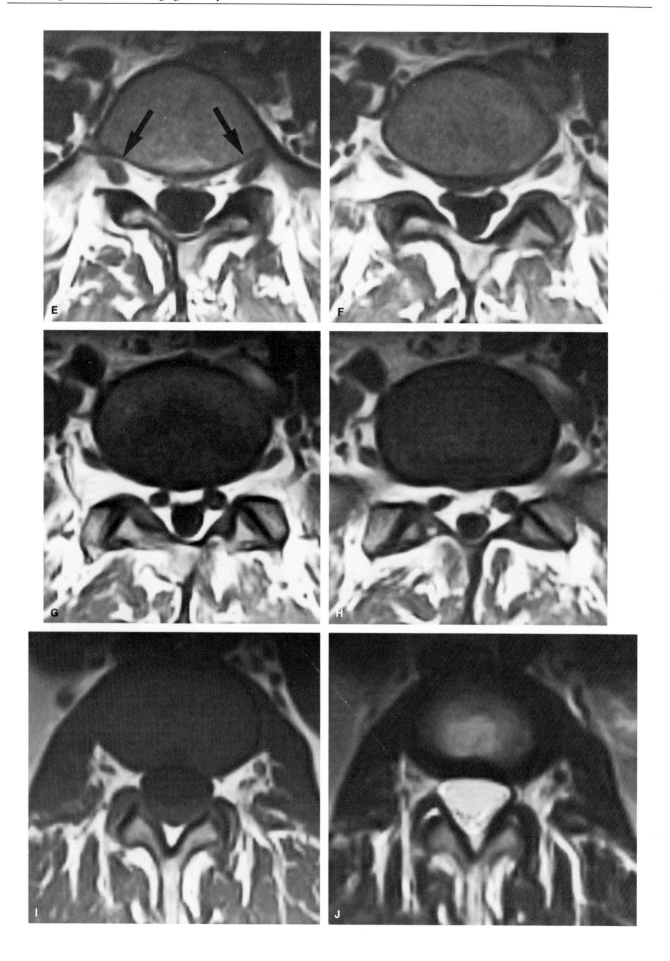

emerge from the thecal sac, which is tapering in dimension. The last section (*H*) is through the disk space itself, a finding apparent when one compares the low signal intensity of the disk to the higher signal intensity of marrow in the vertebral body on more superior cuts.

In a different patient, 3-mm axial (*I*) T1-weighted spin echo (TR/TE = 650/10, 8.4 minute scan time) and (*J*) T2-weighted fast spin echo (TR/TE = 4400/91, 5.0 minute scan time) images at the L3–4 disk space level are compared. The normal hydration of the inner portion of the disk is highlighted due to its high signal intensity on the T2-weighted fast spin echo image. The nerve roots layer posteriorly in the thecal sac and are seen as intermediate signal intensity against a background of low-signal-intensity cerebrospinal fluid on the T1-weighted image and against a background of high signal intensity on the T2-weighted image.

DIAGNOSIS

Normal axial lumbar spine anatomy

DISCUSSION

The bony spinal canal is formed by the vertebral body anteriorly, the pedicles laterally, and the lamina posteriorly. The borders of the intervertebral foramen are the disk and vertebral body anteriorly, the pedicles superiorly and inferiorly, and the facet joints posteriorly.[1] The dorsal root ganglion is 4 to 7 mm in diameter and lies within the fat of the neural foramen.[2] Immediately anterior and ventral is the smaller oval ventral root, which is not usually identified as separate on MR. Lateral to the dorsal root ganglion, the lumbar spinal nerve continues for a short distance as a set of small fascicles, seven to 15 in number. Somewhat more laterally, the fascicles join to form ventral and dorsal rami.

MR Technique

Axial imaging of the lumbar spine is routinely performed using T1-weighted spin echo techniques. The slice thickness should be 3 mm or less to avoid problems with partial volume imaging, with an interslice gap of 10% to 30%. The slices are acquired in groups, with multiple slices at the L3–4, L4–5, and L5–S1 levels. Each group is angled independently to achieve slices parallel to the disk space. Angling of slices is, however, limited by the curvature of the spine, with an exaggerated kyphotic deformity preventing acquisition of cuts parallel to the disk spaces due to slice-to-slice interference posteriorly. The TE ranges from 10 to 20 msec, with shorter TEs providing a greater signal-to-noise ratio and permitting a larger number of slices for a given TR. The TR is typically longer (≈750 msec) than that with sagittal T1-weighted sequences, due to the larger number of slices required. Fields of view from 200 to 280 mm provide adequate in-plane spatial resolution. Application of an anterior saturation slab in the coronal plane is important to decrease motion artifacts from anterior structures that might diminish overall image quality. Although the use of IV contrast media, when introduced in the late 1980s, was primarily limited to the postoperative back, the current trend in the United States is toward using it in most lumbar spine cases to better delineate the disk–thecal sac interface and to highlight epidural venous plexus and scar. The introduction of fast spin echo techniques has now also made possible high-resolution thin-section T2-weighted images, which may become a standard part of future protocols.

Clinical References

1. Yu S, Haughton VM, Rosenbaum AE. MRI and anatomy of the spine. Radiol Clin North Am 1991;29:691–710.
2. Kostelic JK, Haughton VM, Sether L. Proximal lumbar spinal nerves in axial MR imaging, CT, and anatomic sections. Radiology 1992;183:239–241.

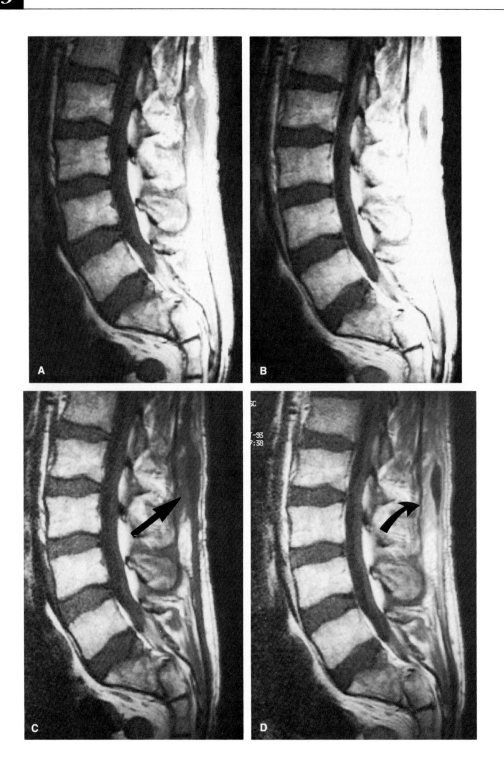

HISTORY

A 34-year-old man with major trauma 1 year before the current scan, which resulted in pelvic and sacral fractures and which required a nephrectomy

FINDINGS

Midline sagittal T1-weighted images before (*A*) and after (*B*) IV contrast administration reveal an old S1–2 fracture. In the soft tissues posterior to L2, a fluid collection is noted. The artifactual high signal intensity of the soft tissues in this region is due to the proximity of the surface coil (used for signal reception) and makes visualization of this abnormality difficult. *A and B* were processed after the exam using an image normalization program, resulting in *C and D*. On these images, the fluid collection (*arrow in C*) within the posterior paraspinous tissues is well depicted, along with the mild enhancement of adjacent tissue (*curved arrow in D*). The fluid collection was presumed to be chronic in nature, unrelated to the patient's current medical problems. Visualization of the sacral fracture is also improved by image normalization.

DIAGNOSIS

Image normalization

DISCUSSION

Surface coil imaging produces high signal intensity from superficially located structures. With selection of an appropriate field of view, these coils provide images with improved resolution and signal-to-noise ratio compared to body coil images. Unlike a circumferential coil, which provides a fairly uniform signal distribution throughout the imaging field, the intensity of the received signal decreases rapidly with increased distance from the coil. Appropriate window settings allow optimal visualization of a portion of the obtained image. In the lumbar spine, for example, correct window width and level settings for the spinal canal and thecal sac result in high signal from the posterior structures, which obscures the posterior muscles and possible abnormalities in the subcutaneous tissues.

The signal fall-off with increasing distance from the coil, however, can be beneficial. The area of interest, adjacent to the surface coil, has high signal intensity and is well visualized. Artifacts from structures further away from the coil are diminished. In a lumbar spine study, for example, the use of a surface coil decreases the artifacts from respiration and vessel pulsation (specifically from the aorta and inferior vena cava).

On T1-weighted images, intensely enhancing tissues, some blood products, certain fluid collections, and high-fat-content tissues, such as the subcutaneous tissues, all have high signal intensity. It can be difficult or impossible to select a window width and level to adequately visualize the vertebrae and canal contents as well as identify lesions in the high-signal-intensity posterior soft tissues. Image normalization is a postprocessing technique that attenuates the signal from tissues that are geometrically closer to the surface coil.

The case presented demonstrates the utility of image normalization with a surface coil.[1,2] With routine window settings, the signal intensity of the tissues nearer the coil is high and the signal decreases with increasing distance from the coil. To optimally visualize the spinal structures as well as the posterior soft tissues, two separate image sets with appropriate window levels and widths would be needed. Image normalization permits simultaneous visualization of the posterior soft tissues and the spinal canal, with optimal windowing throughout the image.

Pitfalls in Image Interpretation

Close inspection of the posterior soft tissues is particularly important in evaluating the pediatric spine. In this population, the use of image normalization could play an important role, with dysraphic spine elements and other abnormalities within the posterior soft tissues better depicted on normalized images. Another use of image normalization is in the postoperative patient in whom the question of infection has been raised. In this instance, a thorough inspection of the posterior soft tissues is important to identify possible infected fluid collections.

Clinical References

1. Axel L, Costantini J, Listerud J. Intensity correction in surface-coil MR imaging. AJR 1987;148:418–420.
2. Lufkin RB, Sharpless T, Flannigan B, Hanafee W. Dynamic-range compression in surface-coil MRI. AJR 1986;147:379–382.

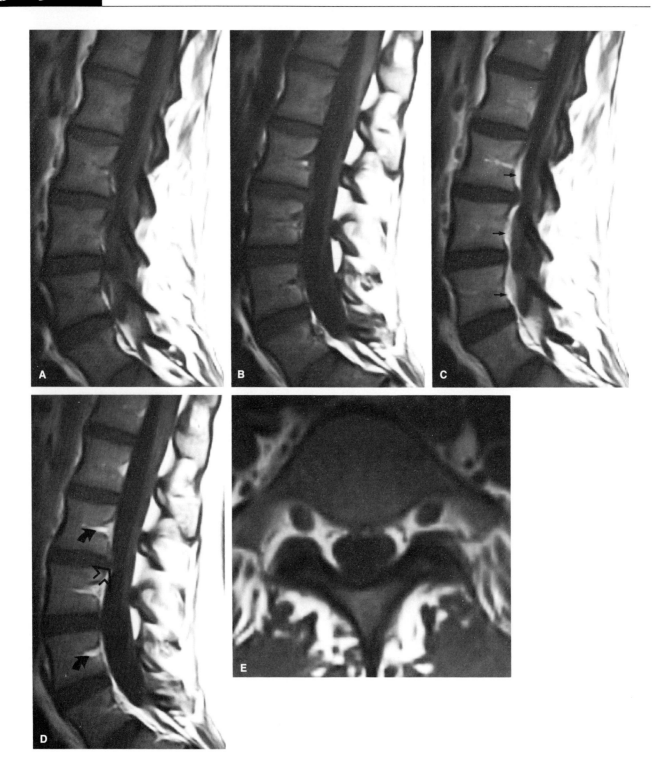

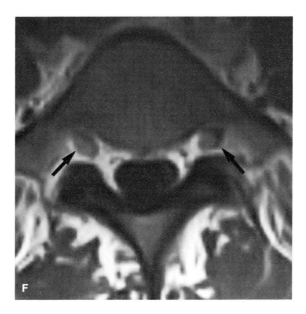

HISTORY

Low back pain

FINDINGS

Precontrast (*A and B*) and postcontrast (*C and D*) T1-weighted sagittal scans are presented. Soft tissue enhancement (*arrows*) is noted at multiple levels posterior to the vertebral bodies, corresponding to the vertebral venous plexus. Enhancement is also noted centrally within the vertebral bodies (*curved arrows*), in the location of the basivertebral vein. Incidental to the discussion—but not the patient—is a right paracentral disk herniation (*open arrow*) at L2–3. There is accompanying dilatation of the adjacent venous plexus.

In a second patient, axial T1-weighted scans at the level of the L5–S1 foramina are compared (*E*) before and (*F*) after contrast administration. The dorsal root ganglia (*arrows*) demonstrate mild uniform enhancement postcontrast.

DIAGNOSIS

Contrast media—normal enhancing structures, lumbar spine

DISCUSSION

Contrast enhancement in the normal spine depends on the vasculature and type of capillary endothelium.[1] Nonfenestrated capillary endothelium, like that within the brain, confines the contrast agent to the intravascular space. An example is the vertebral venous plexus, which has high signal intensity on postcontrast T1-weighted scans due to the high concentration of contrast agent within the blood. (As a side note, another term commonly used to refer to the vertebral venous plexus is "Batson's plexus," based on Batson's original work in the 1940s concerning spread of metastatic disease via this pathway.)[2]

Fenestrated endothelium, present in the dorsal root ganglion, muscle, and marrow, permits contrast to enter the interstitial space, with resultant enhancement of soft tissue. The enhancement of soft tissue is only moderate in degree, with comparison of precontrast and postcontrast scans facilitating recognition. However, the enhancement of normal marrow is particularly difficult to appreciate, due to this tissue's intrinsic high signal intensity on precontrast scans.

The basivertebral veins are consistently well visualized in the lumbar spine, in distinction to the cervical spine. These receive blood from the anterior external vertebral plexus and tunnel through the cancellous bone of the vertebral bodies to converge, typically forming a single vein exiting along the posterior vertebral body surface and draining into the anterior internal (epidural) venous plexus. As in the cervical spine, contrast enhancement in the lumbar spine improves definition of the disk/dural sac interface, due principally to enhancement of the venous plexus.

Clinical References

1. Lee C, Dean BL. Contrast-enhanced MRI of the spine. Top Magn Reson Imag 1991;3:41–73.
2. Onuigbo WI. Batson's theory of vertebral venous metastasis: a review. Oncology 1975;32:145–150.

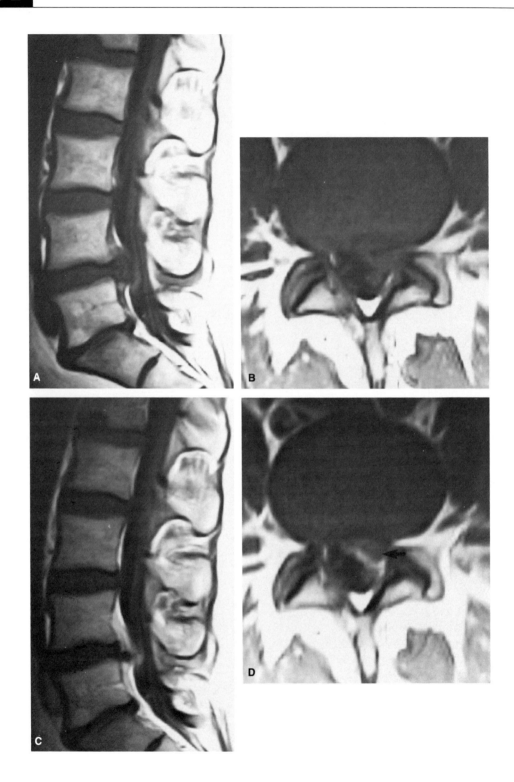

HISTORY

Two patients, the first a 45-year-old with left leg pain and numbness for 5 weeks, and the second a 26-year-old with recurrent right leg pain 6 months after a right L5–S1 microdiskectomy

FINDINGS

Patient #1: On the precontrast (A) sagittal and (B) axial T1-weighted images, abnormal soft tissue is seen anteriorly and to the left of the thecal sac at L4–5. On the corresponding postcontrast (C) sagittal and (D) axial im-

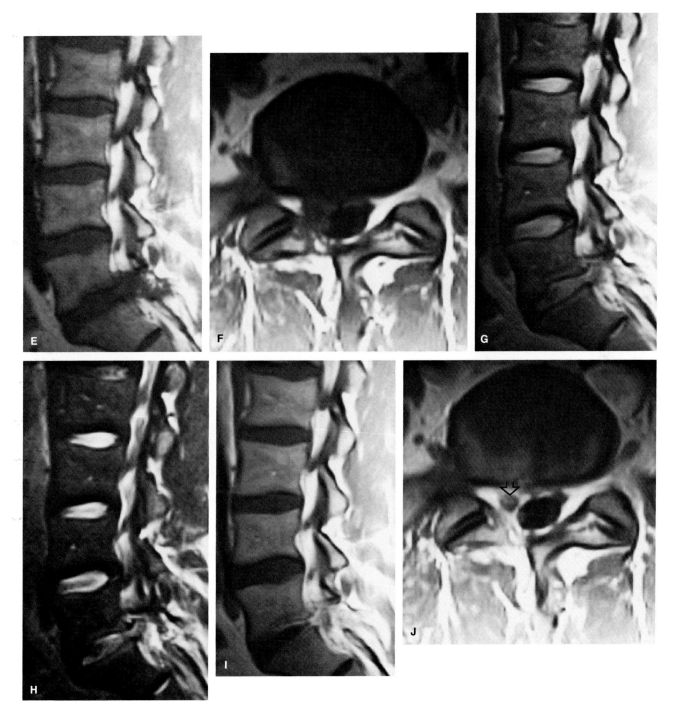

ages, the more peripheral part of the lesion, which corresponds to scar tissue and dilated epidural venous plexus, enhances, but the central part, which corresponds to herniated disk material, does not (*arrow*).

Patient #2: On the precontrast (*E*) sagittal and (*F*) axial T1-weighted images, abnormal soft tissue is seen anteriorly and to the right of the thecal sac at L5–S1. Note is made of postsurgical changes, with partial resection of the right L5 lamina. Sagittal (*G*) proton density and (*H*) T2-weighted images demonstrate apparent contiguity of the L5–S1 disk with this abnormal soft tissue, suggesting the diagnosis of a recurrent disk herniation. However, on the postcontrast (*I*) sagittal and (*J*) axial T1-weighted im-

ages, there is uniform enhancement consistent with postsurgical scar. The right S1 nerve root (*open arrow*), which does not enhance, can be identified on both the sagittal and axial images surrounded by scar tissue.

DIAGNOSIS

Contrast media—indications

Patient #1: L4–5 disk herniation with surrounding granulation tissue and dilated epidural venous plexus; patient #2: postoperative scar at L5–S1

DISCUSSION

In the United States in 1992, intravenous contrast media was used in more than one fourth of all MR spine studies. The high percentage of cases receiving contrast indicates the clinical importance of postcontrast studies, particularly in view of the relatively recent approval of gadolinium chelates for use in the spine.

The scientific literature is replete with studies demonstrating the efficacy of intravenous gadolinium chelate administration in spinal MR. The most widespread use at present is in the postoperative back, for differentiation of scar from recurrent or residual disk herniation. However, recent multicenter studies have demonstrated the indications for contrast administration to be quite broad, including disease in all compartments—intramedullary, extramedullary, and extradural.[1,2] In one such study, intravenous contrast administration was judged to provide additional diagnostic information in 68% of patients with radiologic evidence of significant disease. As early as 1988 (even before approval of gadolinium chelate use for head MR), studies demonstrated contrast administration to be highly efficacious in both intramedullary[3] and intradural extramedullary[4] disease. In the extradural compartment, contrast administration has also been shown to be particularly valuable in the setting of infection. Advantages of contrast use in spinal infection include improved anatomic delineation, increased diagnostic confidence, and the ability to assess disease activity.[5] Recent studies have also demonstrated the efficacy of prospective contrast use in patients with degenerative disease, in particular the "virgin" or unoperated spine.[6] In this setting, contrast administration provides critical additional diagnostic information, including increased conspicuity of disk herniation, improved delineation of the lateral recess and neural foramen, and improved differentiation of disk from venous plexus.

MR Technique

Indications for contrast administration in spine MR are quite broad, including almost all disease categories: trauma, infection, ischemia, neoplasia, demyelination, and degenerative disease (pre- and postoperative). T1-weighted techniques are used for contrast detection. Most protocols include both pre- and postinjection T1-weighted scans, obtained in the same plane, to assist in the identification of abnormal contrast enhancement.

At present the standard dose for a gadolinium chelate is 0.1 mmol/kg, although higher doses (recently approved) hold the potential for further improvements in diagnosis. Fat suppression, although not routinely used at present, is becoming more generally available and can be used to improve contrast visualization by suppressing the bright signal intensity of fat on T1-weighted scans.

Pitfalls in Image Interpretation

The timing of postcontrast scans relative to injection is important, and in most instances scans are performed within the first 10 to 15 minutes. Pitfalls exist with regard to both early and delayed postcontrast imaging. For example, in the first 15 minutes after injection, enhancement of some cord astrocytomas is quite poor, although substantial enhancement can be observed 30 to 45 minutes later. Conversely, imaging after the immediate postinjection time period permits diffusion of contrast into disk material, complicating the differentiation of scar from disk.

Clinical References

1. Runge VM, Bradley WG, Brant-Zawadzki MN, et al. Clinical safety and efficacy of gadoteridol: a study of 411 patients with suspected intracranial and spinal disease. Radiology 1991;181:701–709.
2. Sze G, Brant-Zawadzki MN, Haughton VM, et al. Multicenter study of gadodiamide injection as a contrast agent in MR imaging of the brain and spine. Radiology 1991;181:693–699.
3. Sze G, Krol G, Zimmerman RD, Deck MDF. Intramedullary disease of the spine: diagnosis using gadolinium-DTPA-enhanced MR imaging. AJR 1988;151:1193–1204.
4. Sze G, Abramson A, Krol G, et al. Gadolinium DTPA in the evaluation of intradural extramedullary spinal disease. AJR 1988;150:911–921.
5. Donovan Post MJ, Sze G, Quencer RM, et al. Gadolinium-enhanced MR in spinal infection. J Comput Assist Tomog 1990;14:721–729.
6. West JW, Lee C, Dean BL, et al. The role of gadopentetate dimeglumine in the routine evaluation of the lumbar spine. American Roentgen Ray Society, 91st annual meeting, May 1991.

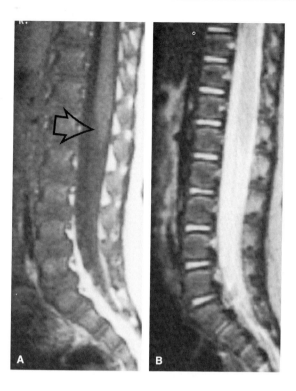

HISTORY

A 9-month-old infant with a questionable sacral dimple

FINDINGS

The sagittal T1-weighted image of the lumbosacral spine (A) reveals low-signal-intensity cerebrospinal fluid filling the thecal sac and surrounding the intermediate-signal-intensity conus medullaris (*open arrow*), which terminates at the L1–2 level. The thecal sac tapers normally in the sacral region. The spine is straight with absence of the adultlike lumbar lordosis. There is no discontinuity of posterior neural arches to indicate spinal dysraphism. The signal intensity of the vertebral bodies is slightly higher than that of the intervertebral disks. The intermediate-signal-intensity vertebral body ossification centers have somewhat flattened anterior and posterior margins with convex superior and inferior margins. They are sandwiched between the slightly lower-signal-intensity cartilaginous end plates. The intervertebral disks appear as low-signal-intensity lines between the end plates. The AP dimension of the ossification centers is visibly less than that of the intervertebral disks. (B) The comparable T2-weighted sagittal image shows high signal intensity in the nucleus pulposus of the intervertebral disks. The vertebral bodies and end plates have a combined rectangular shape and are of intermediate signal intensity, with slightly higher signal in the end plates and lower signal centrally in the ossification centers.

DIAGNOSIS

Normal infant spine

DISCUSSION

The appearance of the developing spinal column is very different from that of the adult spine. The infant spine undergoes a dynamic transformation during the first year. Sze and colleagues have divided the appearance of the infant spinal column into three stages describing signal changes in the ossification centers, vertebral end plates, and intervertebral disks. Stages I, II, and III include patients in their first month of life, 1 to 6 months old, and 7 months or older, respectively. Some variability and overlap exist between the stages.[1]

During the first month, the vertebral bodies are composed predominantly of cartilage. The ossification centers appear oval with low T1 signal intensity. A horizontal, slightly hyperintense signal band, which may be seen coursing through the middle of the ossification center, identifies the developing basivertebral venous plexus. The surrounding cartilaginous end plates have much higher T1 signal intensity than the paraspinous muscles. The intervertebral disks are thin, linear bands with T1 signal isointense to the paraspinous musculature and lower than the end plates. On T2-weighted images, the ossification centers remain of low signal intensity, the end plates demonstrate high signal intensity, and the disks have even higher signal intensity than the end plates.

The spine of infants from about 1 to 6 months old again shows low T1 and high T2 signal intensity in the nucleus pulposus of the intervertebral disk. The oval vertebral bodies demonstrate low to intermediate T1 signal intensity that is comparable to and difficult to differentiate from the signal intensity of the end plates. The T2-weighted images typically show signal nearly isointense to the muscle in the ossification center with slightly lower signal centrally. The end plates have signal intensity slightly higher than the muscles and ossification centers.

In infants 7 months of age and older, the spine begins to assume a more adult appearance. The ossification center becomes progressively more rectangular, with T1 signal intensity hyperintense to the paraspinous muscles and T2 signal slightly greater than the muscles. The end plates demonstrate T1 signal intensity similar to or slightly less than the ossification centers and T2 signal similar to or slightly greater than the ossification centers. The intervertebral disks are nearly isointense to the paraspinous muscles on T1-weighted images, with high T2 signal intensity in the nucleus pulposus.

In addition to the spinal column, MR images of the lumbosacral spine allow evaluation of the distal spinal cord and canal. On sagittal sections, the conus medullaris appears as a mild prominence of the distal cord. The normal conus should terminate above the L3–4 level at birth and should be in a normal adult location, at or above L2–3, by a few months of age.[2] The thecal sac tapers and ends at the S1 or S2 level. The filum terminale is best evaluated on axial images. The filum should be no more than 2 mm in diameter and may normally contain a small amount of fat.

Motion severely degrades the quality of MR images, but obtaining a motionless exam is difficult with infants and young children. Sleep deprivation, swaddling, and feeding the infant just before the study help the patient sleep during the exam. Adequate sedation that lasts the duration of the study is a necessity. However, sedation increases the risk of the study and requires careful monitoring of the patient by trained personnel.

MR Technique

MR is the procedure of choice for evaluation of the pediatric spine due to the lack of ionizing radiation, high sensitivity for soft tissue abnormalities, and multiplanar imaging capabilities. A large segment of the spine can be imaged using an adult spine coil, thin sections, and an appropriate field of view. Very small children may fit inside a head coil, providing an alternative to the use of a dedicated spine coil. Additional coronal or obliquely oriented images are often valuable for better delineation of congenital and neoplastic disease.

Pitfalls in Image Interpretation

Because the appearance of the infant spine is so different from the adult, the novice MR reader may mistake the disks and end plates for the vertebral bodies. T2-weighted images typically demonstrate high signal intensity in the nucleus pulposus of the developing spine at all stages, providing accurate localization of the disks.

Clinical References

1. Sze GS, Barierl P, Bravo S. Evolution of the infant spinal column: evaluation with MR imaging. Radiology 1991; 181:819–827.
2. Wilson DA, Prince JR. MR imaging determination of the location of the normal conus medullaris throughout childhood. AJR 1989;152:1029–1032.

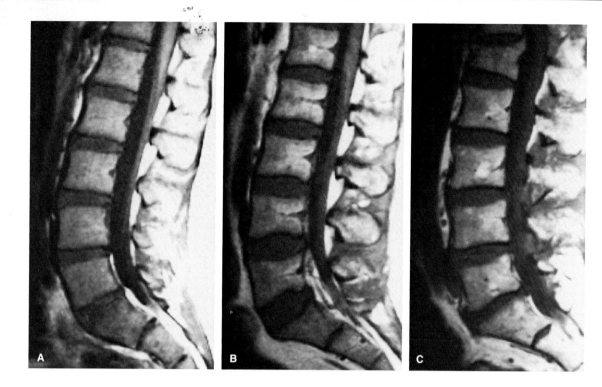

HISTORY

Three patients—a 17-year-old teenage girl, a 37-year-old woman, and a 76-year-old man, all with normal bone marrow for their age

FINDINGS

T1-weighted sagittal scans of the lumbar spine are presented for three patients: (*A*) a 17-year-old, (*B*) a 37-year-old, and (*C*) a 76-year-old. Of note is the preponderance of red marrow (lower signal intensity) in the 17-year-old patient, and the inhomogeneous marrow signal intensity in the 76-year-old patient. The scattered areas of increased signal in the latter patient are the result of replacement of red marrow by yellow marrow.

DIAGNOSIS

Normal vertebral body marrow evolution

DISCUSSION

Normal bone marrow is composed of hematologically active red marrow and hematologically inactive yellow (fatty) marrow.[1] Yellow marrow has increased signal intensity on T1-weighted images and intermediate to slightly hyperintense signal intensity on T2-weighted images. Red marrow signal characteristics come from a lipid and water combination; this results in a less intense T1-weighted signal than that from fatty marrow.

MR changes during growth represent a spectrum that parallels the conversion of red to yellow marrow. At birth, almost the entire marrow space is composed of red marrow. Conversion from red to yellow marrow is first evident in the extremities, specifically in the terminal phalanges. This progresses from the appendicular to the axial skeleton and from the diaphyseal to the metaphyseal regions in long bones.[2]

By about age 25 years, marrow conversion is usually complete and of the adult pattern. Red marrow is mainly concentrated in the axial skeleton (skull, vertebrae, ribs, sternum, and pelvis), and in the proximal appendicular skeleton to a lesser degree (except for the epiphyseal and apophyseal regions, which contain fatty marrow throughout life). Variations of this pattern exist.

The MR appearance of marrow reflects the relative distribution of red marrow, yellow marrow, and trabecular bone. Thus, T1-weighted signal intensity is lower in the spine than in the distal appendicular skeleton throughout life because relatively less red marrow remains in the distal appendicular region than in the spine.

Focal replacement with yellow marrow also occurs (as opposed to diffuse replacement), resulting in spotty areas of increased T1-weighted signal intensity. These focal changes are usually most evident in the posterior elements or in the periphery of the vertebral body, especially adjacent to the end plates. This presumably occurs secondary to decreased vascularity in these regions, prompting the conversion of red marrow to yellow marrow. Focal fatty infiltration increases with age and is said to have an overall prevalence of 60%.

Clinical References

1. Wolf CR, Runge VM. Musculoskeletal system. In: Runge VM, ed. Clinical magnetic resonance imaging. Philadelphia, JB Lippincott, 1990.
2. Vogler JB, Murphy WA. Bone marrow imaging. Radiology 1988;168:679–693.

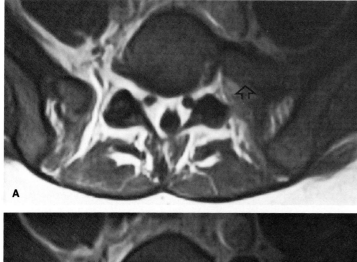

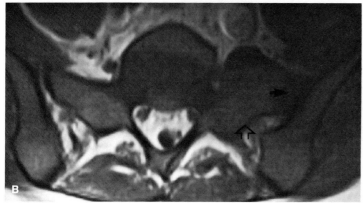

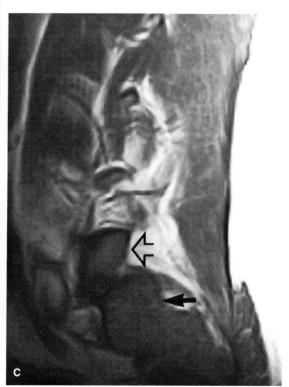

HISTORY

A 24-year-old patient with intermittent left leg pain and numbness

FINDINGS

(A) An axial T1-weighted image through the lower L5 level demonstrates the left pedicle and very large left L5 transverse process (*open arrow*). (B) The adjacent T1-weighted axial image through the L5–S1 disk space again shows the enlarged left L5 transverse process (*open arrow*). There is slightly lower signal intensity at the level of the pseudoarthrosis (*arrow*) between the left L5 transverse process and the sacrum. The signal intensity of the pseudoarthrosis is similar to the posterior L5–S1 disk and lower than the normal marrow signal in the anteroinferior L5 vertebra. Compare the left-sided sacralization to the right side, which shows no transverse process and a normal sacrum. (C) The sagittal T1-weighted image through the left transverse processes demonstrates the large transverse process at L5 (*open arrow*) and the articulation with the sacrum (*arrow*). Plain films (*images not shown*) confirmed these findings.

DIAGNOSIS

Transitional vertebra with partial sacralization of the L5 vertebra

DISCUSSION

A transitional vertebra is a common anomaly of the lumbosacral junction, occurring in 4% to 8% of the population.[1] Although the transverse processes of the lowest lumbar segment may be quite large, most authors agree that classification as a transitional segment requires articulation or fusion of the enlarged transverse process with the sacrum. The abnormality may be unilateral or bilateral, and the transverse process may be fused or form a diarthrodial joint with the sacrum. Incomplete lumbarization or sacralization refers to a unilateral or bilateral articulation forming a diarthrodial joint. Complete lumbarization or sacralization indicates unilateral or bilateral osseous fusion. A mixed pattern indicates fusion on one side with a diarthrodial joint on the contralateral side.[2]

A transitional vertebra is a known cause of back pain. The transitional vertebra typically causes decreased mobility at the affected level. Increased mobility and abnormal stresses imposed on the adjacent spinal levels cause premature degeneration in the disk and facet joints. This is particularly true at the interspace immediately above the transitional vertebra. Disk bulge and herniation, neural foraminal narrowing, and spinal stenosis are more common just above the transitional segment. Degeneration at the articulation between the transverse process and the sacrum is not common and does not correlate well with the location of the patient's back pain.

Midline sagittal MR images demonstrate a variable shape of the body of the transitional vertebra. The body may have a normal square configuration of a lumbar vertebra, a wedge shape of the sacral segments, or an intermediate form. Axial images demonstrate the enlarged transverse processes along with the abnormal articulation or fusion with the sacrum. A unilateral transitional segment is more easily detected due to the obvious asymmetry on the axial image.

Pitfalls in Image Interpretation

Bilateral sacralization may be overlooked on axial images due to the symmetric appearance of the anomalous segment.

Clinical References

1. Elster AD. Bertolotti's syndrome revisited—transitional vertebrae of the lumbar spine. Spine 1989;14:1373–1377.
2. Castellvi AE, Goldstein LA, Chan DPK. Lumbosacral transitional vertebrae and their relationship with lumbar extradural defects. Spine 1984;9:493–495.

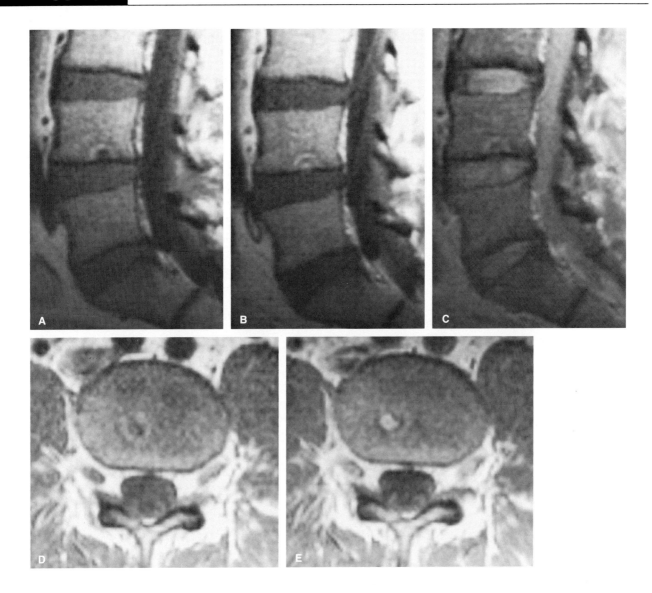

HISTORY

A 39-year-old patient with low back pain

FINDINGS

The sagittal T1-weighted image (*A*) demonstrates a semicircular low-signal-intensity area originating from the vertebral end plate. A thin peripheral rim of increased signal intensity corresponds with focal fatty marrow and type II end plate changes. The sagittal image following intravenous contrast administration (*B*) shows focal enhancement in the low-signal-intensity end plate abnormality. The lesion is again identified on the proton density weighted image (*C*), with increased signal centrally and a peripheral rim of intermediate signal intensity. The intervertebral disks at the L4–5 and L5–S1 levels show slightly decreased signal compared to the other lumbar disks, indicative of early degenerative change. The axial

(*D*) pre- and (*E*) postcontrast images through the end plate demonstrate a circular lesion. Precontrast, the lesion is of low signal intensity centrally with a peripheral rim of intermediate signal intensity. The rim follows fat signal on all imaging sequences, consistent with type II end plate changes. The postcontrast image shows enhancement with a tiny low-signal central focus.

DIAGNOSIS

Schmorl's node of the inferior L4 body

DISCUSSION

A cartilaginous node or Schmorl's node is a prolapse of the nucleus pulposus through the vertebral end plate into the medullary space of the vertebral body. Congenitally weak end plates or any process that weakens the cartilaginous end plate or adjacent bone predisposes to an intravertebral disk herniation. These are more common in athletes and in patients with end plate abnormalities such as Scheuermann's disease.[1] Axial loading of the spine with resultant compression of the nucleus pulposus forces the disk material through a defect in the cartilaginous end plate.

Schmorl's nodes are typically asymptomatic and an incidental finding. They are a common plain film finding in the lumbar spine. On conventional x-ray films, a Schmorl's node appears as a focal depression, contiguous with the vertebral end plate and lined by a sclerotic rim. MR is very sensitive in detecting end plate deformities and abnormal soft tissue structures. A Schmorl's node characteristically has T1 signal intensity lower, and T2 signal intensity higher, than that in the vertebral body marrow.[2] Images following intravenous contrast administration frequently demonstrate enhancement. This enhancement is probably due to the presence of granulation tissue, which develops in response to the herniation. As in the case presented, focal end plate changes are often seen surrounding the herniated disk material.

Herniation through the end plate usually is of no clinical significance, but symptomatic Schmorl's nodes have been reported.[3] The loss of disk material may narrow the disk space and the intervertebral disk may show premature degeneration.

MR Technique

Sagittal MR images demonstrate well the location of a Schmorl's node directly adjacent to the intervertebral disk space.

Pitfalls in Image Interpretation

Metastatic lesions can also appear as focal low-signal-intensity lesions on unenhanced T1-weighted axial images. Sagittal images allow differentiation from a Schmorl's node. A Schmorl's node will be contiguous with the end plate and can show peripheral enhancement. A metastatic lesion is more commonly centrally located with small lesions demonstrating uniform enhancement, including the center of the lesion.

Clinical References

1. Resnick D, Niwayama G. Intravertebral disk herniations: cartilaginous (Schmorl's) nodes. Radiology 1978;126:57–65.
2. Czervionke LF, Daniels DL. Degenerative diseases of the spine. In: Atlas SW, ed. Magnetic resonance imaging of the brain and spine. New York, Raven Press, 1991:795–864.
3. Walters G, Coumas JM, Akins CM, Ragland RL. MRI of acute symptomatic Schmorl's node formation. Pediatr Emerg Care 1991;7:294–296.

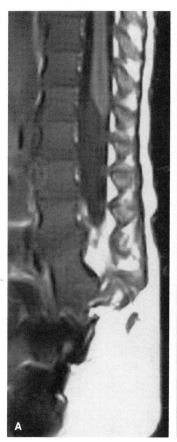

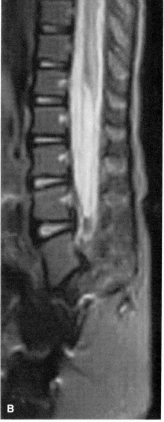

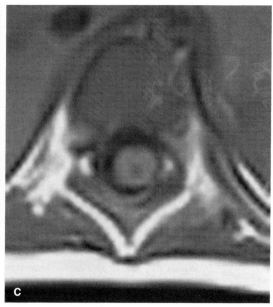

HISTORY

A 21-month-old child with lower extremity sensory and motor deficits

FINDINGS

On the midline sagittal T1-weighted scan (*A*), the cord terminates at the L1–2 level. The contour of the cord terminus is unusual, with the cord ending in a wedge shape (with the dorsal aspect extending further caudally), as opposed to the normal conus medullaris, which displays smooth and gradual tapering. The L5 vertebral body appears dysplastic. Only a portion of S1 is present. A subtle low-signal-intensity line is seen extending the length of the visualized cord, suggesting a small syrinx. The position and shape of the conus, as well as the vertebral body anomalies, are confirmed on the sagittal T2-weighted (TR/TE = 3000/90) scan (*B*). An axial T1-weighted scan just above the level of the cord terminus (*C*) confirms the presence of a dilated central canal (hydromyelia).

DIAGNOSIS

Caudal regression (sacral agenesis)

DISCUSSION

Caudal regression is defined by the absence of sacrococcygeal vertebrae with or without lumbar involvement, and encompasses a wide spectrum of pathology. The level of regression is below L1 in most cases, with agenesis limited to the sacrum in about half of all patients. Unilateral involvement occurs in a minority. Radiographic studies, and in particular MR, are important to rule out surgically correctable lesions.[1] MR accurately depicts the level of regression, the presence of spinal stenosis (below the lowest intact vertebra), and vertebral anomalies.[2] In a study of 13 patients, seven demonstrated a characteristic wedge-shaped cord terminus. The level of the cord terminus varies. Associated anomalies include cord tethering, pulmonary hypoplasia, and renal dysplasia. Neuromuscular abnormalities range from mild distal muscle weakness to complete lower extremity paralysis. There is an association with maternal diabetes.

MR Technique

When a wedge-shaped cord terminus (characteristic for caudal regression) is identified on sagittal scans, the study should be expanded to include the lower lumbar and sacral regions. Midline sagittal T1-weighted images are of greatest use.

When the question of syringohydromyelia is raised, axial T1-weighted images may be required to confirm the presence of a small cavity or syrinx. Partial volume imaging limits the sensitivity of sagittal scans.

Pitfalls in Image Interpretation

Subtle bony abnormalities, such as coccygeal absence or small vertebral anomalies, may be missed by MR and are better identified by plain films or CT. However, these findings are typically of little clinical consequence.

Clinical References

1. Pappas CT, Seaver L, Carrion C, Rekate H. Anatomical evaluation of the caudal regression syndrome (lumbosacral agenesis) with MRI. Neurosurgery 1989;25:462–465.
2. Barkovich AJ, Raghavan N, Chuang S, Peck WW. The wedge-shaped cord terminus: a radiographic sign of caudal regression. AJNR 1989;10:1223–1231.

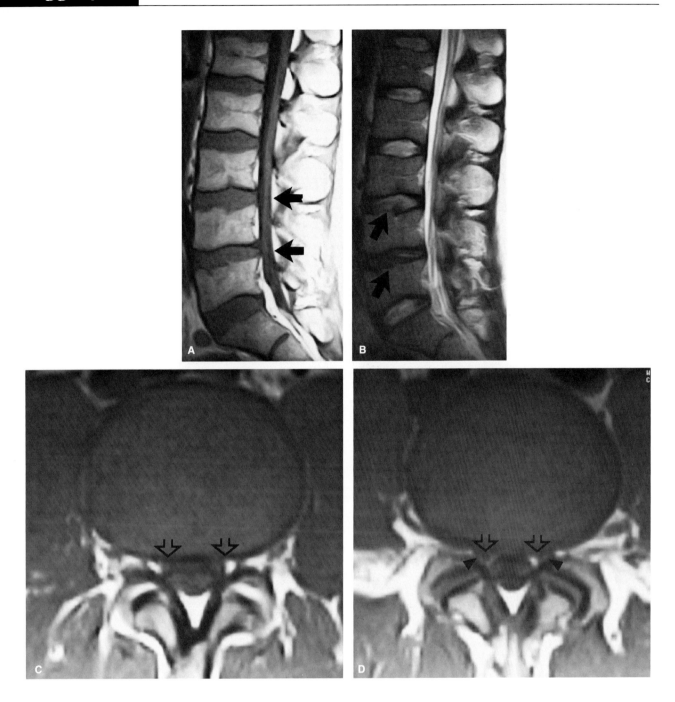

HISTORY

A 35-year-old patient with low back pain and left leg pain and numbness

FINDINGS

(A) The sagittal T1-weighted image demonstrates tapering of the spinal canal from the T12–L1 level extending through the lower lumbar spine. This is most prominent at the L3–4 and L4–5 levels (*arrows*). These findings are confirmed on the sagittal fast spin echo T2-weighted image (B). Diminished signal consistent with disk degeneration is seen at L3–4 and L4–5 (*arrows*). Small posterior spurs are present, further compromising the anteroposterior dimension of the canal. Axial T1-weighted images at the (C) L3–4 and (D) L4–5 levels show narrowing of the canal with deformity of the thecal sac and crowding of the nerve roots. The anteroposterior dimension of the sac measured 9 mm at both levels. The lateral recesses are narrowed bilaterally at the L3–4 and L4–5 levels (*open arrows*), resulting in minimal space for the passage of the nerve roots (*arrowheads*).

DIAGNOSIS

Congenital spinal stenosis

DISCUSSION

Congenital spinal canal stenosis is due to short, thickened pedicles with a decreased interpediculate distance. This results in decreased anteroposterior and transverse dimensions of the spinal canal. Normally, the spinal canal is equal to or slightly greater in anteroposterior dimension than the lower thoracic spinal canal. With spinal stenosis, the canal tapers in the lumbar region, as seen in this case. The lower limit of normal for the anteroposterior canal dimension is 11.5 mm, and the normal lateral recess should be 5 mm.[1] The L4–5 level is the most common site for canal stenosis and tends to be the most severely affected level when the canal is diffusely narrowed.

A congenitally narrow canal predisposes the patient to early symptoms from degenerative disk disease. A disk herniation, disk bulge, or end plate spur can cause canal compromise anteriorly. Thickening or redundancy of the ligamentum flavum, as well as facet hypertrophy, can narrow the canal posteriorly.

Short pedicles may also result in narrowing of the lateral recesses or neural foramina. These areas are best visualized on axial images. The narrowed lateral recess can impinge on the exiting nerve root, producing radicular symptoms. The lateral recess may also be further compromised by degenerative disk disease or hypertrophic changes of the ligamentum flavum or facets. Clinically, canal stenosis typically presents with myelopathic symptoms, but radicular symptoms may result from foraminal narrowing and nerve root impingement.

MR Technique

MR and CT are currently similar in sensitivity and specificity for the diagnosis of spinal stenosis.[2] With future advances in MR, this should become the study of choice due to its superior ability to evaluate soft tissue structures as well as the osseous margins of the spinal canal.

Pitfalls in Image Interpretation

Measurements obtained from MR images may slightly overestimate the degree of stenosis of the osseous spinal canal. This is particularly true with gradient echo imaging sequences. The MR unit should also be checked and carefully calibrated to ensure accuracy.

Clinical References

1. Gaskill MF, Lukin R, Wiot JG. Lumbar disc disease and stenosis. Radiol Clin North Am 1991;29:753–764.
2. Kent DL, Haynor DR, Larson EB, Deyo RA. Diagnosis of lumbar spinal stenosis in adults: a meta-analysis of the accuracy of CT, MR and myelography. AJR 1992;158:1135–1144.

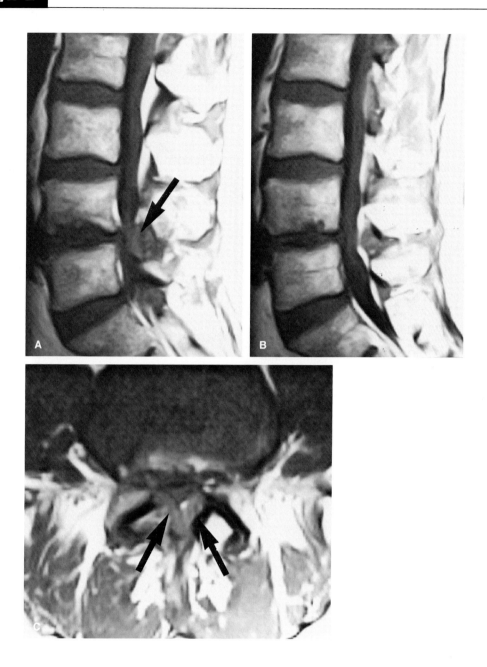

HISTORY

A 68-year-old man with low back pain

FINDINGS

(A) The sagittal T1-weighted image just to the right of midline shows low-signal-intensity cerebrospinal fluid (CSF) filling the thecal sac. A focal segment of intermediate-intensity soft tissue at the L4–5 level is due to volume averaging of the thickened ligamentum flavum (*arrow*). Similar findings are present on the sagittal T1-weighted image just to the left of midline (B), which again demonstrates the segment of intermediate signal intensity centered at L4–5. These images also reveal disk degeneration at L4–5 with disk space narrowing, a disk bulge with associated spurs, end plate irregularities, and adjacent degenerative end plate changes. The axial T1-weighted image at the inferior L4–5 disk level (C) demonstrates severe central stenosis of the spinal canal. The thecal sac is very small and triangular in shape, narrowed anteriorly by the disk bulge and spurs. The intermediate-signal-intensity bands along the posterolateral margins of the sac represent the thickened ligamentum flava (*arrows*). The ligaments measure up to 6 mm thick. The thickened ligaments and facet hypertrophy have obliterated the lateral recesses. A tiny amount of epidural fat is seen in the posterior canal.

DIAGNOSIS

Spinal stenosis with thickened ligamentum flavum

DISCUSSION

Anatomically, the ligamentum flavum is a paired thick fibroelastic band connecting the lamina of adjacent vertebrae throughout the spine. The ligament extends from the anteroinferior aspect of the more superior lamina to the posterosuperior aspect of the inferior lamina. The ligaments are situated in the posterolateral aspect of the spinal canal and become contiguous with the capsule of the facet joint anterolaterally. With degenerative spine disease and disk space narrowing, the ligament becomes fibrotic, thickened, and buckled.[1] It is generally thought that the cells of the ligament do not enlarge. Hypertrophic changes, however, commonly occur in the adjacent facet joints, contributing to the mass effect in this region. These changes produce visible thickening of the ligamentum flavum. The ligament may also calcify and, infrequently, has fat deposits.[2] The normal ligament is about 3 mm thick in the lumbar spine.[3]

Stenosis of the spinal canal has been divided into three types by region of involvement: central, subarticular canal (lateral recess), and foraminal.[4] Prominence and buckling of the ligamentum flavum results in narrowing of the posterolateral spinal canal. This most commonly contributes to narrowing of the lateral recesses of the spinal canal, located between the thecal sac and the neural foramina. Thickening of the ligamentum flavum may also contribute to narrowing of the central canal or the neural foramina. Nerve root impingement may result, producing radicular symptoms.

Pitfalls in Image Interpretation

Calcification of the ligamentum flavum may be missed on an MR study. Conventional spin echo images do not demonstrate calcifications well. Gradient echo techniques better depict calcific deposits. The signal in these regions is low on both spin echo and gradient echo images, unlike the high signal most readers associate with pathology.

Clinical References

1. Stollman A, Pinto R, Benjamin V, Kricheff I. Radiologic imaging of symptomatic ligamentum flavum thickening with and without ossification. AJNR 1987;8:991–994.
2. Grenier N, Kressel HY, Schiebler ML, et al. Normal and degenerative posterior spinal structures: MR imaging. Radiology 1987;165:517–525.
3. Ho PSP, Yu S, Sether L, et al. Ligamentum flavum: appearance on sagittal and coronal MR images. Radiology 1988; 168:469–472.
4. Dorwart RH, Vogler JB, Helms CA. Spinal stenosis. Radiol Clin North Am 1983;21:301–325.

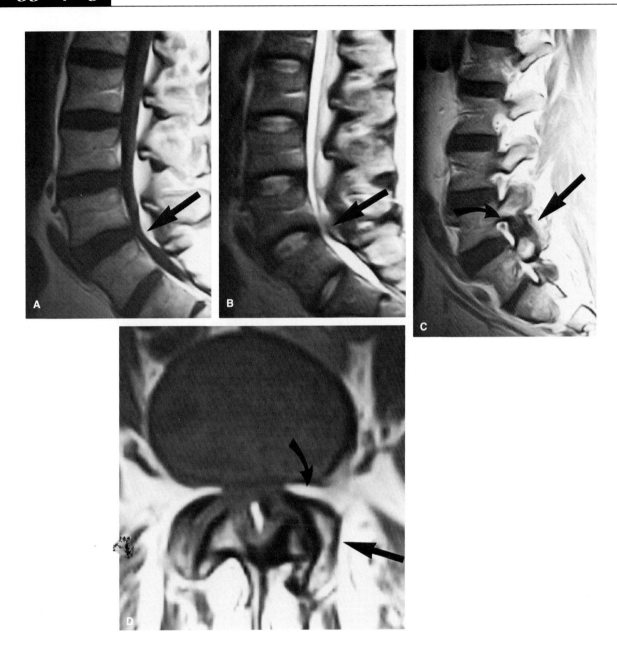

HISTORY

A 45-year-old patient with low back pain and severe left leg pain

FINDINGS

(A) A postinfusion T1-weighted sagittal image reveals prominent narrowing of the lumbar canal (*arrow*) at the L4–5 level. This appearance (*arrow*) is redemonstrated on the fast spin echo T2-weighted sagittal image (*B*). A T1-weighted sagittal image in the plane of the left lumbar facets (*C*) reveals hypertrophy and sclerosis of the left L4–5 facet (*arrow*). The neural foramen (*curved arrow*) remains patent at this level. A similar appearance was present at the right facet joint of L4–5 (*image not shown*). A T1-weighted axial image at the L4–5 level (*D*) confirms the marked facet hypertrophic changes, left greater than right. The superior articulating facet of L5 (*arrow*) is particularly affected. The facet hypertrophy results in bilateral lateral recess stenosis, more severe on the left (*curved arrow*), where the lateral recess measures less than 3 mm wide. Sclerosis of the facet joints is also apparent. The spinal canal is narrowed, measuring 11 mm in anteroposterior dimension. Even more striking is the degree of narrowing of the thecal sac, which measures 4 mm in anteroposterior diameter.

DIAGNOSIS

Severe spinal stenosis and lateral recess stenosis at L4–5 secondary to facet degenerative changes

DISCUSSION

Degenerative changes of the facet joints are one of the most important causes of spinal stenosis. Overgrowth of the articulating facets leads to protrusion of these facets into the spinal canal, with resultant canal distortion and stenosis. Hypertrophy of the superior articulating facet is particularly damaging, as this change is the primary cause of lateral recess stenosis.[1] The lateral recess can be defined as the space between the posterior margin of the vertebral body (with its associated intervertebral disk) and the anterior margin of the superior articulating facet. This space is bounded medially by the thecal sac and laterally by the pedicle. A lateral recess of less than 3 mm is likely to cause symptoms, while a width of 5 mm or greater is invariably normal.[2]

Patients with significant spinal stenosis often present a characteristic clinical picture.[1] These patients typically have a history of prolonged pain in the lower back and buttocks, with pain or paresthesias in the posterolateral aspects of the legs. The pain is usually aggravated by standing or walking. Symptoms improve and may even disappear with sitting or lying down. The symptoms are generally believed to be secondary to nerve root ischemia and thus have been termed "neurogenic claudication." If lateral recess stenosis is also present, the clinical setting may be complicated by severe sciatica. Again, symptoms may be dramatically relieved by rest. This appearance contrasts with disk herniations, in which symptoms are often aggravated by sitting. Objective neurologic deficits and a positive straight leg test are common with disk herniations but are typically minimal in cases of lateral recess stenosis.

MR Technique

Correlation of axial and sagittal images provides an excellent estimation of the effects of facet degenerative changes. The degree of canal deformity and possible lateral recess stenosis are best evaluated on axial images. Sagittal views provide an overview of canal dimensions and vertebral alignment. In addition, possible encroachment on exiting lumbar nerve roots is readily assessed on lateral sagittal images.

Pitfalls in Image Interpretation

Lumbar disk herniations often coexist with degenerative canal stenosis. Failure to recognize lateral recess stenosis is one of the leading causes of persistent symptoms following lumbar diskectomy. Careful evaluation for possible lateral recess or foraminal stenosis should be performed in all patients with suspected lumbar disk disease.

Clinical References

1. Hackney DB. Degenerative disk disease. Top Magn Reson Imag 1992;4:12–36.
2. Ciric I, Mikhael MA, Tarkington JA, Vick NA. The lateral recess syndrome: a variant of spinal stenosis. J Neurosurg 1980;53:433–443.

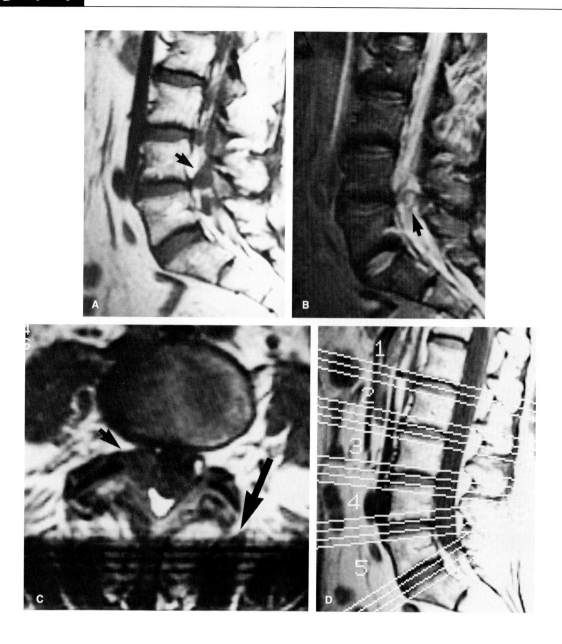

HISTORY

An elderly woman with intermittent low back pain

FINDINGS

Off-midline sagittal (*A*) T1-weighted and (*B*) T2-weighted images reveal a lesion (*small arrow*) within or immediately adjacent to the right L4–5 neural foramen. The mass is isointense with disk material on the T1-weighted image and hyperintense (almost equal to the signal intensity of CSF), with a rim of hypointensity, on the T2-weighted image. On the axial T1-weighted scan (*C*), the mass (*small arrow*) is posterolateral in position relative to the thecal sac and immediately adjacent to the right facet joint. The diagnosis was proven at surgery. Incidental note is made of multiple horizontal low-signal-intensity bands (*large arrow in C*) obscuring anatomic detail in the more dorsal portion of the image. This artifact can be explained by reference to the sagittal scout image (*D*; see MR Technique below).

DIAGNOSIS

Synovial cyst

DISCUSSION

A synovial cyst is an uncommon lesion associated with degenerative facet disease.[1] Clinical symptoms include radicular pain, often sciatic in nature. On CT, a cystic lesion, which may be calcified, is seen adjacent to the facet joint. L4–5 is a common location. Hemorrhage may also occur within a synovial cyst. The appearance of the cyst fluid is variable on MR. Following IV administration of a gadolinium chelate, enhancement of a solid component and the capsule of the cyst can be noted, with delayed enhancement of the cyst itself.[2] Contrast injection can aid in identification of the connection between the cyst and adjacent facet joint, a key to diagnosis. Synovial cysts can compress the thecal sac and contribute to spinal stenosis.

MR Technique

On the sagittal scout (*D*), the five groups of images to be acquired as part of the axial T1-weighted scan are identified. Each set of images is tilted to be parallel with respect to the disk space at that level. More posteriorly, the slices overlap, with the interference between slices leading to the low-signal-intensity bands that obscure the posterior soft tissues on the axial image (*C*). Caution should be used in tilting axial images in patients with exaggerated kyphosis. If too great an angle is applied to different sets of images within the same acquisition, interference between slices can obscure important anatomic detail.

Pitfalls in Image Interpretation

A synovial cyst can mimic clinically a disk herniation. Multiplanar imaging and recognition of the relationship to the adjacent facet joint are important for appropriate diagnosis.

Clinical References

1. Liu SS, Williams KD, Drayer BP, et al. Synovial cysts of the lumbosacral spine: diagnosis by MR imaging. AJR 1990; 154:163–166.
2. Yuh WT, Drew JM, Weinstein JN, et al. Intraspinal synovial cysts—MR evaluation. Spine 1991;16:740–745.

(Images courtesy of Clifford Wolf, MD)

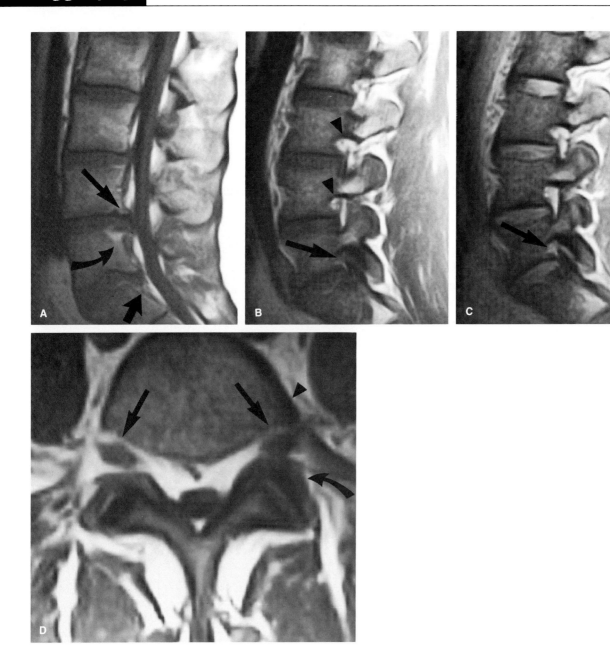

HISTORY

Low back and left lower extremity pain

FINDINGS

(A) The T1-weighted midline sagittal image demonstrates moderate disk bulges and osteophytes (*arrows*) at the L4–5 and L5–S1 levels. Type II end plate disease is noted posteriorly at L4–5 (*curved arrow*). A T1-weighted sagittal image to the left of midline (*B*) reveals a small neural foramen at L5–S1 (*arrow*), which is moderately narrowed secondary to degenerative spurs and hypertrophic facet disease. Only a minimal amount of fat is seen about the exiting L5 nerve root. The more normal keyhole appearance of the fat-filled neural foramina is present at L3–4 and L4–5 (*arrowheads*). A corresponding intermediate T2-weighted sagittal image (*C*) confirms the small left L5–S1 neural foramen (*arrow*). Decreased signal intensity within the L3–4, L4–5, and L5–S1 disks is compatible with disk degeneration. A T1-weighted axial image at the inferior L5 level (*D*) displays the L5 dorsal root ganglia bilaterally (*arrows*). The right dorsal root ganglion is surrounded by fat. The left ganglion is contacted by the hypertrophied superior articulating facet of S1 (*curved arrow*) and a prominent leftward osteophyte (*arrowhead*) arising from the L5 vertebral body.

DIAGNOSIS

Moderate degenerative foraminal stenosis on the left at L5–S1

DISCUSSION

After exiting the lateral recess, the lumbar nerve root enters the neural foramen. The lumbar neural foramina are bounded superiorly and inferiorly by the pedicles, anteriorly by the vertebral bodies and intervertebral disk, and posteriorly by the articulating facets. Degenerative disease in the lumbar intervertebral disks, end plates, and posterior elements may all contribute to stenosis of the neural foramina. Hypertrophy of the superior articulating facet is the most common cause of foraminal narrowing.[1] Lateral disk abnormalities and vertebral osteophytes also often protrude into the neural foramen. Any foraminal degenerative changes are markedly accentuated if the intervertebral disk is narrowed. In such cases, the height of the neural foramen is reduced, and as a result even mild degenerative osteophytes or facet hypertrophy may lead to nerve root compression.

Lumbar foraminal narrowing is most common at L4–5 and L5–S1, where hypertrophic changes of the posterior elements are prevalent. Foraminal stenosis often causes radicular symptoms secondary to direct nerve root compression. Also important in the clinical presentation, however, is pain that emanates directly from the degenerated posterior structures. The facet joints are richly innervated and may be the source of radicular-type pain in the absence of direct nerve root compression.

MR Technique

Sagittal views are optimal for grading the degree of foraminal stenosis. Loss of the usual fat surrounding the exiting nerve root is a sensitive sign of significant foraminal disease. Axial views allow more precise evaluation of the facet joints and of possible coexisting canal stenosis.[2]

Clinical References

1. Hackney DB. Degenerative disk disease. Top Magn Reson Imag 1992;4:12–36.
2. Grenier N, Kressel HY, Schiebler ML, et al. Normal and degenerative posterior spinal structures: MR imaging. Radiology 1987;165:517–525.

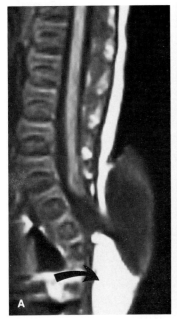 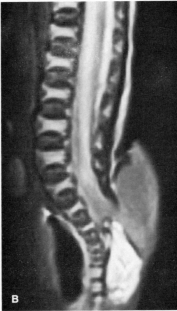 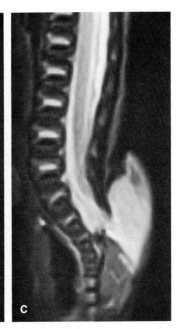

HISTORY

A newborn with a normal neurologic exam and a low lumbosacral mass covered by skin

FINDINGS

(A) The sagittal T1-weighted exam reveals a fluid-filled sac in the lower lumbar region posteriorly that communicates with the thecal sac. The spinal cord extends at least to the lumbosacral junction. Excess fatty tissue is seen posteriorly (*curved arrow*) immediately below the defect. These findings are confirmed on the sagittal proton density (B) and T2-weighted (C) exams, which also demonstrate normal anterior sacral elements. Computed tomography (*images not shown*) demonstrated spinal dysraphism from L4 to S1. The absence of posterior bony elements in this region is confirmed on the sagittal proton density and T2-weighted MR exams.

DIAGNOSIS

Meningomyelocele with tethered cord

DISCUSSION

MRI is the modality of choice for the initial evaluation of suspected spinal dysraphism.[1] With respect to terminology, "spina bifida" refers to an incomplete closure of posterior bony elements. Contents of the spinal canal can extend through such a defect, with the different spinal anomalies categorized according to the tissues within the defect. A simple meningocele contains only dura and arachnoid, without neural tissue. A meningomyelocele contains neural tissue, which accompanies the posterior expansion of the subarachnoid space. At surgery for repair of this neural tube defect (which was performed by primary closure), a single nerve (not seen on MRI or CT) was identified within the fluid-filled sac.

MR Technique

Although both sagittal and axial exams are recommended, T1-weighted sagittal images should be performed first, in case satisfactory sedation cannot be maintained. In such cases, the T1-weighted sagittal exam can often provide sufficient diagnostic information for appropriate patient management.[2]

Pitfalls in Image Interpretation

The normal conus lies between T12 and L2–3, with an average position of L1–2 in children between 0 and 2 years of age. In 19- and 20-year-olds, the conus lies between L1 and L2, with an average position of L1–2. The conus does not ascend throughout childhood, as stated by many authors, but only during the first few months of life.[3] A conus level below L3 is abnormal regardless of age.

Clinical References

1. Altman NR, Altman DH. MR imaging of spinal dysraphism. AJNR 1987;8:533–538.
2. Rindahl MA, Colletti PM, Zee CS, Taber P. MRI of pediatric spinal dysraphism. Magn Reson Imag 1989;7:217–224.
3. Wilson DA, Prince JR. MR imaging determination of the location of the normal conus medullaris throughout childhood. AJR 1989;152:1029–1032.

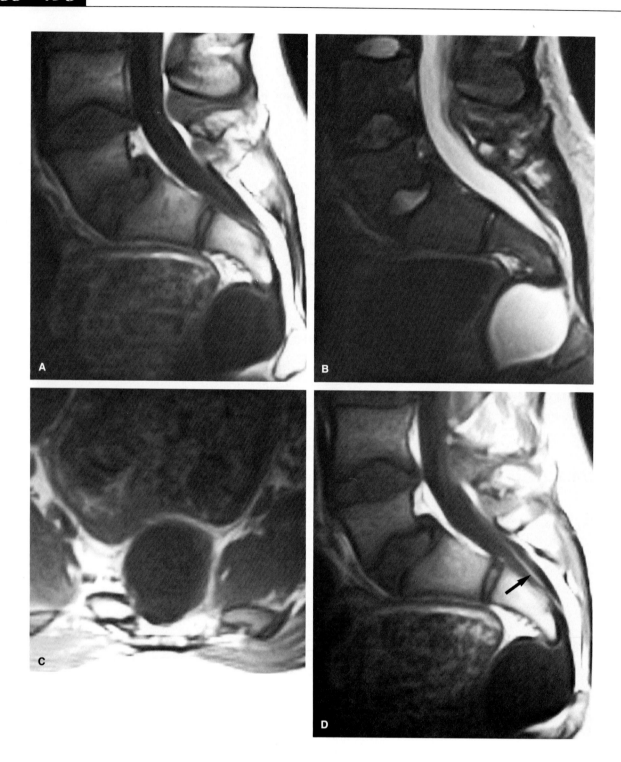

HISTORY

Pelvic mass in a teenage girl

FINDINGS

(A) The T1-weighted sagittal scan reveals a cystic lesion just anterior to the tip of the sacrum. Communication of the cyst with the thecal sac is demonstrated on the T2-weighted (TE = 90) sagittal scan (B). The cyst contents were isointense with cerebrospinal fluid on all pulse sequences. The axial T1-weighted scan (C) again demonstrates the cyst, with associated sacral bony anomalies. The rectum anteriorly is dilated and filled with stool. On closer inspection of the adjacent sagittal (D) T1- and (E) T2-weighted images, the filum terminale (arrow) can be identified entering the cyst. CT confirms the cyst and defect in the posterior arch of the sacrum (F).

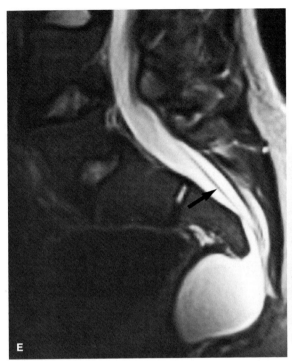

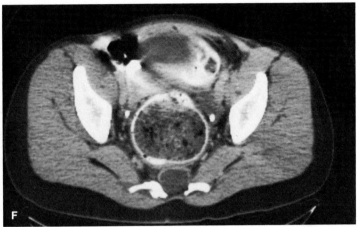

DIAGNOSIS

Anterior sacral meningocele

DISCUSSION

An anterior sacral meningocele is a protrusion of the thecal sac (dura and leptomeninges) through a defect in the sacrum. There is X-linked dominant inheritance. Numerous reports document the superiority of MR over ultrasound, CT, and myelography for preoperative diagnosis.[1-3] The pedicle connecting the thecal sac and the cyst may be obstructed by adhesions, thus giving false negative results on plain film myelography. On plain film, a semicircular erosion of the sacrum ("scimitar sign") is suggestive of an anterior sacral meningocele.

MR Technique

The superiority of MR for diagnosis depends in part on the ability to obtain images in multiple planes. The pedi-cle of tissue that connects (through the sacral defect) the cyst to either a nerve root sleeve or the thecal sac is often best defined on sagittal images. Axial images best define the sacral bony defect.

Pitfalls in Image Interpretation

An anterior sacral meningocele may be mistaken for a prolapsed ovarian cyst or other cystic pelvic lesion. The posterior location of the cyst and associated sacral anomaly permits diagnosis.

Clinical References

1. Chamaa MT, Berney J. Anterior sacral meningocele; value of MRI and abdominal sonography—a case report. Acta Neurochir 1991;109:154–157.
2. Lee KS, Gower DJ, McWhorter JM, et al. The role of MR imaging in the diagnosis and treatment of anterior sacral meningocele—report of two cases. J Neurosurg 1988;69:628–631.
3. Martin B, Boyer de Latour F. MR imaging of anterior sacral meningocele. J Comput Assist Tomog 1988;12:166–167.

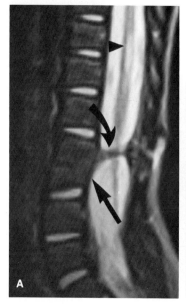

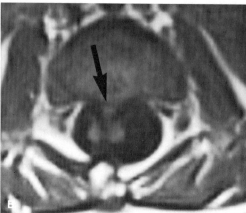

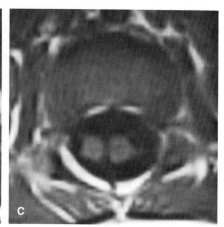

HISTORY

An 18-month-old infant with lower extremity spasticity

FINDINGS

(A) The T2-weighted midline sagittal image demonstrates a segmentation anomaly at L2–3 (*arrow*). A low-signal-intensity band (*curved arrow*) spans the thecal sac at the L2–3 level. A central region of high signal intensity (*arrowhead*) is present within the lower thoracic spinal cord. (B) A T1-weighted axial view at the inferior L2 level reveals splitting of the spinal cord by the previously noted band (*arrow*). Bony dysraphism is identified posteriorly. (C) An additional T1-weighted axial image at a slightly higher level more clearly depicts the separation of the cord into two hemicords.

DIAGNOSIS

Diastematomyelia

DISCUSSION

Diastematomyelia refers to splitting of the spinal cord into two hemicords, each invested by separate layers of pia. Each hemicord contains a central canal, a dorsal horn, and a ventral horn. Diastematomyelia is thought to arise secondary to a persistent accessory neurenteric canal, which prevents fusion of the neural tube in the mid-line. An alternative explanation is that during embryogenesis the paired neural folds turn ventrally rather than fusing in the midline, with resultant formation of two distinct neural tubes.[1]

In about 60% of diastematomyelia patients, the hemicords travel within a single subarachnoid space and dural sac. In the remainder of patients, the arachnoid and dura split into separate sacs. In these latter patients, an osteocartilaginous spur or fibrous band through the dural cleft is almost always present. The spur is typically present at the most inferior aspect of the cleft.

Associated anomalies in diastematomyelia are common. As in this case, vertebral segmentation anomalies, including hemivertebra or butterfly vertebra, are often seen. Spina bifida is usually present. Cutaneous stigmata overlying the spine and orthopedic foot problems, particularly clubfoot, are seen in about half of patients. Symptoms of diastematomyelia are nonspecific, usually related to cord tethering secondary to a septum or a thickened filum terminale.[2]

MR Technique

Detection of possible bony spurs is critical, as resection of the spur, if present, is necessary to improve symptoms of cord tethering. Even large osseous spurs may be inapparent on T1-weighted scans. T2-weighted images are more sensitive for detection of such abnormalities. Still greater sensitivity for bony spurs can be obtained with gradient echo techniques. Gradient echo imaging may be especially useful in patients in whom the septum is seen above the inferior extent of the diastematomyelia. In these patients, a second, often less apparent, spur is likely to be present.[2]

Pitfalls in Image Interpretation

It is not uncommon for a cerebrospinal fluid (CSF) intensity abnormality to project within the spinal cord on sagittal views of diastematomyelia patients. Often the appearance is secondary to the CSF between the two hemicords. However, hydromyelia is present in as many as half of all diastematomyelia patients.[2] Careful

attention to axial images is thus critical for determining the true nature of a central CSF collection.

Clinical References

1. Raghavan N, Barkovich AJ, Edwards M, Norman D. MR imaging in the tethered spinal cord syndrome. AJR 1989; 152:843–852.
2. Barkovich AJ, Naidich TP. Congenital anomalies of the spine. In: Barkovich AJ, ed. Pediatric neuroimaging. New York, Raven Press, 1990:227–271.

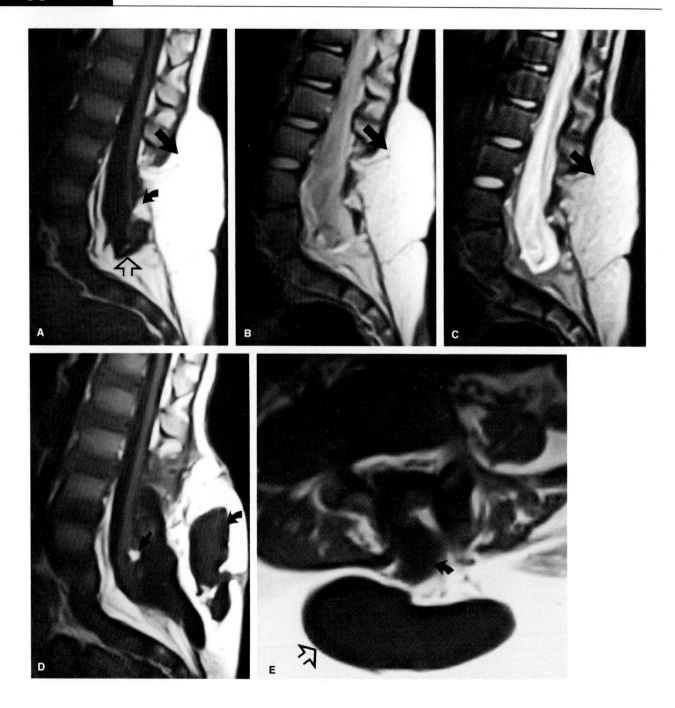

HISTORY

A 5-year-old child who underwent a tethered cord release as a newborn

FINDINGS

A midline T1-weighted sagittal image (*A*) demonstrates a large posterior subcutaneous mass (*arrow*) in the lower lumbar region. The spinous processes in the lower lum-

bar and sacral region are absent. The cord lies in an abnormally low position and terminates within a small extension of thecal sac (*curved arrow*) that lies within the subcutaneous abnormality. The thecal sac has a pouch-like termination (*open arrow*) at the S1 level. The large dorsal mass has signal characteristics compatible with fat on this T1-weighted image. The sacrum is hypoplastic. First and second echo T2-weighted images (*B and C*) again depict the large subcutaneous lesion (*arrow*), which remains isointense to fat. At this time, the patient had developed symptoms of retethering and was taken to surgery for a tether release. On a postoperative T1-weighted sagittal view (*D*), the cord no longer appears adherent posteriorly, although a small fatty lesion (*arrow*) is still present at the dorsal aspect of the distal cord. The distal thecal sac is now quite capacious, and a prominent fluid collection (*curved arrow*) is present within the subcutaneous tissues. A T1-weighted axial view in the lower lumbar region (*E*) redemonstrates the small lesion with the signal characteristics of fat (*arrow*) at the dorsal aspect of the distal cord. The widely separated posterior elements are apparent. A fluid collection (*curved arrow*) contiguous with the thecal sac is present posterior to the distal cord. An additional large fluid collection (*open arrow*) is seen within the subcutaneous tissues. Additional images (*not shown*) demonstrated contiguity of this fluid collection with the intrathecal contents as well.

DIAGNOSIS

Release of tethered cord (secondary to lipomyelomeningocele), with development of a postoperative pseudomeningocele

DISCUSSION

Lipomyelomeningoceles are composed of lipomas that are firmly attached to the dorsal surface of the spinal cord and that herniate through a dysraphic spinal canal. The resultant lesion accounts for about 20% of skin-covered lumbosacral masses and as many as 50% of cases of occult spinal dysraphism.[1] These lesions are thought to lie at the more severe end of a developmental spectrum that begins with intradural lipomas.[2] They are commonly found in the lumbosacral region and are differentiated from myelomeningoceles by the presence of the lipoma that attaches to the dorsal surface of the placode and by the intact layer of skin that overlies these lesions. The superficial aspect of the lipoma usually merges indistinctly with the subcutaneous fat. The tightly adherent deep portion of the lipoma prevents normal developmental closure of the neural tube, thus accounting for the typical myeloschisis at the cord/lipoma interface. The distal cord is almost invariably tethered by the lipoma, terminating in the lower lumbar or sacral canal. Butterfly

vertebrae or other vertebral segmentation anomalies are present in almost half of patients, as are sacral anomalies such as partial sacral agenesis. Maldevelopment of the feet and scoliosis are additional common associated findings.

Lipomyelomeningoceles, because they are skin-covered, occasionally go undetected until adulthood. Typically, however, patients present before 6 months of age with a fluctuant subcutaneous mass. At this early age, neurologic findings may be minimal, but progressive symptoms are the rule if corrective surgery is not performed. Eventual clinical findings include lower extremity weakness, sensory loss, gait disturbances, and urinary incontinence.

MR Technique

During the development of a lipomyelomeningocele, the lipomatous portion may rotate within the meningocele sac, resulting in complex changes in cord and nerve root orientation.[1] Such distortions increase the risk of surgical trauma, particularly when the dorsal roots are rotated into the midline. Careful comparison of sagittal and axial T1-weighted images allows accurate assessment of anatomy in these patients, thus providing valuable guidance for surgical planning.

Pitfalls in Image Interpretation

Postoperative pseudomeningoceles must be differentiated from other postoperative fluid collections such as seromas or abscesses. Demonstration of contiguity of a fluid collection with the subarachnoid space is the key feature that distinguishes pseudomeningoceles from these other etiologies.

Clinical References

1. DeLaPaz RL. Congenital anomalies of the spine and spinal cord. In: Enzmann DR, DeLaPaz RL, Rubin JB, eds. Magnetic resonance imaging of the spine. St. Louis, CV Mosby, 1990:176–236.
2. Naidich TP, McLone DG, Mutluer S. A new understanding of dorsal dysraphism with lipoma (lipomyeloschisis): radiologic evaluation and surgical correction. AJR 1983;140:1065–1078.

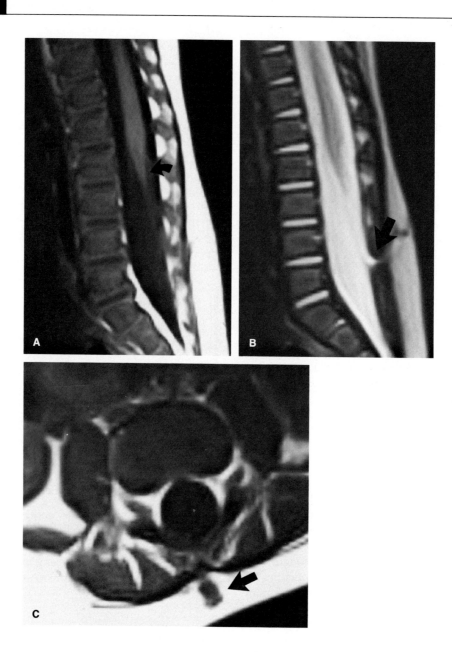

HISTORY

A 9-month-old infant with a 1-day history of fever and vomiting. Physical exam reveals a patch of hair and hyperpigmentation dorsally at the L3–4 level. Drainage has been noted from this region for the past 2 weeks.

FINDINGS

Sagittal (*A*) T1- and (*B*) T2-weighted images of the lumbar spine reveal a sinus tract (*arrow in B*) coursing from the skin to the thecal sac. This abnormality is less apparent on the T1-weighted scan due to the high signal intensity of fat posteriorly, accentuated by proximity to the surface coil. The conus (*curved arrow in A*) lies at L2. A

portion of tract (*arrow*) is also visualized on a single image from the multislice axial T1-weighted scan (*C*).

DIAGNOSIS

Dorsal dermal sinus

DISCUSSION

Cerebrospinal fluid (CSF) cultures were positive and the patient was subsequently placed on IV antibiotics. On surgical exploration, the tract was noted to terminate at the conus medullaris, with the attachment divided and the dermal sinus excised.

A dorsal dermal sinus is an epithelium-lined tract, usually midline, that runs from the skin inwards for a variable distance.[1] Such a tract may terminate in the soft tissue or dura, or extend within the thecal sac. Cord tethering is common. On the skin, there is typically a hairy nevus, hyperpigmented patch, or capillary angioma. About half of patients have an associated dermoid or epidermoid tumor at the termination of the tract. Infection or symptoms of compression (by the tumor mass) lead to clinical presentation.

High-resolution spinal sonography, in addition to MRI, plays an important role in the diagnosis of occult dysraphic lesions in the neonate and infant.[2]

MR Technique

In the setting of infection, contrast enhancement with a gadolinium chelate improves delineation of the sinus tract, in particular the intraspinal portion.[3] Inflammation induces the formation of granulation tissue, which demonstrates marked enhancement following IV contrast administration.

Pitfalls in Image Interpretation

On MRI, the intraspinal portion of a dermal sinus may be poorly visualized, although the subcutaneous tract and possible intramedullary tumor will be well demonstrated.

Clinical References

1. Barkovich AJ, Edwards MS, Cogen PH. MR evaluation of spinal dermal sinus tracts in children. AJNR 1991;12:123–129.
2. Korsvik HE, Keller MS. Sonography of occult dysraphism in neonates and infants with MR imaging correlation. Radiographics 1992;12:297–306.
3. Algra PR, Hageman LM. Gadopentetate dimeglumine-enhanced MR imaging of spinal dermal sinus tract. AJNR 1991;12:1025–1026.

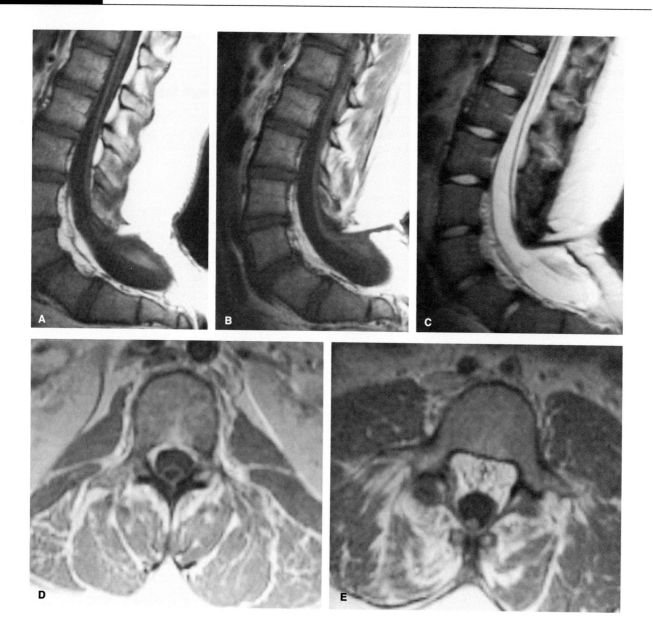

HISTORY

A 16-year-old girl who had myelomeningocele repair at birth. She presents with progressive decreased lower extremity motor function and increasing frequency of urinary tract infections over the past year.

FINDINGS

(*A and B*) On midline sagittal T1-weighted scans (TR/TE = 450/10), the cord is noted to extend to the L4–5 level without a well-defined conus and to tether posteriorly (the neural placode) in soft tissue at the site of the previous myelomeningocele repair. There is an accentuated kyphotic deformity of the lumbar spine. A syrinx is also noted, which begins at the T12 level and extends inferiorly, with its termination not well seen. Normal posterior elements are absent at L4 and lower levels. These findings are confirmed on (*C*) the midline fast T2-weighted sagittal scan (TR/TE = 3500/90), which corresponds in slice position to *A*.

Three axial postcontrast T1-weighted scans are illustrated (*D through F*). On *D*, at the L1 level, the syrinx is seen in cross section, with the cord noted to be immediately adjacent to the posterior dura. On *E*, at the L3–4 level, the cord is again visualized, but without a syrinx. At this level and on *F*, at the L4–5 level, dysraphic abnormalities of the posterior elements are evident. On *F*, the neural placode is noted to extend into the posterior soft tissues.

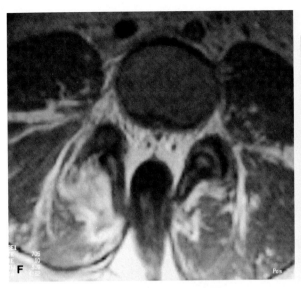

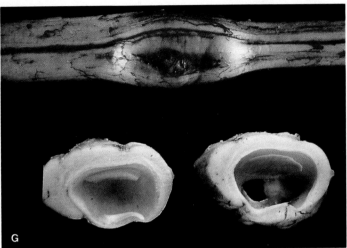

DIAGNOSIS

Tethered cord, with hydromyelia

DISCUSSION

The tethered cord is a congenital anomaly in which the conus medullaris is held in an abnormally low position. In the absence of pathology, the conus reaches the normal adult position (L1–2) by 2 months of age. Three types of cord tethering are described, associated with a short (tight) filum terminale, an intradural lumbosacral lipoma, or diastematomyelia.[1] Tethered cord syndrome can also occur as a delayed consequence of myelomeningocele repair, as in the present case. In this instance, not all children with radiologic evidence of tethering will be symptomatic. Symptoms include gait difficulty, motor and sensory loss in the lower extremities, and bladder dysfunction, and are due to cord ischemia from traction.

The most common presentation at MR is that of a young child with progressive neurologic dysfunction. On imaging, the cord typically extends without change in caliber to the lumbosacral region, tethering posteriorly with an associated lipoma and dysraphism of the posterior spinal elements. MR is particularly valuable in the evaluation of suspected cord tethering.[2] The position of the conus medullaris, thickening of the filum terminale, lesions causing cord traction, and bony dysraphism are all readily visualized.

The patient in this case subsequently underwent a tethered cord release. At surgery, the conus and nerve roots were demonstrated to be scarred and adherent to the dorsal aspect of the thecal sac. This scar was dissected free, with the nerve roots spared that responded to neurostimulation.

MR Technique

In spinal dysraphism, T1-weighted images acquired in sagittal, axial, and coronal planes supply critical diagnostic information by clearly depicting abnormal anatomy and providing differentiation between fat and nervous tissue.[3] In cases where infection is questioned, T2-weighted and postcontrast T1-weighted images can provide important additional information.

Pitfalls in Image Interpretation

Axial images are superior to sagittal images for locating the tip of the conus. On sagittal images, the conus may be difficult to separate from roots of the cauda equina, particularly if the sections are slightly off midline.

Pathologic Correlate

As illustrated by this gross specimen (G), hydromyelia is a focal dilatation of the central spinal canal. The canal remains lined by ependyma. Such lesions are rarely symptomatic.

Clinical References

1. Merx JL, Bakker-Niezen SH, Thijssen HOM, Walder HAD. The tethered spinal cord syndrome: a correlation of radiological features and perioperative findings in 30 patients. Neuroradiology 1989;31:63–70.
2. Raghavan N, Barkovich AJ, Edwards M, Norman D. MR imaging in the tethered spinal cord syndrome. AJR 1989; 152:843–852.
3. Rindahl MA, Colletti PM, Zee CS, Taber P. MRI of pediatric spinal dysraphism. Magn Reson Imag 1989;7:217–224.

(G from Okazaki H, Scheithauer B. Atlas of neuropathology. New York, Gower Medical Publishing, 1988, p. 294. By permission of Mayo Foundation.)

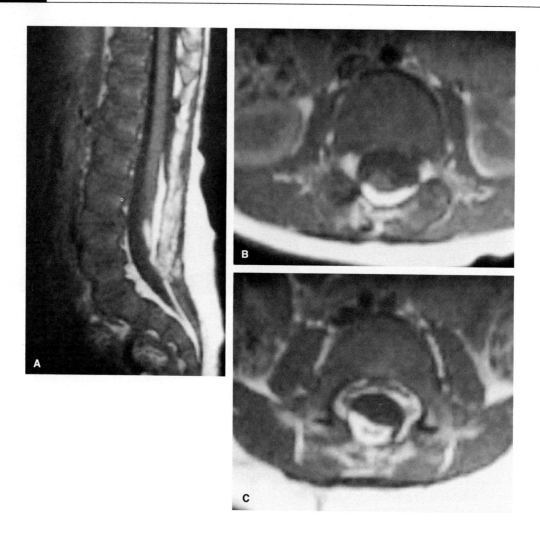

HISTORY

Two patients. The first is a 2-month-old infant noted at birth to have a 3 × 5 cm lipoma over the lower lumbar spine with dimpling centrally. There was normal function of the upper and lower extremities, as well as normal bowel and bladder function. The second patient is an older child who has had a surgical procedure.

FINDINGS

Patient #1: On the midline sagittal T1-weighted scan (A), the conus is noted to extend to L3. Abnormal fatty tissue is present, adherent to the tip of the conus and posterior to the lower cord. On an axial T1-weighted scan through the tip of the conus (B), abnormal fatty tissue is seen immediately adjacent and posterior to the cord. On an axial T1-weighted scan 2 cm lower (C), abnormal fatty tissue is again noted, which encases the cauda equina and filum terminale and is adherent to the posterior dural sac. The posterior spinous elements are absent, and the pedicles are widely spaced. By reference to the sagittal exam, it

can be confirmed that there is absence of normal posterior elements throughout the entire lumbar spine.

Patient #2: (D) Sagittal and (E) axial T1-weighted images reveal a lipoma (*arrow*) involving the neural placode. The cord terminus, although low, is surrounded by cerebrospinal fluid and specifically not tethered posteriorly.

DIAGNOSIS

Tethered cord—variations in appearance: patient #1, with lipoma; patient #2, following surgical release

DISCUSSION

Early diagnosis and surgical treatment of cord tethering can prevent urinary incontinence and other symptoms.[1] The use of synthetic dural grafts decreases the incidence of retethering following corrective surgery.

Lipomas are the most common form of occult spinal dysraphism, and almost always involve the lumbar or

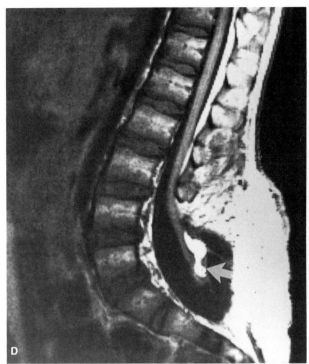

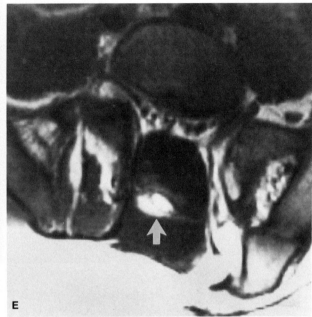

sacral spine. Occult spinal dysraphism and spina bifida occulta are equivalent terms used to label a group of developmental anomalies that demand separate classification from meningoceles and myelomeningoceles. This group includes diastematomyelia, dermal sinus tracts, fibrous bands, dermoids, neurenteric cysts, and lipomas. These lesions, unlike meningoceles and myelomeningoceles, are usually not associated with the Chiari II malformation. A lumbosacral lipoma usually presents at birth, and is most commonly midline. When the patient is an infant, no neurologic deficits may be present; symptoms commonly appear in childhood.

Operative repair is best undertaken soon after diagnosis in patients with occult spinal dysraphism, because these lesions cause progressive neurologic deficits. When surgery is done before symptoms appear, they can be prevented, and if deficits are present, progression can be arrested. The primary aim of surgery is to untether the cord. Lumbosacral lipomas are removed as completely as possible, with attention to freeing the conus from the tethering effect of the lipoma.

In the Chiari II malformation, syrinx cavities can occur at any position along the cord (a tethered cord with an accompanying syrinx is illustrated in 33.1481-1). However, these are most common in the lower thoracic cord or within the distal part of a tethered cord. With the advent of MR, it has been recognized that syringohydromyelia and/or myelomalacia near the conus or point of tether is a relatively common finding, not restricted to patients with Chiari II.[2] Cavity formation may be a result of traction forces and ischemia. Because myelomalacia should precede actual cavitation, and because of the un-

certainty in absolute differentiation of these two entities by MR, the observed focal low-signal-intensity lesion (as visualized on T1-weighted images) has been referred to as syringohydromyelia/myelomalacia.

MR Technique

Axial images are necessary for confident identification of focal syringohydromyelia or myelomalacia near the tip of the conus or within the cord near the point of tethering.

Pitfalls in Image Interpretation

Following successful release of a tether, the level of the cord terminus typically does not change, making interpretation of postoperative scans difficult with regard to possible retethering.[3]

Clinical References

1. Traill MT, Runge VM, Wolpert SM. Dysraphism: MRI strategies. MRI Decisions 1989;2:2.
2. Raghavan N, Barkovich AJ, Edwards M, Norman D. MR imaging in the tethered spinal cord syndrome. AJR 1989; 152:843–852.
3. Brophy JD, Sutton LN, Zimmerman RA, et al. MR imaging of lipomyelomeningocele and tethered cord. Neurosurgery 1989;25:336–340.

(D and E *from Runge VM. Clinical magnetic resonance imaging. Philadelphia, JB Lippincott, 1990, p. 280.)*

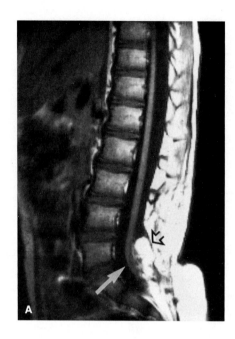

HISTORY

A 7-year-old child several years after surgical release of a tethered cord, who now presents with new onset of incontinence

FINDINGS

One sagittal T1-weighted image (TR/TE = 450/20) is presented. No distinct conus is seen. The cord ends at the L5–S1 level (*arrow*) and appears to be adherent to posterior soft tissue structures. An associated intradural lipoma (*open arrow*) is also noted.

DIAGNOSIS

Tethered cord (retethering)

DISCUSSION

Retethering is a frequent and major complication in children who have been treated surgically for a tethered spinal cord. In one series, three of 20 children demonstrated on long-term follow-up signs of retethering despite appropriate surgery.[1] On MR, the presence of postoperative adhesions is probably the best criteria for diagnosis of spinal cord retethering.

MR Technique

One often notes the use of shorter TRs (400 to 500 msec) for sagittal T1-weighted images, as opposed to longer TRs (600 to 800 msec) for axial images. With current multislice spin echo techniques, the TR imposes a limitation on the number of slices that can be acquired in one scan sequence. Typically, fewer slices are required in the sagittal plane (to image from pedicle to pedicle), thus permitting a shorter TR to be used.

Pitfalls in Image Interpretation

The agreement between operative findings and MR is much higher in primary than in secondary tethered cord syndrome (TCS). In one clinical series, MR suggested cord tethering in 88% of patients with surgically proven primary TCS (with the imaging diagnosis based on a low position of the conus) and in only 69% of secondary TCS (with the imaging diagnosis based on the presence of adhesions).[2]

Clinical References

1. Lagae L, Verpoorten C, Casaer P, et al. Conservative versus neurosurgical treatment of tethered cord patients. Z Kinderchir 1990;45(Suppl 1):16–17.
2. Reichel M, Hamm B, Weigel K, Wolf KJ. Primary and secondary tethered cord syndromes; their nuclear magnetic tomographic diagnosis and comparison with the surgical findings in 40 patients. Rofo 1992;157:124–128.

(Image from Runge VM, ed. Clinical magnetic resonance imaging. Philadelphia, JB Lippincott, 1990, p. 566.)

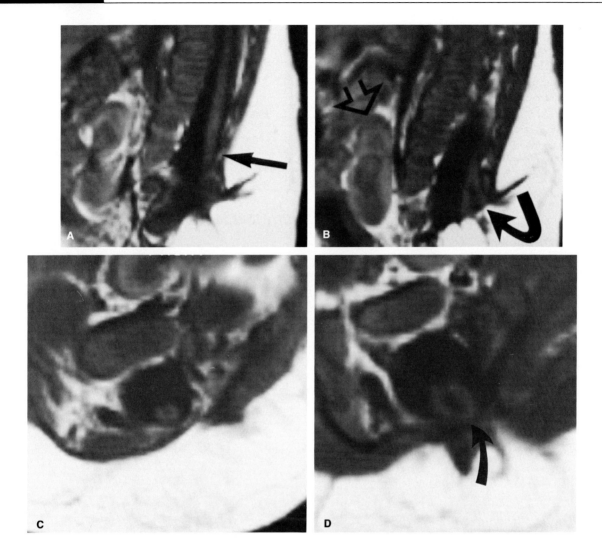

HISTORY

Bony spinal dysraphism by plain film

FINDINGS

(*A and B*) Two adjacent sections from the sagittal T1-weighted exam reveal the spinal cord (*arrow in A*) to extend to the termination of the thecal sac. There is dilatation of the central spinal canal to form a small syrinx (*curved arrow in B*) at the point of tethering posteriorly. Other notable abnormalities include bony spinal dysraphism posteriorly and a pelvic kidney (*open arrow in B*) anteriorly.

(*C and D*) Two axial T1-weighted sections are also presented. At the higher level (*C*), the central syrinx is seen near its origin. A portion of the pelvic kidney is again visualized at the top of the image. The dilatation of the central canal (*curved arrow in D*) becomes progressively greater as the cord approaches the point of tethering.

DIAGNOSIS

Terminal myelocystocele

DISCUSSION

Terminal myelocystocele is a rare congenital cystic dilatation of the caudal central spinal canal.[1] There is trumpet-like flaring of the distal central canal, which is lined by ependyma and surrounded by a meningocele. These cystic structures herniate posteriorly through a bony defect into the subcutaneous tissues. The pia covering the spinal cord is reflected at the junction between the placode and the meninges along the wall of the meningocele, creating a closed CSF cavity that communicates with the central canal. The cyst lined with ependyma is frequently larger than the meningocele, and is thin-walled without internal structures. In the case presented, however, the ependyma-lined cyst is quite small. Associated anomalies of the GI and GU tracts, vertebral bodies, and cloacal exstrophy are common. An association with teratogens such as loperamide hydrochloride and retinoic acid has been postulated.

Dysraphic spine abnormalities with meningeal involvement and posterior fluid collections also occur in the cervical and thoracic regions. Two types are reported: hydromyelia with an associated myelocystocele extending posteriorly into a meningocele, and meningoceles with tethering of the cord to the posterior part of the meningocele sac.[2] The cases with a myelocystocele also demonstrated an associated Chiari II malformation.

MR Technique

Sagittal imaging best visualizes the elements that define a myelocystocele, permitting diagnosis.

Pitfalls in Image Interpretation

On myelography, because the ependyma-lined cyst is separate, only the meningocele may be demonstrated. This may be smaller and at a different level than the mass evident clinically.

Clinical References

1. Peacock WJ, Murovic JA. MR imaging of myelocystoceles—report of two cases. J Neurosurg 1989;70:804–807.
2. Steinbok P, Cochrane DD. The nature of congenital posterior cervical or cervicothoracic midline cutaneous mass lesions—report of eight cases. J Neurosurg 1991;75:206–212.

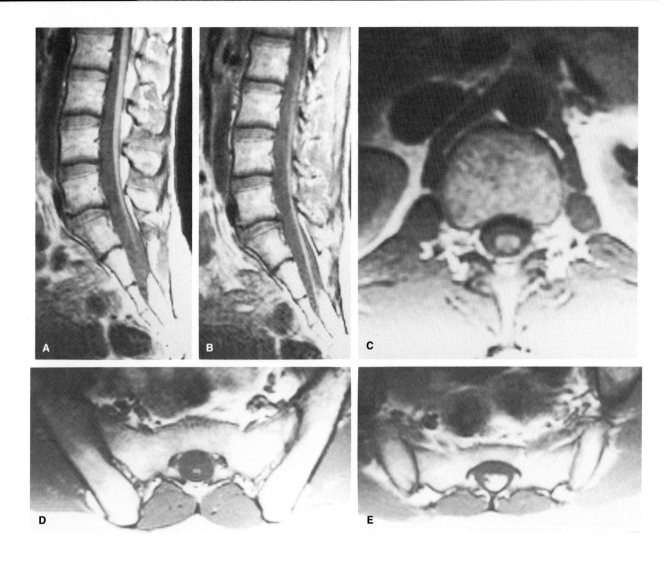

HISTORY

A 23-year-old man with incontinence

FINDINGS

(*A and B*) Sagittal T1-weighted scans reveal a thick linear structure with intermediate signal intensity (isointense with the spinal cord and nerve roots) extending from the terminal portion of the spinal cord to attach caudally to a high-signal-intensity mass (lipoma) at the S3 level. Axial T1-weighted scans are presented at three levels: (*C*) through the terminal portion of the spinal cord, which was low-lying; (*D*) through the thick linear structure previously identified; and (*E*) through the lipoma itself.

DIAGNOSIS

Tight filum terminale

DISCUSSION

The tight filum terminale syndrome represents a complex of deformities associated with a short and thick filum terminale and a low position of the conus medullaris. The age at which symptoms develop is variable. Patients may suffer from difficulty with locomotion, abnormal lower extremity reflexes, bladder dysfunction, sensory changes, orthopedic deformities (e.g., clubfoot), back pain, and radiculopathy. Adults most frequently present with radiculopathy.

The normal filum measures 2 mm or less in maximum diameter.[1] The normal position of the conus medullaris varies with age, but usually reaches the adult level of L1–L2 by 2 months of age and generally should not be below the L2–L3 level by age 12 years.[2] In the tight filum syndrome the conus medullaris is almost always low-lying, being tethered by the filum. Decreased T1-weighted signal intensity is not uncommonly seen in the central portion of the spinal cord, due to either myelomalacia or hydromyelia.

Transection of the filum or of associated fibrous adhesions, as well as removal of a spinal lipoma (as in this case), may result in remission of pain and improvement of sensorimotor deficits, or slow the progression of symptoms.[3]

Clinical References

1. Raghaven N, Barkovich AJ, Edwards MSB, Norman D. MR imaging in the tethered spinal cord syndrome. AJNR 1989;19:27–36.
2. Barkovich AJ, Naidich TP. Congenital anomalies of the spine. In: Barkovich AJ, ed. Pediatric neuroimaging. New York, Raven Press, 1990.
3. Maiuri F, Gambardella A, Trinchillo G. Congenital lumbo-sacral lesions with late onset in adult life. Neurological Research 1989;11:238–244.

(Images courtesy of Mark Osborne, MD)

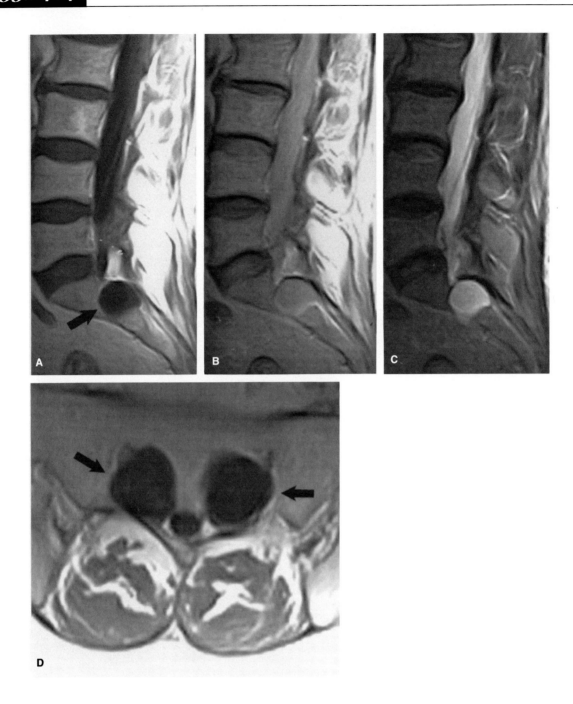

HISTORY

A 65-year-old woman with low back pain

FINDINGS

(A) The preinfusion T1-weighted sagittal image reveals an oval area of low signal intensity (*arrow*) posterior to the S1–2 level just to the right of midline. On (B) the proton density weighted and (C) the heavily T2-weighted sagittal images, the signal intensity of the mass follows the signal intensity of cerebrospinal fluid (CSF). Chemical shift artifact is noted on B and C above and below the lesion (along the readout axis), at the interface with surrounding fat. There is no abnormal contrast enhancement on the postinfusion axial image (D), which demonstrates bilateral perineural cysts at this level (*arrows*). Adjacent axial images (*not shown*) revealed continuity with the thecal sac.

DIAGNOSIS

Large perineural cysts

DISCUSSION

Spinal meningeal cysts are actually diverticula of the meningeal sac, nerve root sheath, or arachnoid, most likely of congenital origin. Nabors and associates classified these into three general categories.[1] Type I and II spinal meningeal cysts are extradural, the former without and the latter with spinal nerve root fibers. Type III cysts are intradural. Type I cysts include extradural arachnoid cysts and sacral meningoceles, type II include Tarlov perineural cysts and spinal nerve root diverticula, and type III include intradural arachnoid cysts.

Tarlov perineural cysts, also known as nerve root sleeve cysts, occur as a focal dilatation of the nerve root sleeve. Tarlov cysts are the same lesion as spinal nerve root diverticula.[1] As noted above, they are classified as type II spinal meningeal cysts, defined as extradural meningeal cysts that contain spinal nerve fibers. The associated nerve roots may lie within the wall of the cyst or may pass through the cyst.[2] The cysts communicate with the thecal sac and are therefore filled with freely flowing CSF. Communication of the cyst with the subarachnoid space may be demonstrated by CT following intrathecal administration of contrast.

The cysts are most commonly identified in the sacral area, where they are often quite large. They are frequently multiple and bilateral, and occur anywhere along the spine on the dorsal nerve roots. An expanding cyst can result in erosion and scalloping of the adjacent vertebral body or pedicle as well as enlargement of the neural foramen. These are usually asymptomatic but can cause symptoms, which include bowel or bladder problems and sciatic pain.

On MR imaging, a Tarlov cyst appears as a round to oval mass in the spinal canal or neural foramen. The signal intensity is homogeneous and can follow the signal of CSF or have slightly different signal intensity on T2-weighted images due to higher protein content of the cyst fluid compared to CSF, and lack of CSF pulsations in the cyst. The cysts do not enhance with intravenous MR contrast administration. This is an important differential point to distinguish a Tarlov cyst from a neurinoma; the latter is a lesion that enhances intensely.

Clinical References

1. Nabors MW, Pait TG, Byrd EB, et al. Updated assessment and current classification of spinal meningeal cysts. J Neurosurg 1988;68:366–377.
2. DeLaPaz RL. Congenital anomalies of the spine and spinal cord. In: Enzmann DR, DeLaPaz RL, Rubin JB. Magnetic resonance of the spine. St. Louis, CV Mosby Company, 1990: 225–230.

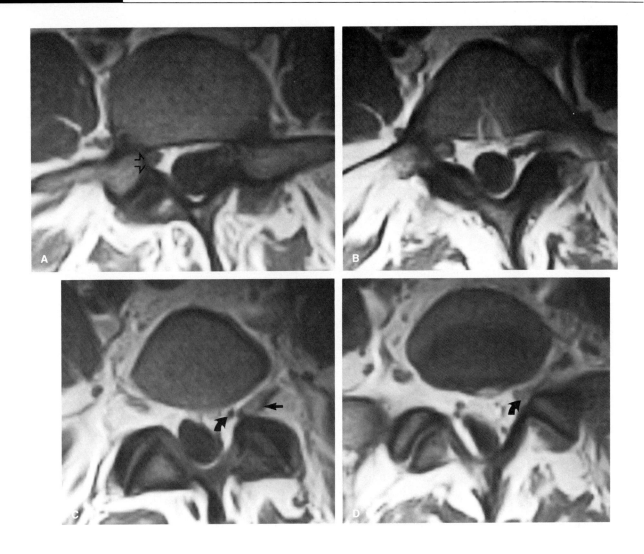

HISTORY

A 33-year-old morbidly obese woman with migratory lower extremity pain

FINDINGS

(*A through E*) Three-millimeter-thickness axial postcontrast T1-weighted images are displayed from the mid-L5 vertebral body level to mid-S1. For simplicity, only every other section from the actual exam has been printed. On *A*, although the right L5 nerve root (*open arrow*) has already exited from the thecal sac, a large abnormal nerve root sleeve is noted on the left. (*B*) On the next lower section, two separate nerve roots can be identified on the left. (*C*) At the level of the L5–S1 foramen, the enhancing dorsal root ganglion of L5 (*arrow*) can be differentiated from the more medial (and lower-signal-intensity) S1 nerve root sheath (*curved arrow*). On *D and E*, the low-

est two sections, the S1 nerve root on the left (*curved arrows*) is noted to remain within the bony spinal canal and to descend in a more normal position relative to the right S1 nerve root.

DIAGNOSIS

Conjoined nerve root

DISCUSSION

Anomalies of the lumbosacral nerve roots are seen in 1% to 3% of the population, usually involving the L5 and S1 roots unilaterally.[1] Three types were described by Cannon in 1961. Type 1 anomalies (conjoined root) are by far the most common. In this anomaly, two nerve roots arise from a single dural sheath (root sleeve), but exit separately in the appropriate foramina. In type 2 anoma-

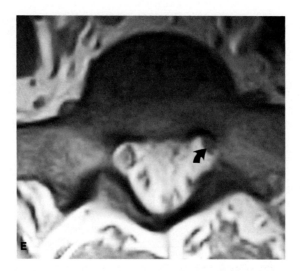

lies, two nerve roots exit through a single foramen. In this situation, there may be one foramen without a nerve root, or all foramina may be occupied—with one foramen containing two roots. In type 3, two adjacent nerve roots are connected by an anastomotic root.

Although these anomalies are rare, their recognition is important because of the potential for failed back surgery when these accompany a disk herniation. Without adequate decompression by foraminotomy or pedicle excision, symptomatology persists in a high number of patients. In the absence of accompanying pathology, most patients with anomalies of the lumbosacral nerve roots are asymptomatic, although radicular pain has been described.

Pitfalls in Image Interpretation

Without intrathecal contrast, a conjoined nerve root can be mistaken on CT for herniated disk material.[2] This distinction should not present difficulty on MR due to superior soft tissue contrast.

Clinical References

1. Neidre A, MacNab I. Anomalies of the lumbosacral nerve roots. Spine 1983;8:294–299.
2. Torricelli P, Spina V, Martinelli C. CT diagnosis of lumbosacral conjoined nerve roots. Neuroradiology 1987;29:374–379.

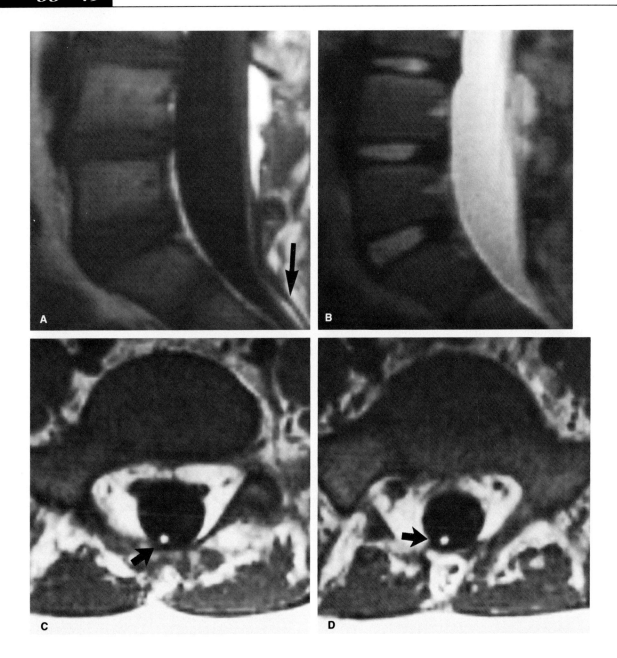

HISTORY

Noncontributory

FINDINGS

(A) The midline sagittal T1-weighted image demonstrates linear high signal intensity (*arrow*) within the filum ter-minale, as it runs along the posterior aspect of the thecal sac, at the level of the sacrum. Just cephalad, at the L5–S1 level, the filum also appears slightly hyperintense. (*B*) The corresponding heavily T2-weighted image is grossly normal. The conus was normal in location (*images not shown*). Two adjacent axial T1-weighted images through S1 (*C and D*) identify the filum in cross section (*arrows*), with abnormal hyperintensity. The filum measured between 1 and 2 mm in diameter. Note is also made of mild bony dysraphism posteriorly.

DIAGNOSIS

Fatty filum terminale

DISCUSSION

The filum terminale is a thin connective tissue strand. It has an intradural component that extends from the tip of the conus medullaris to the distal tip of the thecal sac, and a contiguous extradural component that runs from the distal thecal sac to insert on the first coccygeal segment. The normal filum measures 2 mm or less in diameter at the L5–S1 level. It has uniform caliber and demonstrates intermediate to low signal intensity on all imaging sequences, similar to the adjacent nerve roots. Because of this, the normal filum may be difficult to differentiate from a nerve root.

A small amount of fat may be identified within the filum and has been reported to occur in 1% to 5% of cases.[1] This often results in mild fusiform dilatation of the affected segment. This may be an incidental finding in an asymptomatic patient with the conus medullaris in normal position, at or above the L2–3 level, and no other evidence of spinal cord tethering. The fatty filum may, however, be associated with cord tethering. Therefore, patients with evidence of fat in the filum should receive careful evaluation of the spinal cord and conus to rule out a possible tethered cord.

MR Technique

Fat within the filum demonstrates high T1 signal intensity. The fat will become less apparent on T2-weighted images as the signal from the surrounding CSF increases. The diameter of the filum is best assessed, and fat best detected, on axial images. The fat signal may be missed or diminished on sagittal images due to volume averaging with the surrounding low-signal CSF.

A thin fatty film may not be well demonstrated on sagittal images of the spine. Similarly, the level of the conus medullaris is often difficult to define on sagittal images. Axial sections are more sensitive in detecting small collections of fat in the filum terminale and provide more accurate localization of the conus.[2]

Clinical References

1. Okumura R, Minami S, Asato R, Konishi J. Fatty filum terminale: assessment with MR imaging. J Comput Assist Tomog 1990;14:571–573.
2. Raghavan N, Barkovich AJ, Edwards M, Norman D. MR imaging in the tethered spinal cord syndrome. AJR 1989; 10:27–36.

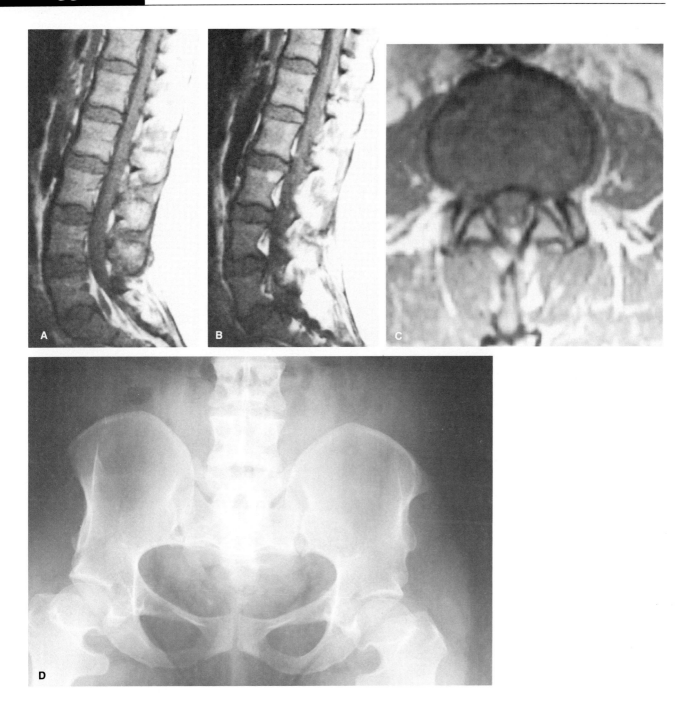

HISTORY

A 30-year-old woman with short stature and low back pain

FINDINGS

(*A and B*) T1-weighted sagittal images of the lumbar spine reveal an accentuated lumbar lordosis with a horizontally oriented sacrum. There is scalloping of the posterior aspect of vertebral bodies L3 through L5. The AP diameter of the spinal canal is less than normal. (*C*) The T1-weighted axial image through the L2–3 disk demonstrates spinal canal narrowing in both the AP and lateral dimensions. (*D*) A plain film of the pelvis reveals the "champagne glass" appearance of the flattened iliac wings, as well as the horizontal acetabula.

DIAGNOSIS

Achondroplasia

DISCUSSION

Achondroplasia is an autosomal dominant disorder of enchondral bone formation that results in premature synostosis of vertebral ossification centers. The laminae are thickened and the pedicles shortened. Vertebral bodies are reduced in height with hypertrophy of the intervertebral disks. These abnormalities combine to create a spinal canal that is narrowed in both the transverse and AP directions.[1,2] The intervertebral disks are reportedly predisposed to herniate due to their hypertrophy, which may create significant problems in an already narrowed spinal canal. Degenerate bone spurs and ligamentous hypertrophy also have an exaggerated effect in these patients.

In childhood, neurologic deficits in achondroplasia are usually the result of constriction of the foramen magnum and cervical canal narrowing, which may lead to communicating hydrocephalus.

Clinical References

1. Fortuna A, Ferrante L, Acqui M, et al. Narrowing of the thoracolumbar spinal canal in achondroplasia. J Neurosurg Sci 1989;33:185–196.
2. Giglio G, Passariello R, Pagnotta G, et al. Anatomy of the lumbar spine in achondroplasia. Basic Life Sci 1988;48:227–239.

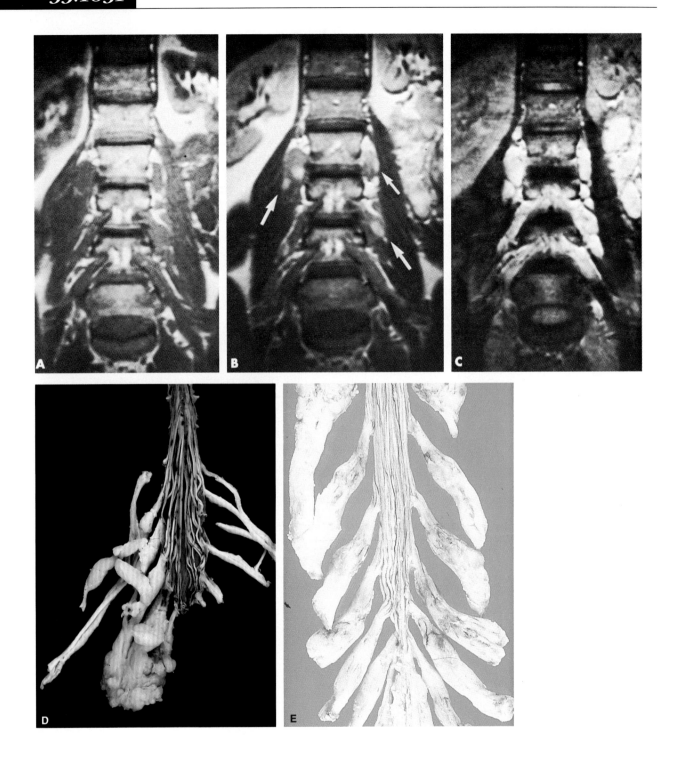

HISTORY

Asymptomatic, with multiple subcutaneous nodules

FINDINGS

Multiple large paraspinal soft tissue masses, with heterogeneous yet marked contrast enhancement (*arrows*), are noted in the lumbar region on (*A*) precontrast and (*B*) postcontrast T1-weighted coronal scans. These lesions are markedly hyperintense on the T2-weighted scan (*C*).

DIAGNOSIS

Plexiform neurofibromas (neurofibromatosis type 1)

291

DISCUSSION

Neurofibromatosis types 1 and 2 are distinct clinical entities—the disease genes are on different chromosomes (17 versus 22)—that both produce multiple neurofibromas.[1] MR with gadolinium enhancement has supplanted other techniques for visualization of brain, spinal, and peripheral nerve tumors in both disorders. Café-au-lait spots and iris hamartomas (Lisch nodules) are signs of neurofibromatosis type 1. Acoustic neuromas, usually bilateral, are characteristic for neurofibromatosis type 2. Both diseases are autosomal dominant.

Spinal manifestations in neurofibromatosis include bony dysplasia, dural ectasia, lateral meningoceles, and spinal cord and extradural lesions. A solitary lesion may involve an individual nerve outside the spinal canal, or multiple nerves may be involved in a plexiform manner. Lesions that on MR are slightly hyperintense to muscle on T1-weighted images and markedly hyperintense on T2-weighted images are characteristic for neurofibromas.[2]

MR Technique

Screening of the entire spine is recommended in both neurofibromatosis type 1 and 2 because of the propensity to develop clinically significant intradural disease, which may be asymptomatic.[3] Lesions involving the paraspinal region are best displayed on coronal T2-weighted images.

Pathologic Correlate

Neurofibromas can involve major nerve trunks, spinal nerves, and cranial nerves. Of solitary lesions involving peripheral nerves, only 10% are associated with neurofibromatosis. Neurofibromas typically spread longitudinally within a nerve, producing fusiform enlargement. Plexiform neurofibromas are the result of enlargement and lengthening of multiple nerve fascicles—they resemble a bag of worms—and are diagnostic of neurofibromatosis. Two examples of neurofibromas, both in patients with neurofibromatosis, are illustrated (D and E). In the first, the involvement of the right sacral area is plexiform in nature. In the second, involvement is bilateral but not plexiform.

Clinical References

1. Mulvihill JJ, Parry DM, Sherman JL, et al. NIH conference: neurofibromatosis 1 (Recklinghausen disease) and neurofibromatosis 2 (bilateral acoustic neurofibromatosis), an update. Ann Intern Med 1990;113:39–52.
2. Burk DL, Brunberg JA, Kanal E, et al. Spinal and paraspinal neurofibromatosis: surface coil MR imaging at 1.5T. Radiology 1987;162:797–801.
3. Egelhoff JC, Bates DJ, Ross JS, et al. Spinal MR findings in neurofibromatosis types 1 and 2. AJNR 1992;13:1071–1077.

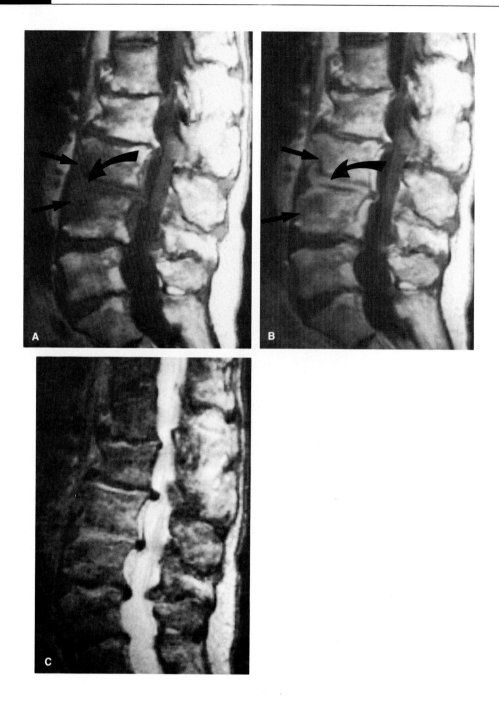

HISTORY

A 95-year-old woman with a 2-week history of low back pain and sharp pain radiating down both legs. The patient was unable to walk due to the pain. Past history revealed a febrile illness 2 months before admission secondary to a urinary tract infection.

FINDINGS

(A) The sagittal preinfusion T1-weighted image shows abnormal decreased signal intensity in the anterior portion of the inferior L3 and superior L4 vertebral bodies (*arrows*). The signal intensity of the intervertebral disk (*curved arrow*) is indiscernible from that of the adjacent anterior vertebrae. Thickening of the adjacent paraspinous soft tissue is also demonstrated along the anterior margin of the spine. (B) The postinfusion T1-weighted image reveals enhancement within the vertebral bodies (*arrows*), disk (*curved arrow*), and paraspinous soft tissue. (C) On the sagittal T2-weighted image, high signal intensity is seen in the involved vertebrae, disk, and soft tissue mass. (D) The anteroposterior plain film of the lumbar spine shows ill-defined end plates and sclerosis of the vertebral bodies adjacent to the L3–4 disk space.

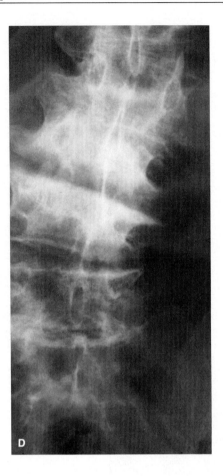

Severe degenerative changes and scoliosis are also present.

DIAGNOSIS

Osteomyelitis and disk space infection

DISCUSSION

Spondylitis and disk space infection can occur secondary to hematogenous seeding by an arterial or venous route. The infection involves the disk space as well as the adjacent vertebral bodies and paraspinous soft tissues. Extraspinal involvement may also produce an epidural abscess. The plain film findings of decreased height of the intervertebral disk space, poorly defined vertebral body end plates, and sclerotic changes in the adjacent vertebrae are seen late in the process. This is particularly true in older patients with underlying severe degenerative changes in the spine.

Infection within the marrow space, with resultant edema and inflammatory changes, produces decreased T1 signal intensity. The signal intensity of the vertebral end plates thus becomes similar to the signal intensity of the intervertebral disk. On T2-weighted images, the increased water content produces increased signal intensity in inflamed tissues. Increased T2 signal intensity is also seen in the intervertebral disk. A combination of these findings is necessary to accurately diagnose a disk space infection.[1] The finding of an enhancing paraspinous soft tissue mass should raise the suspicion of infection.

MR Technique

In osteomyelitis, MR has been shown to be as sensitive and accurate as radionuclide imaging.[1] Intravenous contrast administration adds an additional dimension and should be used in evaluation of patients with suspected disk space infection.

Pitfalls in Image Interpretation

High T2 signal intensity in the vertebral body end plates is not specific for infection. Increased T2 signal intensity may also be seen with type I end plate changes, a degenerative process, or other causes of marrow edema such as trauma.

Clinical Reference

1. Ross JS. Inflammatory disease. In: Modic MT, Masaryk TJ, Ross JS. Magnetic resonance imaging of the spine. Chicago, Year Book Medical Publishers, 1989:173–177.

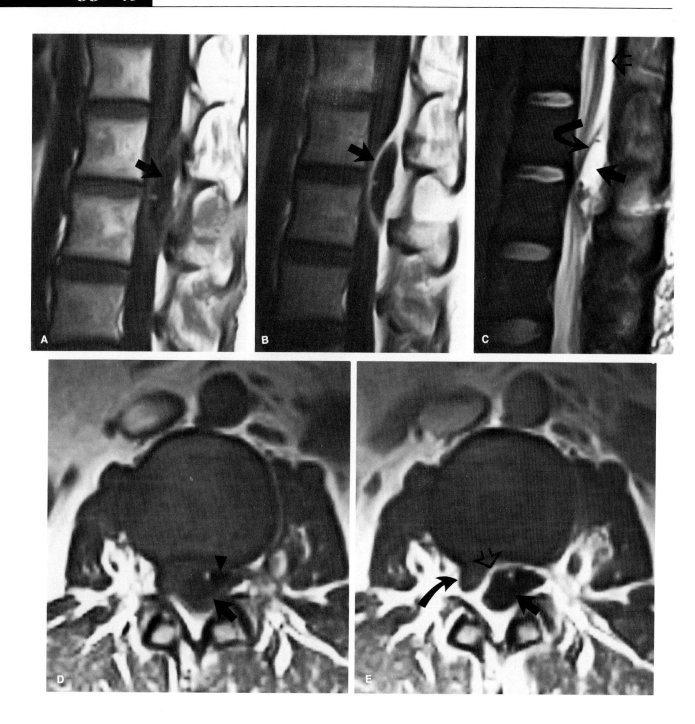

HISTORY

A 33-year-old woman with intractable pain due to a severe right leg injury. An indwelling epidural catheter for pain management was placed 1 month before the current admission. The patient presented with a tender, indurated subcutaneous mass at the site of the epidural catheter, as well as severe back and right leg pain.

FINDINGS

(*A*) The noncontrast sagittal T1-weighted image reveals an abnormal fluid collection (*arrow*), accompanied by a small amount of soft tissue, within the left posterior epidural space. These findings are confirmed on the postinfusion sagittal T1-weighted image (*B*), which also reveals peripheral contrast enhancement (*arrow*). On the sagittal T2-weighted image (*C*), the fluid collection (*arrow*) is slightly hyperintense to CSF within the thecal sac (*open arrow*). The curvilinear low-signal dura (*curved arrow*) separates the epidural fluid and subarachnoid space. The axial preinfusion T1-weighted image (*D*) confirms the epidural location of the fluid (*arrow*). A gas bubble is seen (*arrowhead*) slightly laterally within this collection. In retrospect, the gas bubble can be noted on the sagittal T2-weighted scan as a region of signal void at the most caudal extent of the fluid collection. The axial postinfusion T1-weighted scan (*E*) well demonstrates the enhancing dural interface (*open arrow*). The epidural collection is larger than the thecal sac (*curved arrow*), which is displaced anteriorly and to the right.

DIAGNOSIS

Inflammatory epidural fluid collection

DISCUSSION

An inflammatory reaction consisting of granulation tissue and fluid may produce sufficient mass effect to cause cord compression and neurologic symptoms. The reaction may be due to an infectious or noninfectious cause. Images obtained after the administration of intravenous contrast demonstrate enhancement of the inflammatory mass. In addition, the enhancement frequently provides information to allow localization in the epidural or intradural space.[1]

The patient illustrated underwent a subsequent laminectomy at the catheter site. The pathologic evaluation reported predominantly neutrophilic infiltration of the surgical specimen. No definite organism was cultured.

Pitfalls in Image Interpretation

The enhancing soft tissue in this case represents granulation tissue. Enhancement within soft tissue can be due to inflammation alone and does not necessarily represent infection.

Clinical Reference

1. Sandhu FS, Dillon WP. Spinal epidural abscess: evaluation with contrast-enhanced MR imaging. AJNR 1991;12:1087–1093.

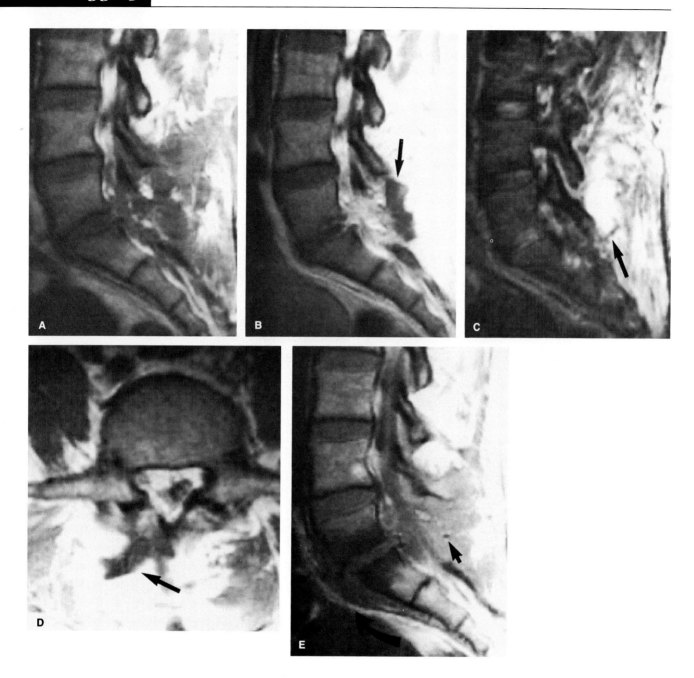

HISTORY

A 42-year-old patient with persistent back pain following right L5–S1 laminotomy and microdiskectomy

FINDINGS

On the initial postoperative study, obtained 5 weeks after surgery, the T1-weighted sagittal image (A) reveals irregularly decreased signal intensity in the posterior soft tissues to the right of midline, at the site of the right L5–S1 laminectomy. Much of this area enhances following contrast administration (B), indicating the presence of granulation tissue. Mild enhancement is present at the posterior margin of the L5–S1 intervertebral disk. A more posterior component (*arrow*), which has signal characteristics compatible with fluid, does not enhance. On the T2-weighted sagittal image (C), the nonenhancing portion (*arrow*) becomes very high in signal intensity, again compatible with fluid. A postinfusion T1-weighted axial image at the inferior L5 level (D) confirms the small fluid collection (*arrow*). Moderate enhancing granulation tissue is present about the right S1 nerve root and anterior to the thecal sac on the right. No evidence for recurrent disk herniation is seen on this study.

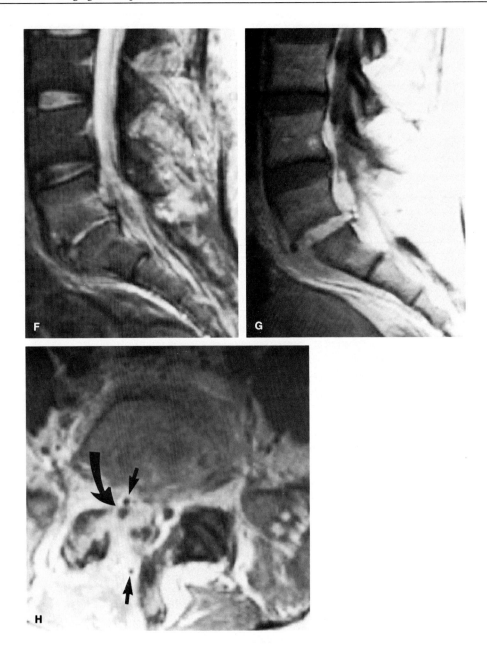

The patient's severe back pain persisted despite rest and analgesics. A second MR was obtained 10 weeks postoperatively. The T1-weighted sagittal image (*E*) now demonstrates prominently decreased signal intensity at the end plates adjacent to the L5–S1 disk. The end plates are indistinct, and the intervertebral disk appears narrowed. A large amount of abnormal soft tissue intensity is present in the prevertebral region (*curved arrow*). Small foci of signal void (*short arrow*), compatible with susceptibility artifact, are identified within the spinal canal and in the posterior soft tissues. Because these foci of susceptibility were not present on the initial postoperative study, they probably represent gas bubbles rather than metallic fragments. On the T2-weighted sagittal view

(*F*), the affected end plates are of abnormal high signal intensity. The L5–S1 intervertebral disk, despite being quite narrowed, is of higher signal intensity than the other lumbar disks. The postcontrast T1-weighted sagittal image (*G*) reveals intense enhancement of the L5–S1 disk and the abnormal prevertebral soft tissues. The adjacent L5 and S1 end plates also enhance. The right laminotomy defect is well seen on the postcontrast T1-weighted axial image at L5–S1 (*H*). Abnormal enhancement is present about the right side of the thecal sac, surrounding the right S1 nerve root (*curved arrow*), within the right L5–S1 facet, and within the right paraspinal musculature. Several foci of susceptibility artifact (*small arrows*) are again noted.

DIAGNOSIS

Severe postoperative diskitis at L5–S1

DISCUSSION

Diskitis is a relatively rare postoperative complication, occurring in 1% to 3% of back surgery patients.[1] Any invasive procedure including diskography, myelography, and chemonucleolysis may predispose patients to diskitis. Diskitis in such cases is typically secondary to direct inoculation of the disk space. *Staphylococcus aureus* is the most commonly cultured organism in these patients and was the causative organism in the current case.

The typical clinical presentation of postoperative diskitis is severe back pain developing 1 to 4 weeks after surgery. Pain is often accompanied by muscle spasms, and a positive straight leg raise test is frequently present. Fever and wound infections are seen in a small minority of patients, and the white blood cell count is generally only minimally elevated. In light of these nonspecific findings, it is not surprising that delays in diagnosis of diskitis are quite common.

The typical MR appearance of diskitis consists of abnormally decreased signal intensity within the vertebral end plates on T1-weighted scans, with increased signal intensity noted on T2-weighted images. These signal abnormalities are usually in the form of horizontal bands that involve one third to one half of the vertebral body.[2] The vertebral end plates are often indistinct, and the disk itself demonstrates increased signal intensity on T2-weighted scans. Following contrast administration, enhancement of the affected disk space, posterior annulus, and adjacent vertebral end plates is commonly seen. In severe cases, enhancing soft tissue masses contiguous to the disk space may be present, usually in the prevertebral region.

The development of gas within the soft tissues, although seen infrequently, is another highly suggestive sign of infection. In the current example, a small fluid collection was present near the laminectomy site on the initial follow-up study. We have observed such collections in a number of patients who eventually developed diskitis.

Small fluid collections, presumably seromas, are frequently present immediately after surgery. The presence of fluid collections in the later postoperative period is worrisome. Such fluid collections may serve as a nidus for bacterial growth and the eventual development of diskitis.[3]

MR Technique

Intravenous contrast allows improved diagnostic confidence in distinguishing normal postoperative changes from those of diskitis. Although the posterior annulus may normally enhance, enhancement of the disk itself is not a normal postoperative finding. Decreased signal intensity in the end plates on T1-weighted images and enhancement of these areas postcontrast has been described as the single most reliable indicator of postoperative diskitis.[2] Severe type I end plate changes may be similar in appearance, but should be present preoperatively. Additionally, patients with end plate degenerative changes almost always have degenerated, low-signal-intensity disks on T2-weighted images. Diskitis patients typically demonstrate increased signal intensity within the disk on T2-weighted scans.

Pitfalls in Image Interpretation

Even after appropriate antibiotic therapy is instituted, MR findings of diskitis may progress.[2] In particular, enhancement of the disk space and adjacent end plates may become more severe, despite relief in symptomatology. Caution should thus be exercised in attributing progressive MR findings to failure of antibiotic therapy.

Clinical References

1. Fernand R, Lee CK. Postlaminectomy disk space infection: a review of the literature and a report of three cases. Clin Orthop 1986;209:215–218.
2. Boden SD, Davis DO, Dina TS, et al. Postoperative diskitis: distinguishing early MR imaging findings from normal postoperative disk space changes. Radiology 1992;184:765–771.
3. Duncan V, Lee C, Runge VM, et al. The role of postoperative seromas in the development of infection in the failed back syndrome. AJR 1993;160S:48.

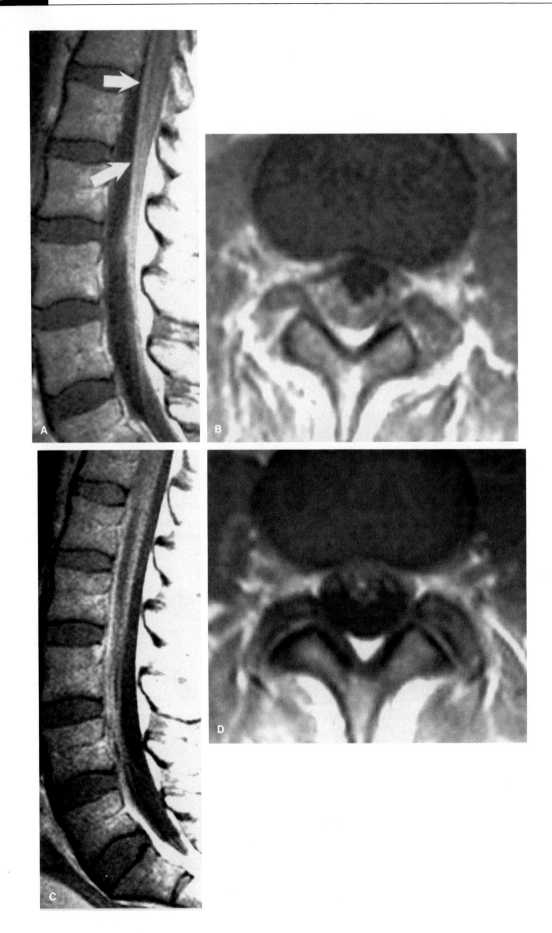

HISTORY

Severe back pain, nausea, and photophobia 1 week after hysterectomy with epidural anesthesia

FINDINGS

Precontrast T1- and T2-weighted sagittal images were unremarkable (*images not shown*). (*A*) Following gadolinium chelate administration, prominent enhancement (*white arrows*) of the lumbar nerve roots and the surface of the conus is noted. (*B*) A postcontrast T1-weighted axial image at the L2–3 level confirms the marked enhancement of the nerve roots within the cauda equina. These also appear mildly thickened, but retain their usual position within the dependent portion of the thecal sac. The patient returned for follow-up after 1 month of antibiotic therapy. Her back pain remained severe at this time. (*C*) A postcontrast T1-weighted sagittal image reveals persistent enhancement of the lumbar nerve roots. The nerve roots now lie anteriorly within the thecal sac. (*D*) A postcontrast axial image at L3–4 demonstrates marked clumping of the enhancing, anteriorly positioned lumbar nerve roots.

DIAGNOSIS

Spinal meningitis with progression to arachnoiditis

DISCUSSION

Cultures in this patient revealed *Staphylococcus aureus* as the causative organism. The patient's original meningeal symptoms improved after intravenous antibiotic therapy, but her back pain persisted, presumably secondary to the development of arachnoiditis. This case illustrates just one of the many possible etiologies of spinal arachnoiditis. In the modern era, infection is an uncommon cause of arachnoiditis. Previous surgery, often for disk herniation, is probably the leading cause of arachnoiditis. Other etiologies include prior trauma, hemorrhage, Pantopaque, and the irritant effects of intrathecal steroids and anesthetics. Arachnoiditis is thought to arise as part of the body's normal reparative process after meningeal injury. Initially, a minimal inflammatory cellular exudate is present in association with a prominent fibrinous exudate. This fibrinous exudate eventually results in collagenous adhesions that obliterate the nerve root sheaths and cause nerve root clumping.

Ross and colleagues have described three different appearances of arachnoiditis on MR imaging.[1] In patients with the mildest disease, prominent conglomerations of nerve roots were noted centrally within the thecal sac. A second group of patients demonstrated adherence of nerve roots to the periphery of the thecal sac. The third group, thought to be the most seriously effected, demonstrated increased soft tissue within the thecal sac, which filled the majority of the thecal sac. Individual nerve roots were indiscernible in the latter group.

MR Technique

Enhancement of clumped nerve roots may allow easier detection of arachnoiditis because of improved CSF–nerve root contrast.[2] Enhancement of moderate and severe cases of arachnoiditis, however, is variable and inconsistent. The greatest utility of contrast enhancement may be in cases of early nerve root inflammation,[3] in which nerve root clumping may not be present. The current case is such an example. At the time of the initial study, the only definite abnormalities were found on postcontrast images.

Pitfalls in Image Interpretation

The appearance of mild nerve root clumping can be seen normally at the L2 or L3 levels.[1] The diagnosis of arachnoiditis thus requires demonstration of abnormal nerve roots at multiple contiguous levels. Caution should also be exercised in cases of severe spinal stenosis, in which the altered dimensions of the spinal canal may result in the false impression of nerve root clumping.

Clinical References

1. Ross JS, Masaryk TJ, Modic MT, et al. MR imaging of lumbar arachnoiditis. AJR 1987;149:1025–1032.
2. Johnson CE, Sze G. Benign lumbar arachnoiditis: MR imaging with gadopentatate dimeglumine. AJR 1990;155:873–880.
3. Sklar EML, Quencer RM, Green BA, et al. Complications of epidural anesthesia: MR appearance of abnormalities. Radiology 1991;181:549–554.

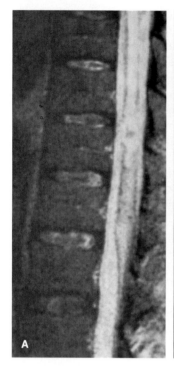
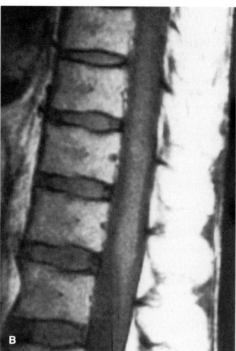
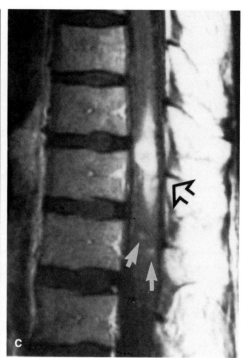

HISTORY

A 57-year-old man with progressive lower extremity weakness and paresthesias, as well as bowel and bladder dysfunction, for 3 months

FINDINGS

(*A*) The T2-weighted (TE = 80) sagittal scan reveals diffuse abnormal hyperintensity of the lower cord and conus. (*B*) The precontrast T1-weighted sagittal scan is unremarkable. (*C*) On the postcontrast T1-weighted scan, an enhancing intramedullary mass (*open arrow*) is identified at T11, with two additional small enhancing lesions (*small arrows*) within the conus. Head CT (*images not shown*) revealed two ring enhancing lesions with surrounding edema in the right frontal and left parietal lobes. Diagnosis was by biopsy of both the intracerebral and spinal cord lesions.

DIAGNOSIS

Histoplasmosis

DISCUSSION

Central nervous system (CNS) involvement by *Histoplasma capsulatum* is rare, except with disseminated disease, despite the prevalence of infection (an estimated 40 million Americans). Histoplasmosis is a systemic fungal infection, most common in the Mississippi, Ohio, and St. Lawrence River drainages. Most infections are respiratory, with the disseminated form seen most frequently in infants, the elderly, and immunocompromised patients. CNS involvement can take the form of granulomas, meningitis, cerebritis, or spinal cord involvement.[1]

Pitfalls in Image Interpretation

With regard to diagnosis, the presence of multiple enhancing lesions on either CT or MR is nonspecific. The preliminary diagnosis in this patient before biopsy was metastatic neoplasm. Multiple enhancing lesions can also result from infection (with hematogenous spread), ischemia, and trauma. Other fungal infections reported in an intramedullary location include *Cryptococcus neoformans*, *Candida*, and *Aspergillus fumigatus*.[2]

Clinical References

1. Desai SP, Bazan C, Hummell W, Jinkins JR. Disseminated CNS histoplasmosis. AJNR 1991;12:290–292.
2. Bazan C, New PZ. Intramedullary spinal histoplasmosis—efficacy of gadolinium enhancement. Neuroradiology 1991; 33:190.

(A through C *from Desai SP, Bazan C, Hummell W, Jinkins JR. Disseminated CNS histoplasmosis. AJNR 1991;12:290, with permission.*)

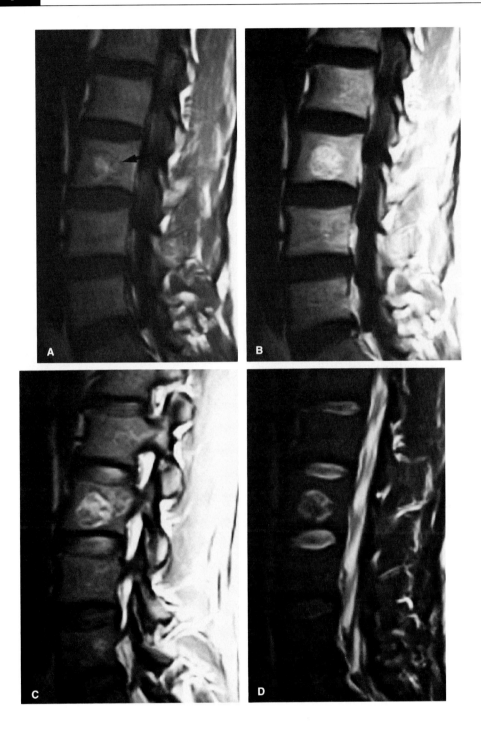

HISTORY

A 44-year-old patient with low back pain

FINDINGS

A round, mottled area of increased signal intensity (*arrow*) is seen in the central portion of the L3 vertebral body on the sagittal T1-weighted image (*A*). The post-infusion T1-weighted image (*B*) reveals mild abnormal enhancement. The lesion also exhibits high signal intensity on the sagittal (*C*) intermediate and (*D*) heavily T2-weighted images. Mottled signal intensity is demonstrated with interspersed areas of very low signal intensity on all imaging sequences, corresponding with prominent trabeculae.

DIAGNOSIS

Hemangioma of the vertebral body

DISCUSSION

Hemangiomas are benign neoplasms that are frequent incidental findings on magnetic resonance studies of the spine. In a large autopsy study, hemangiomas were found in 11% of patients.[1] Hemangiomas are most commonly solitary but may be multiple. They vary greatly in size and may be confined to a small area within the vertebral body or may involve the entire vertebral body. The lesion may also extend outside the margins of the vertebral body, causing mass effect on adjacent structures. If the extension is in a posterior direction, the mass can compromise the spinal canal. Although uncommon, weakening of the involved vertebra can occur and result in a fracture.

Hemangiomas typically appear as focal areas of high signal intensity within the vertebral bodies on T1-weighted images. The signal intensity remains high on T2-weighted images. This is at least partially explained by the histologic content—a mixture of angiomatous tissue and adipose tissue between prominent trabeculae. The fat content accounts for the high-intensity T1 signal.[2] Frequently, a reticular pattern of low signal intensity is seen representing the thickened trabecula, with more prominent vertical trabeculae.

MR Technique

Certain MR techniques either accentuate or attenuate signal from fatty tissues. These can be used to help differentiate tissue composition. Chemical shift artifact at fat–water interfaces may also confirm the presence of fat in a lesion.

Pittfalls in Image Interpretation

Another common incidental finding on spinal MR studies is focal fatty replacement or fat islands within the vertebrae. These areas follow fat signal on all imaging sequences. Therefore, the signal intensity is high on T1-weighted images, similar to hemangiomas. Focal fat collections, however, show progressively decreased signal intensity on the first and second echo of T2-weighted spin echo sequences.

Clinical References

1. Masaryk TJ. Neoplastic diseases of the spine. Radiol Clin North Am 1991;29:829–845.
2. Ross JS, Masaryk TJ, Modic MT. Vertebral hemangiomas: MR imaging. Radiology 1987;165:165–169.

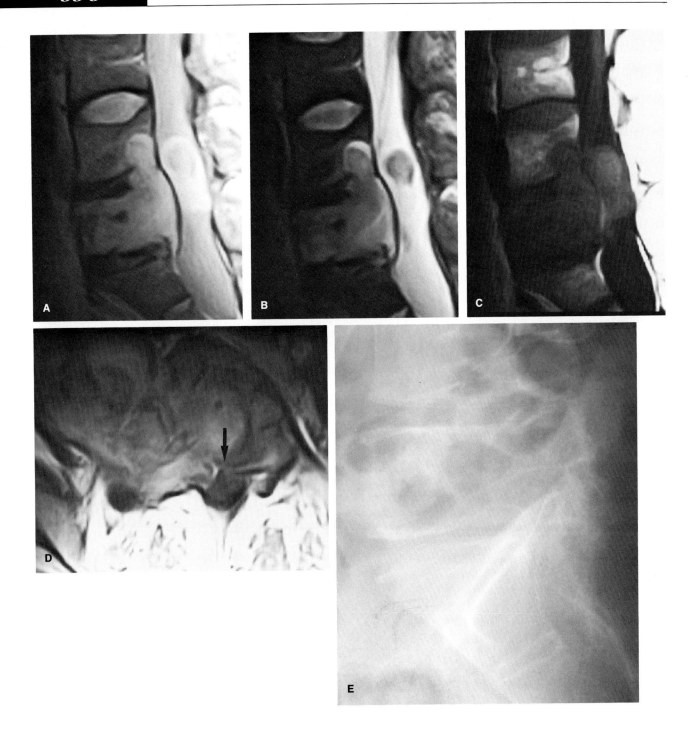

HISTORY

A 42-year-old man, now wheelchair-bound, with chronic lower extremity pain

FINDINGS

On the intermediate and heavily T2-weighted sagittal images (*A and B*), an extensive soft tissue mass with relatively high signal intensity is demonstrated within the L5 vertebral body. The mass extends into the spinal canal and continues through the posterior L4–5 intervertebral disk to involve the posteroinferior L4 vertebral body. The nerve roots of the cauda equina are displaced anteriorly by the lesion. The mass is somewhat inhomogeneous and is of lower signal intensity on the second echo of the T2-weighted scan, although peripheral areas of high signal intensity are noted. A very low-signal-intensity rim is present at the posterior margin of the lesion. On the T1-weighted sagittal precontrast image (*C*), the lesion is of intermediate signal intensity. Extent of the lesion posteriorly into the spinal canal is again well demonstrated. On the T1-weighted sagittal postcontrast image (*image not shown*), somewhat inhomogeneous enhancement of the abnormality was noted. The T1-weighted postcontrast axial image at the L5 level (*D*) reveals the extensive paraspinal involvement by this large enhancing lesion, and also well demonstrates the encroachment upon the spinal canal (*arrow*). The intraspinal component seen on the sagittal views was above this level. Thin, low-signal-intensity borders are present about the lesion, most prominently on the left in this image. A lateral radiograph of the lower lumbar spine (*E*) reveals mild sclerosis and loss of height of the L5 vertebral body. The posterior cortex of L5 is absent.

DIAGNOSIS

Malignant nerve sheath tumor

DISCUSSION

This case is presented for discussion of giant cell tumors. The appearance is consistent with such a lesion and also illustrates the importance of differential diagnosis.

With the exception of the sacrum, giant cell tumors of the spine are relatively rare, accounting for 1.3% to 9.3% of giant cell tumors.[1] The peak incidence is between 20 and 40 years, with a female predominance. Vertebral giant cell tumors appear to have a better prognosis than those located elsewhere, with relatively low rates of recurrence following resection. The most common clinical presentation is local pain, although intraspinal extension may result in symptoms of cord or nerve root compression.

On MR, giant cell tumors are somewhat lobular and exhibit fairly homogeneous, intermediate signal intensity on T1-weighted images and mixed signal intensity on T2-weighted scans. T2-weighted images frequently demonstrate bright patches within the lesion, thought to represent areas of hemorrhage or cystic degeneration.[2] A low-signal-intensity rim may be present about the lesion on both T1- and T2-weighted scans, secondary to resid-

ual, expanded bone or a sclerotic reaction at the tumor margin.[3] Although rare, a giant cell tumor may cross the joint space.

MR Technique

Enhancement has been noted in giant cell tumors following iodinated contrast administration.[1] In light of the highly vascular nature of these lesions, enhancement with paramagnetic contrast media would be expected. MR provides valuable guidance for surgical resection of vertebral giant cell tumors, on the basis of both ready access to multiplanar imaging and superior depiction of soft tissue extent.

Pitfalls in Image Interpretation

The differential diagnosis for vertebral giant cell tumor includes principally osteoblastoma, aneurysmal bone cyst, and metastatic disease. As illustrated by the present case, other less common lesions may also mimic a giant cell tumor. Compared with giant cell tumors, osteoblastomas are more common in the posterior elements and are generally less lobular in appearance. Aneurysmal bone cysts may appear very similar to giant cell tumors but are typically found in a younger age group. Metastatic disease is differentiated by clinical history and the presence of multiple lesions. Additionally, the extension through the posterior intervertebral disk noted in the current case would be very unusual for metastatic disease.

Clinical References

1. Bidwell JK, Young JWR, Khalluff E. Giant cell tumor of the spine: CT appearance and review of the literature. J Comput Tomog 1987;11:307–311.
2. Tehranzadeh J, Murphy BJ, Mnaymneh W. Giant cell tumor of the proximal tibia: MR and CT appearance. J Comput Assist Tomog 1989;13:282–286.
3. Golfieri R, Baddeley H, Pringle JS, et al. Primary bone tumors: MR morphologic appearance correlated with pathologic examinations. Acta Radiologica 1991;32:290–298.

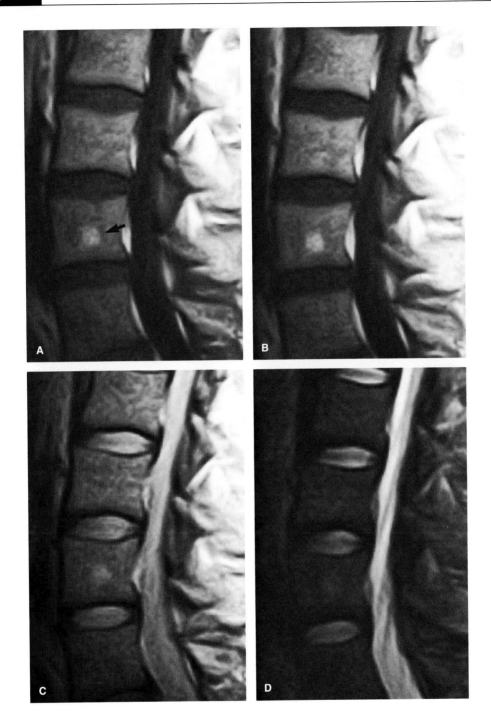

HISTORY

A 39-year-old patient with low back pain

FINDINGS

(A) The precontrast T1-weighted image shows a round area of increased signal (*arrow*) centrally in the L3 vertebral body. (B) The sagittal image following infusion of paramagnetic contrast reveals no change, with no evi-dence of enhancement. The (C) intermediate and (D) heavily T2-weighted images (TE = 30 and 80 respectively) demonstrate continued high signal in the lesion compared with the surrounding marrow. The lesion demonstrates progressively diminished signal intensity with greater T2 and less T1 weighting.

DIAGNOSIS

Focal fat deposits in the vertebral marrow

DISCUSSION

The differential diagnosis of focal high signal intensity on the T1-weighted images includes focal fat deposition, hemangioma, and type II end plate changes. Focal fat deposits should follow fat signal on all imaging sequences, with high T1 signal intensity and progressively decreased signal on the intermediate and heavily T2-weighted images. In contrast, hemangiomas typically demonstrate intermediate to high signal on T2-weighted images. Hemangiomas characteristically demonstrate mild enhancement on postinfusion images, not seen with focal fat. If the vascular component in the hemangioma is small, it may be difficult or impossible to differentiate from focal fat. However, this differentiation is not important because neither of these lesions is of clinical significance. Type II end plate changes are differentiated from focal fat deposition only by their location adjacent to degenerated intervertebral disks, and histologically by the presence of enlarged bony trabeculae. The end plate changes abut the disk space, whereas focal fat is usually located more centrally in the vertebral body.

Focal fatty changes are probably produced by focal ischemia in the marrow and subsequent fatty replacement of the hematopoietic elements. This can occur at any level in the spine and is frequently detectable in multiple vertebrae. The deposits are typically rounded and range up to 15 mm in diameter. Focal fat is more common in older individuals and has been detected in over 90% of MR studies on individuals in the fifth and sixth decades.[1]

MR Technique

Focal fat in the marrow may produce a chemical shift artifact with characteristic signal changes along the frequency encoding axis. Signal from the fat deposits can be diminished by the use of fat-suppression techniques when other significant pathology is suspected.

Clinical Reference

1.   Hajek PC, Baker LL, Goobar JE, et al. Focal fat deposition in axial bone marrow: MR characteristics. Radiology 1987; 162:245–249.

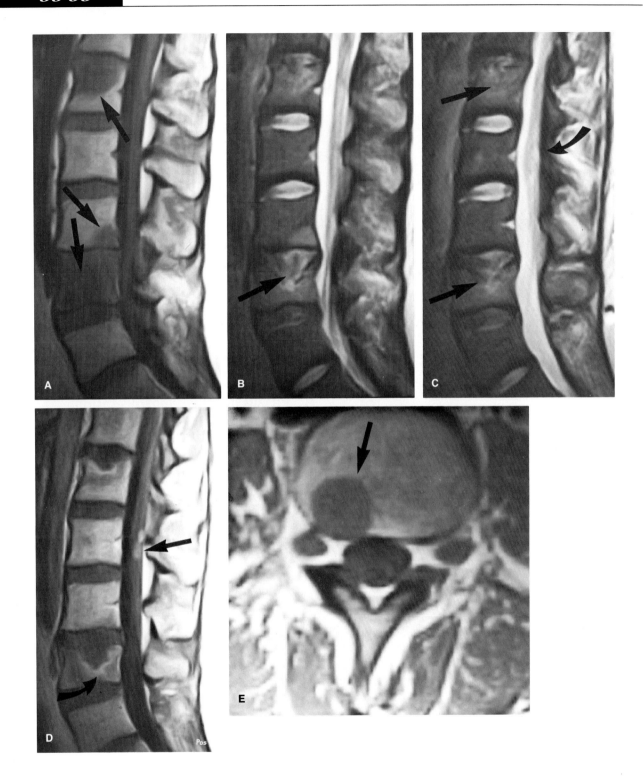

HISTORY

A 35-year-old woman with breast cancer and increasing
pain and numbness in the legs

FINDINGS

(A) The T1-weighted midline sagittal image demonstrates
areas of abnormally decreased signal intensity within the

L1, L3, and L4 vertebral bodies (*arrows*). The superior end plate of L4 is ill defined. The affected regions are of increased signal intensity on the corresponding T2-weighted sagittal view (*B*). On this image, it is apparent that disk material has herniated into the superior end plate of L4 (*arrow*) and that loss of height of the L4 vertebral body has occurred. An additional T2-weighted sagittal image slightly to the left of midline (*C*) redemonstrates the L1 and L4 vertebral lesions (*arrows*). Additionally, a subtle, ill-defined area of increased signal intensity is noted within the spinal canal at the L2 level (*curved arrow*). (*D*) A postinfusion T1-weighted sagittal image at this position reveals nodular enhancement within the spinal canal at L2 (*arrow*). The vertebral body lesions at L1 and L4 are less conspicuous postcontrast, although the deformity of the superior end plate of L4 (*curved arrow*) is more clearly defined. A precontrast T1-weighted axial image at the L3 level (*E*) confirms the small lesion within the posteroinferior L3 vertebral body (*arrow*).

DIAGNOSIS

Vertebral and leptomeningeal metastases

DISCUSSION

The vertebral column is the most common site of skeletal metastatic disease. Lung cancer is the most frequent cause of metastatic disease to the spine. Other common etiologies, in order of decreasing frequency, include breast, prostate, renal cell, and hematologic malignancies.[1]

The classic plain film finding of vertebral metastatic disease is an absent pedicle, and for years many thought that the pedicle was particularly vulnerable to metastatic disease. The conspicuity of an absent pedicle on plain films is primarily because the pedicle is the site of the most compact bone within the vertebra; as a result, loss

of bone in the pedicle is more apparent than in the vertebral body. MR studies have demonstrated that in actuality the vertebral body is almost always the initial site of spinal metastatic disease, with pedicle involvement occurring secondarily.[2] Furthermore, as seen at L3 in the current case, when early vertebral body metastatic disease is present, it is usually the posterior vertebral body that is first affected. This pattern of involvement is secondary to the proximity of the posterior vertebral body to the vertebral venous plexus, making this region of the vertebral body more susceptible to tumor emboli.

MR Technique

Leptomeningeal metastases to the cauda equina, as seen in the current case, may cause clinical symptoms suggestive of conus or severe thecal sac compression. Cord or thecal sac compression is generally well visualized on noncontrast scans. Administration of intravenous contrast, however, is necessary to achieve maximum sensitivity for spinal leptomeningeal disease.[3]

Pitfalls in Image Interpretation

A Schmorl's node may appear as a low-signal-intensity abnormality within the vertebral body on T1-weighted images, and could be confused with a metastatic lesion. Correlation of axial and sagittal views should allow demonstration of the typical location and contiguity to the disk of a Schmorl's node.

Clinical References

1. Ratanatharathorn V, Powers WE. Epidural spinal cord compression from metastatic tumor: diagnosis and guidelines for management. Cancer Treat Rev 1991;18:55–71.
2. Asdourian PL, Weidenbaum M, DeWald RL. The pattern of vertebral involvement in metastatic vertebral breast cancer. Clin Orthop 1990;250:164–170.
3. Jahre C, Sze G. MRI of spinal metastases. Top Magn Reson Imag 1988;1:63–70.

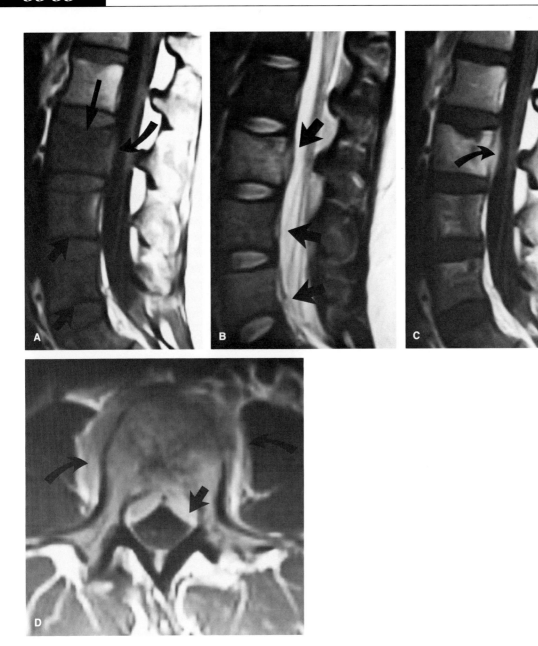

HISTORY

A 34-year-old woman with breast carcinoma and increasing back pain

FINDINGS

(*A*) The T1-weighted midline sagittal image demonstrates abnormally low signal intensity replacing the normal marrow signal of L3, L4, and L5 (*arrows*). A small amount of abnormal soft tissue (*curved arrow*) is noted posterior to the L3 vertebral body. (*B*) On the corresponding T2-weighted sagittal view, the affected vertebral bodies are of abnormal increased signal intensity. (*C*) Following contrast administration, there is inhomogeneous lesion enhancement; thus, the abnormalities within L3, L4, and L5 become less apparent. The soft tissue posterior to L3 (*curved arrow*) also enhances. (*D*) A postinfusion T1-weighted axial view confirms the abnormal enhancing epidural tissue (*arrow*). Moderate deformity of the thecal sac is present bilaterally. Additional enhancing tissue (*curved arrows*) is now apparent surrounding the entire L3 vertebral body.

DIAGNOSIS

Metastatic breast carcinoma with epidural extension at L3

DISCUSSION

Most cases of epidural compression of the spinal cord or cauda equina are a result of a vertebral metastasis with secondary bony collapse or erosion involving the epidural space. Epidural tumor may also result from spread through the neural foramen of paraspinal lesions; this pattern of spread is more common in pediatric patients. Epidural metastases in the absence of adjacent bony or paraspinal lesions are exceedingly rare. Early detection of epidural lesions is critical, as delays in diagnosis result in a much lower likelihood that the patient will recover losses of neurologic function.

Most patients with epidural lesions will have cord or cauda compression at only one level. However, about a fifth of patients will have compression at two or more sites at some time during their disease.[1] MR's superior soft tissue contrast and ability to evaluate large areas of the spine in multiple planes make it ideally suited for evaluation of epidural lesions. Myelography of patients with multilevel disease may require administration of contrast above and below affected levels, and intervening disease is often inaccessible. Additionally, these very ill patients may have considerable difficulty tolerating a myelographic study. Computed tomography cannot detect multiple levels of compression unless extensive scans are performed, and intrathecal contrast is still necessary for clear delineation of the extent of intraspinal disease.

MR Technique

Sagittal images provide a survey of the area of interest in evaluating vertebral metastatic disease. From these images, areas of suspected intraspinal tumor extension can be selected for axial examination. The use of paramagnetic contrast allows excellent delineation of enhancing tumor from a compressed spinal cord or cauda equina.

Pitfalls in Image Interpretation

A disk fragment may mimic epidural metastatic disease on unenhanced MR images. Epidural metastases generally enhance following contrast administration, whereas disk fragments do not. However, if delayed postcontrast scans are obtained, disk fragments may enhance.

Clinical Reference

1. Ratanatharathorn V, Powers WE. Epidural spinal cord compression from metastatic tumor: diagnosis and guidelines for management. Cancer Treat Rev 1991;18:55–71.

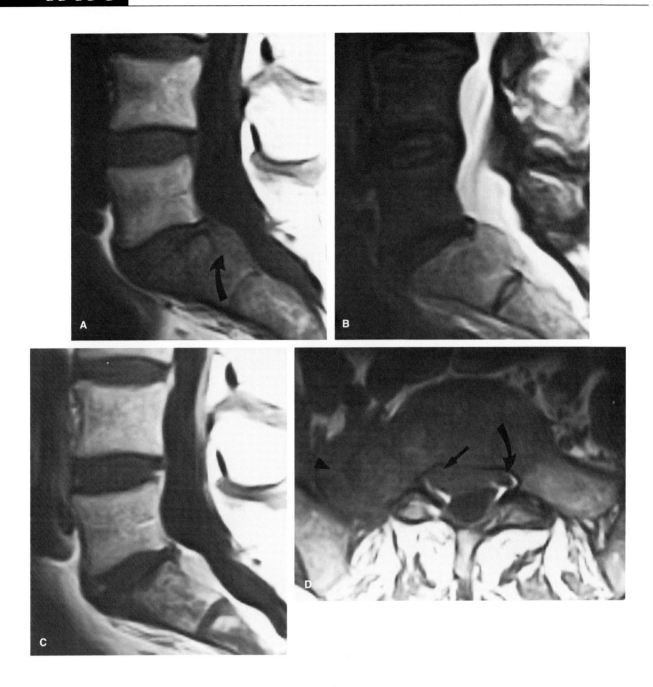

HISTORY

A 79-year-old patient with lung cancer and right S1 radiculopathy

FINDINGS

(A) The T1-weighted midline sagittal image demonstrates abnormally decreased signal intensity throughout the sacrum, most prominent at the S1 level. Epidural soft tissue involvement is apparent at both S1 and S2 (*curved arrow*). These abnormalities are of increased signal intensity on the corresponding T2-weighted sagittal view (*B*). Irregular enhancement of the sacrum is apparent on the postinfusion T1-weighted sagittal image (*C*). The epidural disease demonstrates homogeneous enhancement. (*D*) A precontrast T1-weighted axial image at the S1 level confirms the abnormal signal intensity within the sacrum. The epidural soft tissue mass distorts the thecal sac and severely compresses the right S1 nerve root (*arrow*). The normal left S1 nerve root (*curved arrow*) is unaffected. Expansion of the right sacral ala with paraspinal extension (*arrowhead*) is also apparent.

DIAGNOSIS

Sacral metastases with epidural tumor causing severe right S1 nerve root compression

DISCUSSION

Epidural metastatic disease in the lumbar region may result in symptoms related to compression of the conus or cauda equina. Pain is the initial complaint in the vast majority of cases.[1] In mild cases, such as the current example, compression of a single nerve root may occur, with resultant radiculopathy that mimics the symptoms of disk herniation. More extensive lesions result in lower extremity motor impairment, which usually precedes sensory deficits. Autonomic dysfunction is generally a late finding. However, in rare cases, tumors that compress the conus cause autonomic dysfunction in the absence of motor or sensory deficits.

The mass effect caused by epidural tumor extension has in the past been demonstrated with myelography. The risks of intrathecal contrast, however, are significant. In patients with high-grade block, lumbar puncture below the level of tumor may result in acute neurologic deterioration in as many as 24% of patients.[2] Additionally, lesions above a level of block are easily missed. MR allows accurate, noninvasive evaluation of the extent of epidural lesions. Simultaneous evaluation of the vertebral bodies and paraspinal regions is also obtained.

MR Technique

The extent of epidural tumor may be underestimated on noncontrast MR, as tumor may be poorly delineated from CSF on both T1- and T2-weighted scans. Epidural tumor extending into the spinal canal typically enhances intensely following paramagnetic contrast administration. As a result, the extent and effect of these lesions is often much more conspicuous on postcontrast studies.[2]

Clinical References

1. Ratanatharathorn V, Powers WE. Epidural spinal cord compression from metastatic tumor: diagnosis and guidelines for management. Cancer Treat Rev 1991;18:55–71.
2. Kamholtz R, Sze G. Current imaging in spinal metastatic disease. Semin Oncol 1991;18:158–169.

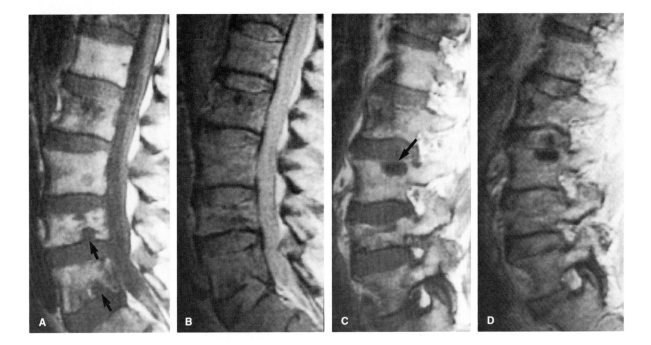

HISTORY

A 64-year-old man with prostate carcinoma and severe low back pain

FINDINGS

(*A*) A T1-weighted midline sagittal image reveals irregularly decreased signal intensity within multiple lumbar vertebral bodies, most prominent at L2. Mild loss of vertebral body height is present at L2 and L4. No significant canal stenosis is identified. Schmorl's nodes are noted at the inferior end plates of L4 and L5 (*arrows*). Following contrast administration, there was subtle enhancement of the vertebral lesions (*images not shown*). The lesions remain low in signal intensity on the intermediate T2-weighted sagittal scan (*B*). A T1-weighted sagittal view to the left of midline (*C*) reveals an additional well-defined low-signal-intensity lesion at the superior end plate of L3 (*arrow*). This abnormality remains very low in signal intensity on the corresponding intermediate T2-weighted view (*D*). A plain lateral radiograph of the lumbar spine (*E*) demonstrates sclerotic lesions within multiple lumbar vertebral bodies. The well-defined lesion at the superior end plate of L3 is clearly visualized.

DIAGNOSIS

Osteoblastic metastases from prostate carcinoma

DISCUSSION

The axial skeleton is the most common site of hematogenous metastatic disease in patients with prostate carcinoma. The metastases are in large part secondary to the rich pelvic venous drainage to the vertebral column through Batson's plexus. MR is an extremely sensitive modality for detection of vertebral lesions in patients with prostate carcinoma. On T1-weighted images, prostate metastases are generally of low signal intensity. T2-weighted signal characteristics are variable and depend on the osteoblastic activity of the metastatic lesions.[1] In lytic prostate metastases, high signal intensity will be present on T2-weighted images. The more common osteoblastic lesions are of low signal intensity on T2-weighted scans, with the degree of low signal intensity related to the extent of the lesion's osteoblastic activity.

The vast majority of osteoblastic metastatic lesions are secondary to prostate carcinoma. Other malignancies that may result in blastic metastases include medulloblastoma, carcinoid tumor, lymphoma, and bladder carcinoma. Lung and breast carcinoma are most often lytic but, particularly when treated, may be osteoblastic.

MR Technique

As many as one fourth of patients with cord compression secondary to prostate carcinoma may present with two sites of compression.[2] Studies limited to one region of the spine may miss significant abnormalities, resulting

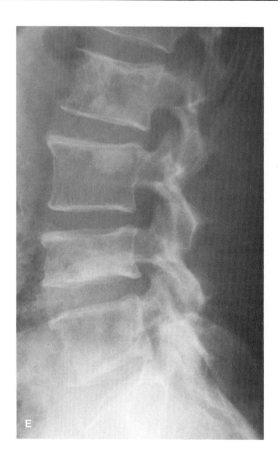

in inadequate or insufficient therapy. In patients with suspected metastatic disease, a sagittal scout view that includes the entire spine (from C1 to the sacrum) is thus very helpful for detecting areas of gross metastatic involvement.

Pitfalls in Image Interpretation

Paget's disease, like prostate carcinoma, is frequently found in elderly males and may even coexist with prostate carcinoma. The sclerotic lesions of Paget's disease may be falsely interpreted as osteoblastic metastases on MR. Plain film demonstration of the typical cortical

thickening of Paget's disease and correlation with the patient's history provide the keys to diagnosis in this situation.

Clinical References

1. McCarthy P, Pollack HM. Imaging of patients with stage D prostatic carcinoma. Urol Clin North Am 1991;18:35–53.
2. Flynn DF, Shipley WU. Management of spinal cord compression secondary to metastatic prostatic carcinoma. Urol Clin North Am 1991;18:145–152.

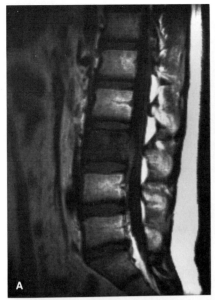
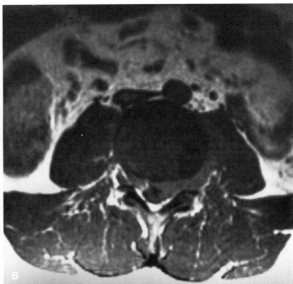
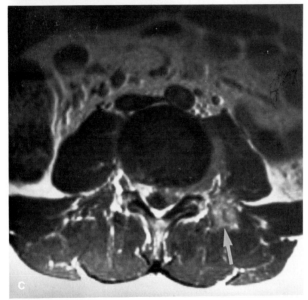

HISTORY

A teenager previously treated for Ewing's sarcoma

FINDINGS

(A) The sagittal T1-weighted image reveals marrow replacement with metastatic tumor at the L3 level. Both (B) the precontrast and (C) the postcontrast T1-weighted axial images well demonstrate extradural tumor extension. However, only the postcontrast image delineates abnormal soft tissue extension into the paraspinal musculature (*arrow*).

DIAGNOSIS

Metastatic Ewing's sarcoma with soft tissue extension

DISCUSSION

Tumor involvement of a vertebral body is best detected on MR by replacement of normal marrow fat. The characteristic low signal intensity of metastatic lesions allows differentiation from high-signal-intensity normal yellow and red marrow on nonenhanced T1-weighted images.[1] Gadolinium chelate-enhanced MR is not routinely used for the evaluation of bony metastatic disease, although enhancement within metastatic lesions can confirm their presence in difficult cases. However, many lesions become isointense to or more difficult to discern from surrounding bone marrow after the administration of contrast.[2] An exception to this rule is the patient with soft tissue neoplastic involvement. Contrast administration in this instance can be valuable for recognition or better delineation of soft tissue tumor extent.

Pitfalls in Image Interpretation

Although contrast administration can be useful for delineation of soft tissue tumor involvement, unenhanced T1-weighted images must be acquired for the evaluation of bony metastatic disease.

Clinical References

1. Runge VM. Contrast media. In: Runge VM. Clinical magnetic resonance imaging. Philadelphia, JB Lippincott, 1990.
2. Sze G, Krol G, Zimmerman RD, Deck MD. Malignant extradural spinal tumors: MR imaging with Gd-DTPA. Radiology 1988;167:217–223.

(A through C from Runge VM. Clinical magnetic resonance imaging. Philadelphia, JB Lippincott, 1990, p. 544.)

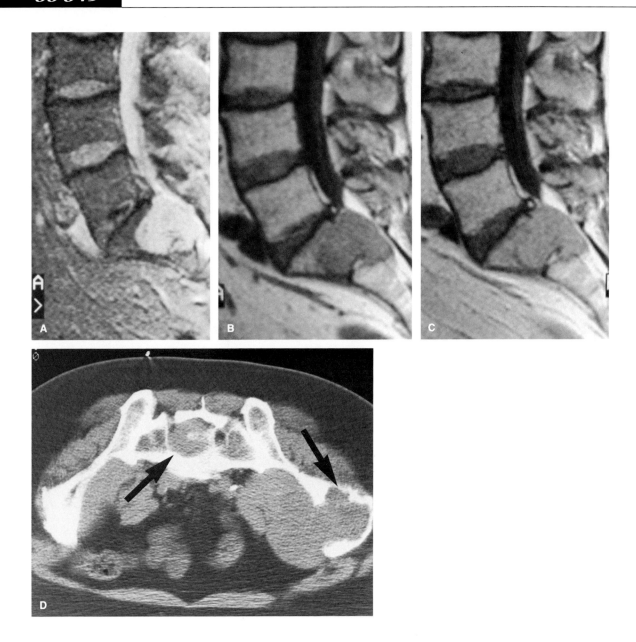

HISTORY

A 64-year-old man with a 2-year history of back and leg pain, now worse

FINDINGS

(A) The sagittal T2-weighted exam reveals a high-signal-intensity lesion involving S1, with expansion posteriorly compromising the terminal spinal canal. The lesion is well seen on (B) precontrast and (C) postcontrast T1-weighted images, being of slightly lower signal intensity than normal marrow precontrast and demonstrating slight but uniform enhancement postcontrast. (D) CT was subsequently performed (in the prone position) for bi-opsy of the S1 lesion. At CT, an additional lesion was noted involving the right iliac crest, with both sites (arrows) biopsied.

DIAGNOSIS

Plasmacytoma

DISCUSSION

Plasma cell myeloma, which includes both multiple my-eloma and plasmacytoma, is a malignant disease of plasma cells. A wide spectrum of disease is seen.[1,2] In some patients, there is a single plasmacytoma of bone, with local radiation therapy curative. Others are asymptomatic, with the disease recognized only by laboratory studies. Some patients with low levels of myeloma protein and no bone lesions demonstrate a stable clinical course with little change over years. In some patients with higher levels of myeloma protein, early chemotherapy can be required to prevent or treat complications.

As previously stated, myeloma can present as a single lesion of bone, a plasmacytoma. Laboratory studies, indicative of disseminated myelomatosis, in these patients may be either positive or negative. Many patients, if followed for years, develop additional lesions; in others, a solitary lesion has been followed for 20 to 30 years without demonstration of dissemination. Solitary plasmacytoma is rare and can simulate radiologically giant cell tumor. The spine and pelvis are common locations. The lesion is typically osteolytic and may be expansile. The diagnosis should be considered in an elderly patient with involvement of a single vertebral body.

Pitfalls in Image Interpretation

The appearance in this case is by no means specific for a plasmacytoma. Much more common, with involvement of two sites, would be metastatic disease from such primaries as breast and lung.

Clinical References

1. Dimopoulos MA, Moulopoulos A, Delasalle K, Alexanian R. Solitary plasmacytoma of bone and asymptomatic multiple myeloma. Hematol Oncol Clin North Am 1992;6:359–369.
2. Moulopoulos LA, Varma DGK, Dimopoulos MA, et al. Multiple myeloma: spinal MR imaging in patients with untreated newly diagnosed disease. Radiology 1992;185:833–840.

(Images courtesy of Clifford Wolf, MD)

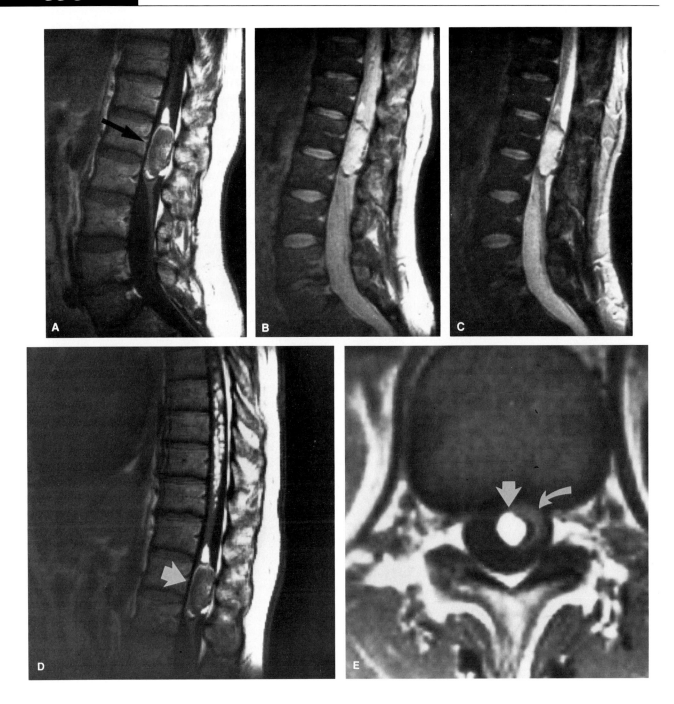

HISTORY

A 43-year-old patient with no prior significant medical history who presents with long tract and conus signs. A hairy patch and dermal sinus were noted on physical exam in the sacral area. Plain films revealed spina bifida.

FINDINGS

Sagittal (A) T1-weighted and (B and C) T2-weighted (TE = 45, 90) images reveal an intramedullary soft tissue mass (*arrow*) at the L1–2 level that contains fatty elements. The cord continues below the mass, with tether-ing demonstrated at the L5 level (*image not shown*). On the sagittal T1-weighted thoracic spine exam (D), the mass (*arrow*) is again noted, with additional intramed-ullary high signal intensity extending superiorly. The ax-ial T1-weighted exam (E) confirms the intramedullary lo-cation of this abnormal high-signal-intensity tissue (*arrow*) in the midthoracic region, with associated cord deformity (*curved arrow*).

DIAGNOSIS

Dermoid tumor, with associated cord tethering and li-pomatous infiltration

DISCUSSION

A clear distinction has not always been made in the literature between dermoid and epidermoid cysts, with reference to both by the term "pearly tumors." Pathologically, dermoid and epidermoid cysts are distinct entities, with the presence of hair or other skin elements defining a dermoid. Both tumor types arise due to inclusion of ectodermal elements at the time of neural groove closure, which occurs between the third and fifth weeks of development. These tumors are so rare that their true incidence cannot be reasonably assessed. In the spinal canal, most lesions occur in the lumbosacral region, with dermoids more common. A dermoid can be either intra- or extramedullary. Dermoids vary in size, and appear as well-defined rounded lesions. The cyst characteristically contains a thick yellow material composed of desquamated epithelium and sebaceous gland secretions. A frequent associated feature is the presence of a dermal sinus. Spinal dysraphism is frequently present. Incomplete surgical resection is often the case, with very slow regrowth.[1]

In the scientific literature, a similar case of an epidermoid tumor with extensive intramedullary fat extending over a long cord segment has been reported.[2] Rupture of such a lesion can result in free fat droplets within the intracranial subarachnoid space, similar to rupture of an intracranial dermoid.

The distinction between dermoid cysts and teratomas, which are composed of tissues from all three germinal layers, has not always been clear in the scientific literature. In the spinal canal, except for the sacrococcygeal form, teratomas are quite rare. Lesions may be solid or cystic. The sacrococcygeal form commonly undergoes malignant transformation.

Clinical References

1. Graham DV, Tampieri D, Villemure JG. Intramedullary dermoid tumor diagnosed with the assistance of MRI. Neurosurgery 1988;23:765–767.
2. Barsi P, Kenez J, Varallyay G, Gergely L. Unusual origin of free subarachnoid fat drops: a ruptured spinal dermoid tumor. Neuroradiology 1992;34:343–344.

(A through E from Runge VM. Clinical magnetic resonance imaging. Philadelphia, JB Lippincott, 1990, pages 251 and 564.)

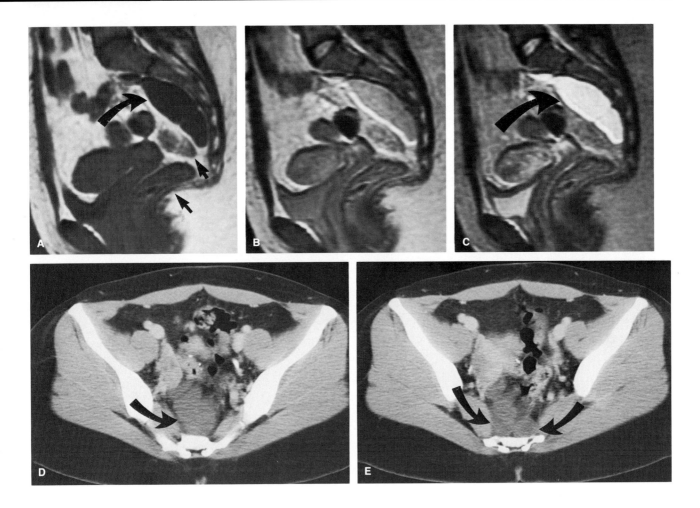

HISTORY

A 25-year-old woman with a pelvic mass on ultrasound

FINDINGS

On the sagittal T1-weighted image just off the midline (A), a low-signal-intensity mass (*curved arrow*) is identified just anterior to the sacrum without an intervening plane of fat. Parts of the rectosigmoid colon and rectum (*short arrows*) are identified anterior to the mass. On the proton density weighted image (B), chemical shift artifact is seen between the mass and anterior fat, identifying its contents as fluid in nature. On the T2-weighted image (C), the lesion (*curved arrow*) is strikingly hyperintense. Septations within the mass give the appearance of haustra. On CT (D and E), the mass (*curved arrows*) is distinct from bowel, with the latter identified by air and dilute contrast. The lesion was surgically resected.

DIAGNOSIS

Lymphangioma

DISCUSSION

Lymphangiomas are believed to be congenital lesions, caused by obstruction of lymphatic drainage.[1] Three fourths occur in the neck (posterior triangle), 20% in the axilla, and 5% elsewhere, including specifically the retroperitoneum. Lesions of the neck and axilla are more common in children under age 2, while those of the retroperitoneum are more common in older children and adults.[2]

Lymphangiomas are usually asymptomatic, with treatment by surgical resection. Accurate definition of the full extent of the lesion is critical, with recurrence common following incomplete resection. Symptoms, when present, may be caused by mass effect or due to rupture, hemorrhage, or infection. The signal intensity characteristics on MR are that of fluid, with low intensity on T1-weighted images (similar to muscle) and high intensity on T2-weighted images. Fibromuscular septae and/or fat may be present between the abnormal fluid spaces. Hemorrhage within the cysts can occur, altering signal intensity characteristics.

Pitfalls in Image Interpretation

Other diagnoses that should be considered in the case of a presacral mass include tailgut cyst, rectal duplication, epidermal cyst, teratoma, and neuroblastoma.[3] Tailgut cyst is a rare congenital lesion, seen as a well-defined retrorectal mass, that is more common in women and typically presents in middle age. A tailgut cyst may be asymptomatic or come to medical atten-

tion due to infection. Duplications are typically anterior to the rectum. With an epidermal cyst (or anal gland cyst) there will usually be an associated cutaneous defect. The lack of a sacral defect or bony invasion makes the diagnosis of a meningocele or chordoma unlikely.

Clinical References

1. Siegel MJ, Glazer HS, St Amour TE, Rosenthal DD. Lymphangiomas in children: MR imaging. Radiology 1989;170:467–470.
2. Hovanessian LJ, Larsen DW, Raval JK, Colletti PM. Retroperitoneal cystic lymphangioma: MR findings. Magn Reson Imag 1990;8:91–93.
3. Johnson AR, Ros PR, Hjermstad BM. Tailgut cyst: diagnosis with CT and sonography. AJR 1986;147:1309–1311.

(Images courtesy of Clifford Wolf, MD)

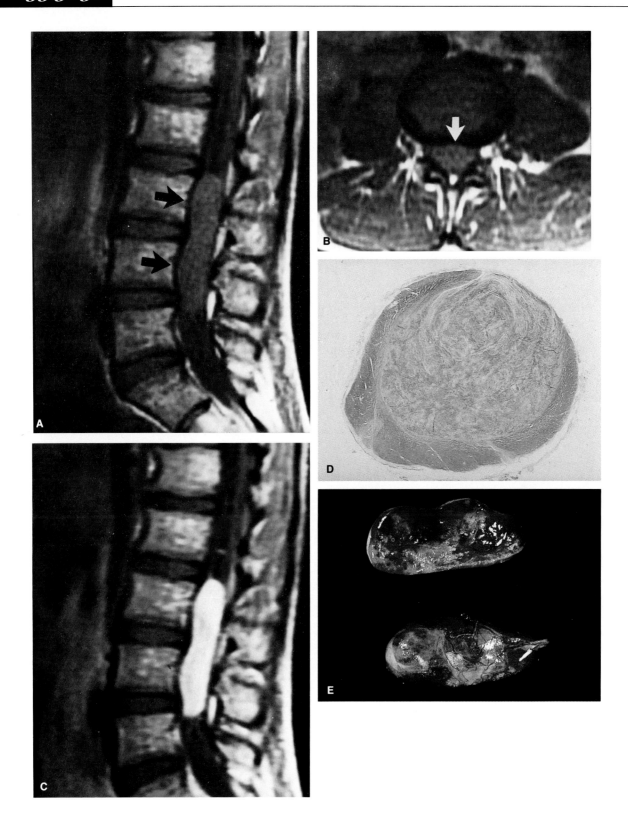

HISTORY

A 21-year-old patient with lower extremity numbness for 3 months and recent onset of back pain

FINDINGS

(*A*) The sagittal T1-weighted scan reveals an intermediate-signal-intensity intradural mass (*arrows*) extending from L2–3 to L4–5. On both sagittal and axial T1-weighted scans (*B*), the lesion (*white arrow in B*) was noted to occupy essentially the entirety of the spinal canal. On the T2-weighted scan (*image not shown*), the mass was hyperintense but of slightly lower signal intensity than cerebrospinal fluid. There is marked uniform enhancement on the postcontrast sagittal T1-weighted scan (*C*). The posterior margins of the L3 and L4 vertebral bodies appear slightly scalloped.

DIAGNOSIS

Ependymoma

DISCUSSION

Ependymomas of the filum terminale often present with nonspecific clinical symptoms, including low back pain and radiculopathy. Moderate motor deficits, sensory loss, and sphincter dysfunction are, however, common.[1] Long-term disease-free survival can be achieved with resection alone using microsurgical technique.[2]

Ependymomas of the spinal canal are slow-growing, well-circumscribed benign tumors. They constitute 60% to 70% of all spinal cord tumors, occur predominantly in the third to sixth decades of life, and in most cases arise in the conus region, cauda equina, or filum terminale. Focal enlargement of the cord on MRI, limited to a few spinal levels, favors the diagnosis of an ependymoma over that of an astrocytoma. Tumoral hemorrhage is not uncommon.

MR Technique

Intravenous contrast administration is suggested in the examination of intramedullary tumors for improved tumor visualization and differentiation of solid tumor from cysts and cord edema.[3] In postoperative ependymomas, contrast enhancement can be critical for the identification of residual tumor and local recurrence.

Pitfalls in Image Interpretation

It is difficult to separate the various intramedullary tumor types on the basis of MR morphology and signal characteristics alone.

Pathologic Correlate

An ependymoma situated at T10 is illustrated in cross section (*D*). This lesion is relatively central in location, due to its origin within the central canal. Spinal ependymomas are usually well demarcated and lend themselves to total resection. Myxopapillary ependymomas (*E*) are a special variant that arise in the lumbosacral region. A common location is the filum terminale, where they form sausage-shaped lesions. Myxopapillary tumors are highly vascular and covered by a delicate capsule that is subject to rupture.

Clinical References

1. Rivierez M, Oueslati S, Philippon J, et al. Ependymoma of the intradural filum terminale in adults, 20 cases. Neurochirurgie 1990;36:96–107.
2. McCormick PC, Torres R, Post KD, Stein BM. Intramedullary ependymoma of the spinal cord. J Neurosurg 1990;72:523–532.
3. Li MH, Holtas S. MR imaging of spinal intramedullary tumors. Acta Radiol 1991;32:505–513.

(A through C from Runge VM. Magnetic resonance imaging: clinical principles. Philadelphia, JB Lippincott, 1992, p. 200. D and E from Okazaki H, Scheithauer B. Atlas of neuropathology. New York, Gower Medical Publishing, 1988, pages 93 and 95. By permission of Mayo Foundation.)

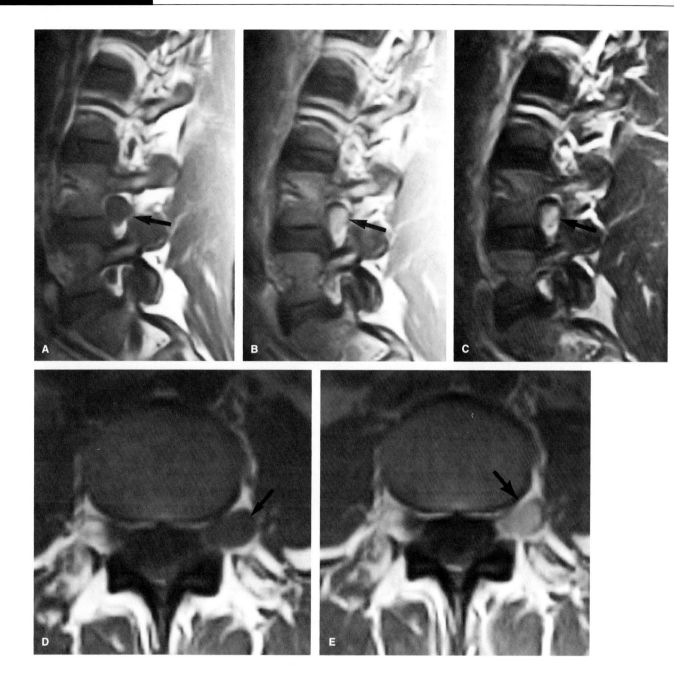

HISTORY

A 36-year-old patient with left leg pain

FINDINGS

(A) The T1-weighted sagittal view to the left of midline reveals a 1.5-cm lesion (*arrow*) within the left L4–5 neural foramen. The lesion is of relatively low signal intensity, similar to that of the intervertebral disks, but appears separate from the L4–5 disk. On the corresponding intermediate and heavily T2-weighted images (*B and C*),

the lesion (*arrows*) is of mildly increased signal intensity relative to the spinal cord. The lesion is fairly homogeneous in appearance on the T2-weighted scan. (*D*) A T1-weighted axial image at the L4–5 level redemonstrates the abnormality (*arrow*), which fills the left neural foramen. (*E*) Following contrast administration, homogeneous enhancement of the abnormality (*arrow*) is identified. The exiting L5 nerve root is well seen on the right but is inapparent on the left. (*F*) An additional postinfusion T1-weighted axial image at the dorsal root ganglia level clearly depicts the right-sided dorsal root ganglion (*arrow*). On the left, the enhancing mass completely envelops the expected location of the ganglion. No normal

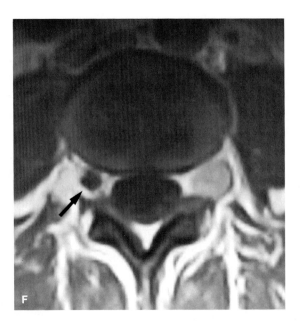

left dorsal root ganglion can be identified. A similar, but much smaller, enhancing nodule was also identified encompassing the exiting left S1 nerve root (*image not shown*).

DIAGNOSIS

Neurofibromas

DISCUSSION

Schwannomas and neurofibromas are the most common tumors to arise from the nerve root sheaths. Although both of these lesions arise primarily from Schwann cells, neurofibromas are distinguished by abundant connective tissue and by the presence of nerve cells within the substance of the tumor.[1] Nerve sheath tumors are most often intradural extramedullary in location, but about a third of cases are purely extradural, and mixed intradural extradural lesions are not uncommon. Intramedullary nerve sheath tumors are very rare.

Distinguishing schwannomas and neurofibromas may be difficult, but several characteristics are helpful in the differential. Schwannomas are typically solitary lesions, while multiplicity of lesions strongly favors neurofibromas. Neurofibromas tend to infiltrate the nerve during growth, thus resulting in fusiform enlargement of the nerve. Schwannomas, in contrast, usually are well-circumscribed lesions located eccentrically in relation to the nerve.[2] The nerve of origin is frequently engulfed by neurofibromas, whereas in schwannomas, the displaced nerve often remains evident. In the current case, a presumptive diagnosis of neurofibroma was made based on the multiplicity of lesions and the pattern of involvement of the lumbar nerve roots.

Additional imaging characteristics, although less reliable, may be helpful in the differentiation of the two lesions. Schwannomas are often very heterogeneous on T2-weighted images. Neurofibromas are generally more homogeneous in appearance, although in some cases the lesions are of higher signal intensity peripherally than centrally. This "target" appearance on T2-weighted images is thought to be characteristic of neurofibromas.[2,3]

MR Technique

Axial images are critical for demonstrating the relationship of nerve sheath tumors to the exiting lumbar nerve roots. Possible canal compromise is also best assessed in the axial plane.

Pitfalls in Image Interpretation

Foraminal neurofibromas are occasionally mistaken for lateral disk herniations. The signal characteristics of a neurofibroma may be very similar to those of an extruded disk herniation. The characteristic enhancement of neurofibromas, however, allows confident discrimination between these two lesions. Herniated disk material should not enhance.

Clinical References

1. Russel DS, Rubinstein LJ. Pathology of tumors of the nervous system, 5th ed. Baltimore, Williams & Wilkins, 1989:560.
2. Suh JS, Abenoza P, Galloway HR, et al. Peripheral (extracranial) nerve tumors: correlation of MR imaging and histologic findings. Radiology 1992;183:341–346.
3. Sakai F, Sone S, Kiyono K. Intrathoracic neurogenic tumors: MR-pathologic correlation. AJR 1992;159:279–283.

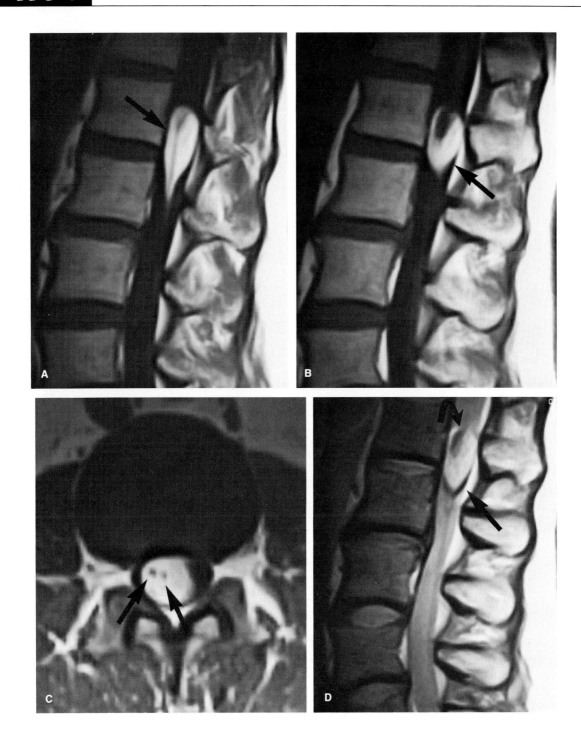

HISTORY

A 48-year-old man with difficulty voiding

FINDINGS

(*A and B*) T1-weighted sagittal images demonstrate a large, hyperintense mass (*arrow*) that fills the spinal canal at the L1–2 level. The spinal cord terminates within the upper portion of the abnormality. The conus is nor-

mal in position and lies at T12–L1. (*C*) The T1-weighted axial view reveals the intradural location of the mass. Lumbosacral nerve roots (*arrows*) appear to course through the lesion. The abnormality remains hyperintense on (*D*) the intermediate T2-weighted sagittal image, but is of lower signal intensity on (*E*) the second echo. A dark border (*arrow*) at the inferior margin of the lesion and a high-signal-intensity rim (*curved arrow*) at the superior aspect of the lesion are compatible with chemical shift artifact. The mass, with its accompanying chemical shift artifact, is again noted on the fast spin echo

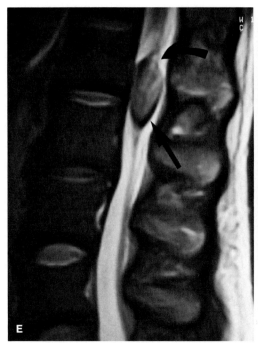

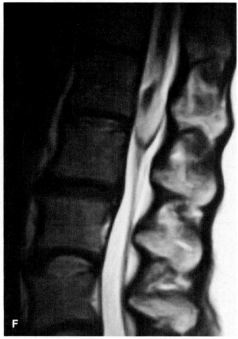

T2-weighted view (*F*). The lesion is isointense to fat on all imaging sequences.

DIAGNOSIS

Intradural lipoma

DISCUSSION

Intradural lipomas lie at the more benign end of a developmental spectrum that includes lipomyelomeningocele.[1] With intradural lipomas, the dorsal spinal defect, if present, is minimal. Intradural lipomas and lipomyelomeningocele are thought to result from premature separation of cutaneous ectoderm from neuroectoderm.[2] As a result, surrounding mesenchyme enters the exposed neural tube, impeding closure of the neural folds. This mesenchyme later differentiates into fat.

Intradural lipomas account for about 1% of intraspinal tumors and are somewhat more common in men. Intradural lipomas are most common in the thoracic region but may arise anywhere along the spinal axis, including the conus and cauda equina. Most of these lesions occur along the dorsal aspect of the cord, but about a fourth are located laterally or anterolaterally. Patients with cervical or thoracic intradural lipomas often present with a history of slowly developing, ascending monoparesis or paraparesis with cutaneous and deep sensory loss. Lumbosacral intradural lipomas may cause flaccid lower extremity paresis and sphincter dysfunction.[2]

MR Technique

Sagittal MR scans allow accurate assessment of the cephalocaudal extent of intradural lipomas. Axial images are vital for demonstration of the relationship of the lesions to the spinal cord and nerve roots, thus providing valuable surgical guidance.

Pitfalls in Image Interpretation

An intradural lipoma, because of its high signal intensity on T1-weighted images, may be confused with hemorrhage by the novice MR reader. The fat characteristics of a lipoma, however, are reliably diagnosed by noting the isointensity of the lesion to fat on all sequences and by noting the presence of chemical shift artifact. This artifact occurs only at fat–water interfaces in the frequency encoding direction, and appears as artifactual high signal intensity at one margin of a lipoma and signal void at the other margin.[3]

Clinical References

1. Naidich TP, McLone DG, Mutluer S. A new understanding of dorsal dysraphism with lipoma (lipomyeloschisis): radiologic evaluation and surgical correction. AJR 1983; 140:1065–1078.
2. Barkovich AJ, Naidich TP. Congenital anomalies of the spine. In: Norman D, ed. Contemporary neuroimaging. Volume I: pediatric neuroimaging. New York, Raven Press, 1990:227–271.
3. DeLaPaz RL. Congenital anomalies of the spine and spinal cord. In: Enzmann DR, DeLaPaz RL, Rubin JR, eds. Magnetic resonance of the spine. St. Louis, CV Mosby, 1990;176–236.

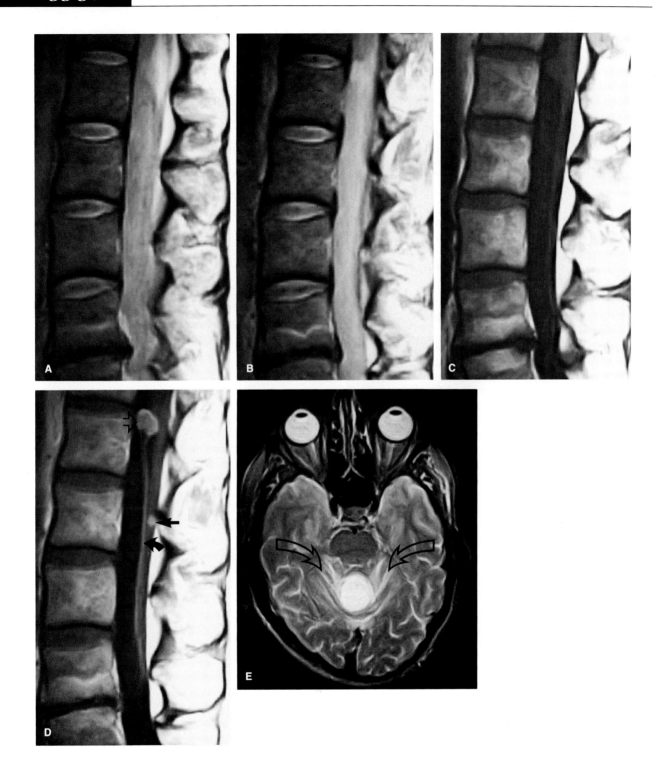

HISTORY

An elderly man with lung carcinoma

FINDINGS

On the midline sagittal T2-weighted (TE = 45) image (A), abnormal high signal intensity is noted within the conus, consistent with edema. On the adjacent T2-weighted section (B), a large intradural extramedullary mass is just barely evident, anterior to the conus. The lesion is slightly hyperintense relative to cerebrospinal fluid (CSF). The abnormality is also visualized, although poorly, on the precontrast T1-weighted scan (C). Following intravenous contrast administration (D), the lesion demonstrates intense enhancement (*open arrow*). Other findings noted on the postcontrast scan include abnormal

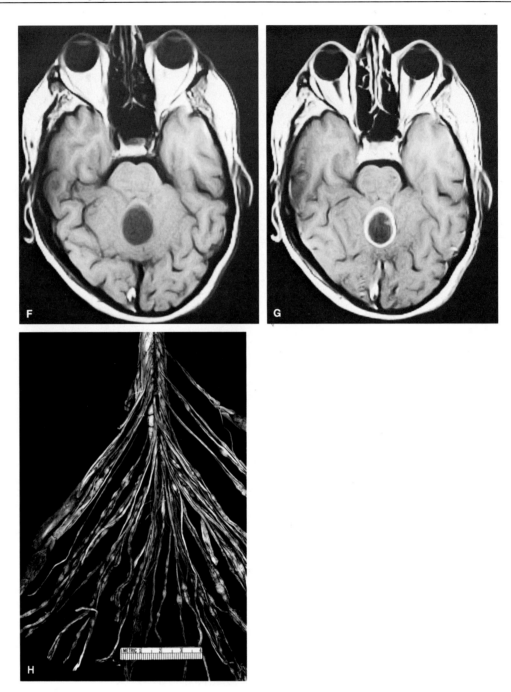

enhancement of a nerve root (*curved arrow*) caudal to the mass and identification of a second lesion (*arrow*) at the L2 level.

A head MR exam, obtained 7 months earlier, is also presented. On (*E*) the T2-weighted scan (TE = 90), a midline cyst with signal intensity slightly greater than CSF is noted in the superior cerebellum. There is a small amount of surrounding brain edema (*curved open arrows*). On the precontrast T1-weighted scan (*F*), the signal intensity characteristics of the lesion (slightly higher than CSF) are also not consistent with CSF. Postcontrast, abnormal rim enhancement is noted (*G*).

DIAGNOSIS

Lumbar leptomeningeal metastases

DISCUSSION

This patient presented initially with a solitary cystic cerebellar metastasis and subsequently developed leptomeningeal metastatic disease. About one third of patients with parenchymal metastases to the brain or spine will also have leptomeningeal disease. The latter is not surprising, given the high incidence of breast and lung carcinoma. These two tumor types not uncommonly metastasize to the brain, and are also the most common visceral neoplasms to spread to the subarachnoid space. Leptomeningeal involvement per se portends a particularly poor prognosis. In this patient, at L1 there was intramedullary tumor extension with resultant cord edema, in addition to the leptomeningeal involvement. The varied appearance of leptomeningeal metastatic disease, which can include both large and small nodules, intramedullary extension, and coating of nerve roots, is also illustrated.[1]

Pathologic Correlate

In meningeal carcinomatosis, there is diffuse involvement of the leptomeninges, most often along the posterior aspect of the cord or its termination. Spinal nerve dysfunction commonly results due to direct nerve infiltration. Deposits can be discrete and nodular, although this appearance is less common, as illustrated here along the cauda equina in a specimen from a patient with disseminated lung carcinoma (H).

Clinical Reference

1. Yousem DM, Patrone PM, Grossman RI. Leptomeningeal metastases: MR evaluation. J Comput Assist Tomog 1990; 14:255–261.

(H *from Okazaki H, Scheithauer B. Atlas of neuropathology. New York, Gower Medical Publishing, 1988, p. 168. By permission of Mayo Foundation.)*

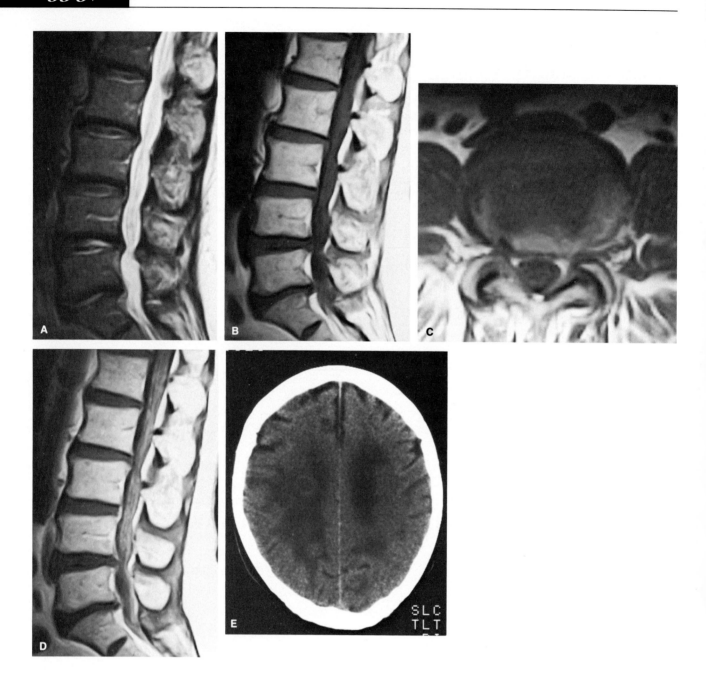

HISTORY

An 83-year-old man with small cell carcinoma of the lung diagnosed 1 year ago and treated with chemotherapy and radiation therapy. The patient is now admitted with a 2-week history of low back pain, leg weakness, and mental status changes.

FINDINGS

On (A) the sagittal T2-weighted exam, there is diffuse disk degeneration, with narrowing of the thecal sac at multiple levels on the basis of degenerative disease. The lumbar nerves within the thecal sac appear prominent on both the T2-weighted and (B) precontrast T1-weighted images. A suggestion of nerve root thickening is also raised on the basis of (C) the axial precontrast T1-weighted exam. (D) Postcontrast, there is striking abnormal enhancement of the cauda equina and lumbar nerves, which now also appear somewhat "beaded." (E) Head CT reveals two lesions surrounded by edema, consistent with intracranial metastatic disease.

DIAGNOSIS

Lumbar leptomeningeal metastases

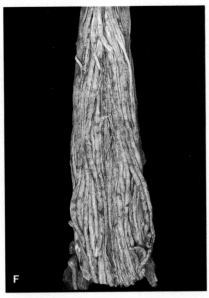

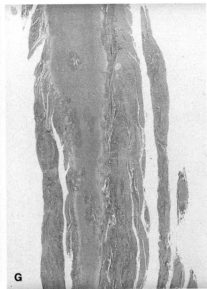

DISCUSSION

Contrast-enhanced MR has been shown to be superior to CT myelography for the diagnosis of leptomeningeal metastases, with MR being the procedure of choice. Although CT myelography may reveal only nonspecific cord irregularity or intrathecal filling defects, contrast-enhanced MR provides specific recognition of small tumor nodules and thickening of nerve roots due to tumor seeding.[1]

MR Technique

Two types of leptomeningeal metastases are poorly depicted on unenhanced MR—small tumor nodules and coating of nerve roots with tumor cells. Both are well seen against a background of normal CSF and uninvolved nerve structures on scans following IV gadolinium chelate administration, mandating contrast use when leptomeningeal seeding is suspected.

Pitfalls in Image Interpretation

In immunosuppressed patients, an infectious meningitis can mimic neoplastic leptomeningeal involvement on MR. For example, cytomegalovirus polyradiculopathy in AIDS has been reported with diffuse leptomeningeal enhancement.[2] Other etiologies, including tuberculosis, toxoplasmosis, and syphilis, should be considered. Sarcoidosis can also produce a similar picture, although cord involvement typically dominates.

Pathologic Correlate

In (*F*) a fresh pathologic specimen, leptomeningeal metastases to the cauda equina (a favorite location) from lung carcinoma are well seen as red hypervascular patches along the nerve roots. (*G*) The cut section more readily shows the extent of infiltration, with ropy thickening of nerve roots by blue-stained tumor cells. Note also the tumor extent within the cord.

Clinical References

1. Blews DE, Wang H, Kumar AJ, et al. Intradural spinal metastases in pediatric patients with primary intracranial neoplasms: Gd-DTPA-enhanced MR vs CT myelography. J Comput Assist Tomogr 1990;14:730–735.
2. Bazan C, Jackson C, Jinkins JR, Barohn RJ. Gadolinium-enhanced MRI in a case of cytomegalovirus polyradiculopathy. Neurology 1991;41:1522.

(F and G from Okazaki H, Scheithauer B. Atlas of neuropathology. New York, Gower Medical Publishing, 1988, p. 168. By permission of Mayo Foundation.)

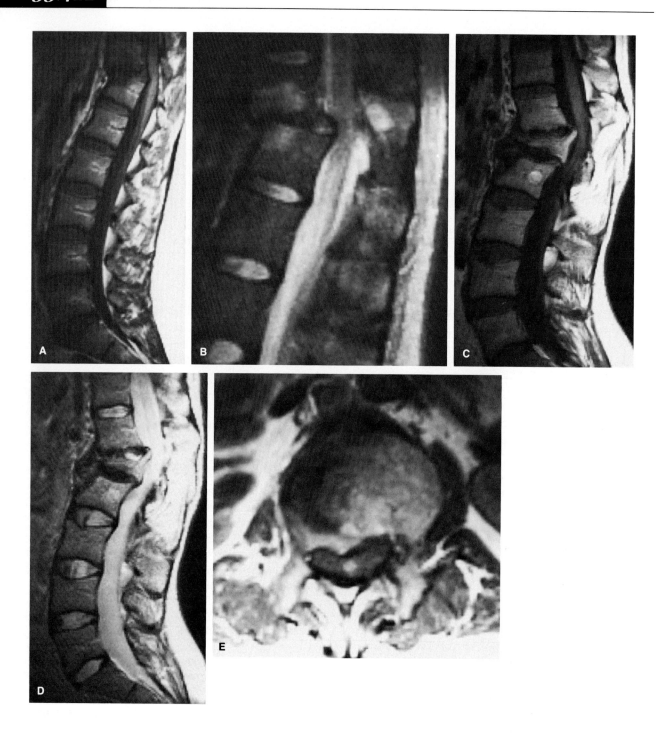

HISTORY

Two patients, the first (who, incidentally, has no neurologic deficit) 5 months and the second several years after a motor vehicle accident

FINDINGS

Patient #1: Sagittal (*A*) T1-weighted and (*B*) T2-weighted images of the lumbar spine are presented. There is an-

terior subluxation of T11 on T12, with relative preservation of the shape of each vertebral body. There is also abnormal low signal intensity on the T1-weighted exam, with corresponding high signal intensity on the T2-weighted exam, anteriorly in the inferior portion of T11 and the superior portion of T12, compatible with marrow edema. There is impingement on the lower cord by the T11–12 disk and the superior posterior margin of T12.

Patient #2: Sagittal (*C*) T1-weighted and (*D*) T2-weighted images, together with (*E*) an axial T1-weighted image at the L1 level, are presented. L1 is wedge-shaped, with abnormal anterior angulation of the spine at this level. The marrow signal intensity is normal. Secondary degenerative changes (osteophytes) are prominent at T12–L1 and L1–L2. There is impingement on the thecal sac and the tip of the conus by bone, best seen on the axial exam. There was also abnormal hyperintensity within the conus on the T2-weighted exam, consistent with myelomalacia, although this is not well seen in *D*.

DIAGNOSIS

Flexion injury (motor vehicle accident)

DISCUSSION

The term "seat belt syndrome" refers to a combination of abdominal and skeletal injuries that occur with seat belt use.[1] The following discussion will be restricted to skeletal injuries. With a two-point restraint system (lap belt), the principal injury is lumbar spine fracture (the Chance fracture). With a three-point restraint system (lap belt and shoulder strap), fractures of the clavicles, ribs, sternum, and lumbar spine can occur. Fractures of the lumbar spine are less common with three-point restraint systems than with a lap belt alone.

With an unrestrained occupant, flexion occurs with the fulcrum centered on the posterior half of the vertebral body. This results in compression of the anterior vertebral body, and in more severe injury distraction of posterior elements. Moderate forces result in stable in-juries, while severe forces can result in unstable injuries, with neurologic deficits common. Such injuries occur most commonly at the thoracolumbar junction. The injury in the first patient could be considered to be of this type, with the anterior compression only mild in degree, a not uncommon situation. The injury in the second patient is also likely of this type, although more severe in degree, and at a lower level than typical.

With a restrained occupant, especially those wearing lap belts alone, characteristic fractures (the Chance fracture and variations thereof) are reported principally at L2 and L3. There may be involvement of one or two levels. Because the fulcrum is centered on the anterior abdominal wall (due to the seat belt), this is a distraction injury, with typically little or no anterior vertebral body compression. Neurologic deficits are uncommon. With a purely ligamentous disruption, the injury may be unstable and have only subtle radiographic findings: a mild increase in the disk space height posteriorly, splaying of the spinous processes, and widening of the facet joints.

With the widespread implementation of three-point restraint systems, Chance fractures have become less common. They are still seen, however, particularly in children and back-seat passengers; in both of these situations the use of a lap belt alone is still common.

Clinical Reference

1. Hayes CW, Conway WF, Walsh JW, et al. Seat belt injuries: radiologic findings and clinical correlation. Radiographics 1991;11:23–26.

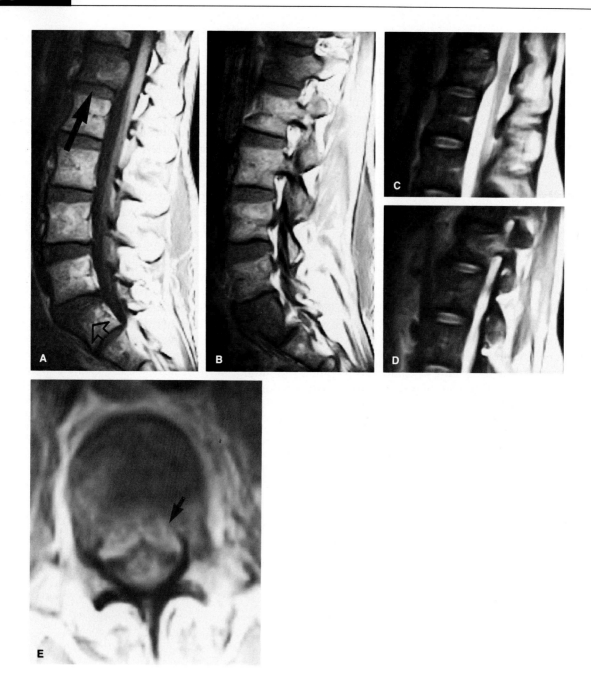

HISTORY

A 51-year-old man with lung carcinoma and sudden onset of back pain

FINDINGS

(*A*) The sagittal T1-weighted image demonstrates mild compression of the L1 vertebral body (*arrow*) with a somewhat indistinct superior end plate. Abnormal low signal intensity fills the L1 body, with extension poste-

riorly into the spinal canal causing moderate canal narrowing. Low signal intensity is also revealed in the S1 body (*open arrow*). (*B*) A right parasagittal T1-weighted image reveals extension of the abnormal low signal into the L1 pedicle with no significant expansion of the pedicle. Mild depression of the superior L1 end plate is present. Greater involvement is seen in the S1 vertebra, which is nearly filled by low signal intensity. (*C*) The midline sagittal fast spin echo T2-weighted image displays heterogeneous high signal intensity in the L1 vertebra, including the posterior extension. (*D*) The right parasagittal T2-weighted image again exhibits abnormal signal extending into the right L1 pedicle. (*E*) The T1-weighted axial image following intravenous contrast administration displays enhancement of the epidural lesion (*arrow*), but no definite compression of the spinal cord. Patchy enhancement is also present in the L1 body and pedicles.

DIAGNOSIS

Pathologic compression fracture

DISCUSSION

Vertebral compression fractures may result from abnormal stresses or weakening of the vertebral body. In the absence of trauma, the MR reader must have a high suspicion for an underlying process that caused weakening of the vertebral body. In some patients with abnormal sensation or insensitivity to pain, the traumatic event may not be easily recalled. Many vertebral body fractures in the elderly are simply due to insufficiency of the bone secondary to senile osteoporosis. This is especially common in postmenopausal females. However, pathologic fractures due to metastatic disease are also more common in the elderly population. The lack of an appropriate history may complicate the clinical diagnosis of a pathologic fracture.

The most common primary neoplasms to metastasize to the bone are lung, breast, prostate, and renal carcinoma. The primary lesion may be unknown at the time of the MR study. Important points that can be obtained from the MR study are the extent of the tumor within the vertebrae, presence of cortical breakthrough or epidural extension of tumor, canal stenosis, spinal cord compression, or additional metastatic lesions. These items may determine appropriate staging and guide the surgeon or radiation therapist in the selection of an appropriate treatment technique.

A pathologic fracture typically has low T1 and high T2 signal intensity, with complete replacement of the marrow signal.[1] Most acute benign compression fractures also have areas of low T1 and high T2 signal, but reveal areas of preserved normal marrow signal within the vertebral body. Old benign compression fractures demonstrate marrow signal isointense to the normal vertebrae. Patients with metastatic disease frequently have multiple lesions in the vertebral bodies and posterior neural arches. Metastatic lesions in the vertebrae typically appear as focal rounded to oval areas of decreased signal intensity on the precontrast T1-weighted images. The metastases may show extension into the pedicles. On images obtained after administration of intravenous contrast, the metastases show variable enhancement. On postcontrast T1-weighted images, they often become less obvious or may even become indistinguishable from the normal fatty marrow signal.

Conventional spin echo techniques can differentiate most compression fractures as benign or pathologic. Chemical shift techniques provide images with selective fat or water signal. Chemical shift images evaluate the degree of marrow replacement better than conventional spin echo images. Fat-suppression techniques demonstrate to better advantage the marrow edema that accompanies benign compression fractures and metastatic lesions.[2] Images obtained after administration of intravenous contrast may reveal enhancement of the epidural extension of the lesion and allow detection of meningeal carcinomatosis.

MR Technique

Neoplastic involvement of the vertebral bone marrow is most easily detected on sagittal precontrast T1-weighted images, which usually demonstrate low-signal-intensity lesions infiltrating the high T1 signal of the fatty marrow. These images also provide comparison with the normal marrow signal of other vertebrae.

Pitfalls in Image Interpretation

Metastatic lesions are more difficult to detect in younger patients who have low T1 signal in their normal hematopoietic vertebral marrow. Diffuse marrow processes also make the diagnosis of an underlying marrow abnormality difficult due to the lack of normal marrow for comparison.

Clinical References

1. Yuh WTC, Zachar CK, Barloon TJ, et al. Vertebral compression fractures: distinction between benign and malignant causes with MR imaging. Radiology 1989;172:215–218.
2. Baker LL, Goodman SB, Perkash I, et al. Benign versus pathologic compression fractures of vertebral bodies: assessment with conventional spin-echo, chemical-shift, and STIR MR imaging. Radiology 1990;174:495–502.

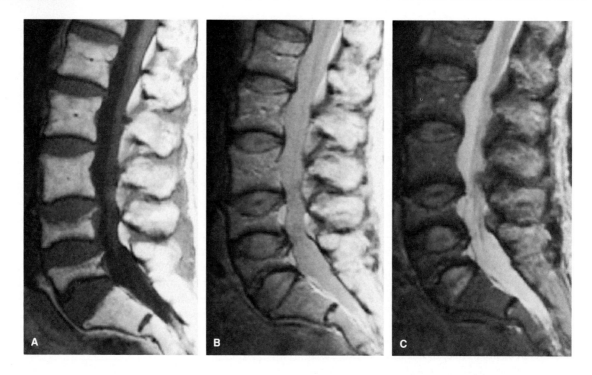

HISTORY

A 72-year-old white woman with osteoporosis

FINDINGS

Midline sagittal images through the lumbar spine demonstrate compression fractures of the L4 and L5 vertebral bodies. The T1-weighted image (*A*) manifests relatively uniform high signal intensity in the aforementioned vertebral bodies, a finding consistent with the preservation of normal bone marrow. The (*B*) first and (*C*) second echoes from the T2-weighted exam also demonstrate homogeneous signal, which is isointense to the remainder of the vertebral bodies.

DIAGNOSIS

Senile osteoporotic compression fractures

DISCUSSION

Normal marrow has a characteristic signal intensity and appearance on both T1- and T2-weighted sequences, which can be used to distinguish benign from malignant processes. Most nontraumatic benign deformities demonstrate normal bone marrow throughout the compressed vertebral body.[1] The remainder of these fractures typically have incompletely preserved bone marrow in a regular pattern. Malignant compression deformities, on the other hand, most often show complete or near-complete replacement of normal bone marrow. This malignant replacement is most easily identified as abnormal hypointensity on T1-weighted images. Less often, malignant vertebral body fractures demonstrate incomplete replacement, with an irregular pattern of replacement. Presumably, the vast majority of vertebral metastases do not result in a compression fracture until infiltration of the entire body has occurred, secondary to structural bone weakening. In benign nontraumatic compression fractures, the bone marrow is displaced following the vector of the compression force rather than the random replacement seen with a malignant process. This results in a more predictable bone marrow pattern with a smooth margin. Conversely, when marrow is incompletely lost secondary to a malignant process, areas of replacement are typically ill-defined and irregular. Secondary features that favor a benign fracture include other coexisting benign fractures and intact pedicles. Secondary features that favor malignancy include the presence of other metastatic lesions, pedicle involvement, and intact vertebral disks, together with the absence of vertebral body fragmentation.

In difficult cases, contrast enhancement with a gadolinium chelate may be helpful. Metastatic compression fractures should show contrast enhancement, while osteoporotic compression fractures may not.[2]

Clinical References

1. Yuh WT, Zachar CK, Barloon TJ, et al. Vertebral compression fractures: distinction between benign and malignant causes with MR imaging. Radiology 1989;172:215–218.
2. Nelson KL, Runge VM. Lumbar spine. In: Runge VM. Clinical magnetic resonance imaging. Philadelphia, JB Lippincott, 1990.

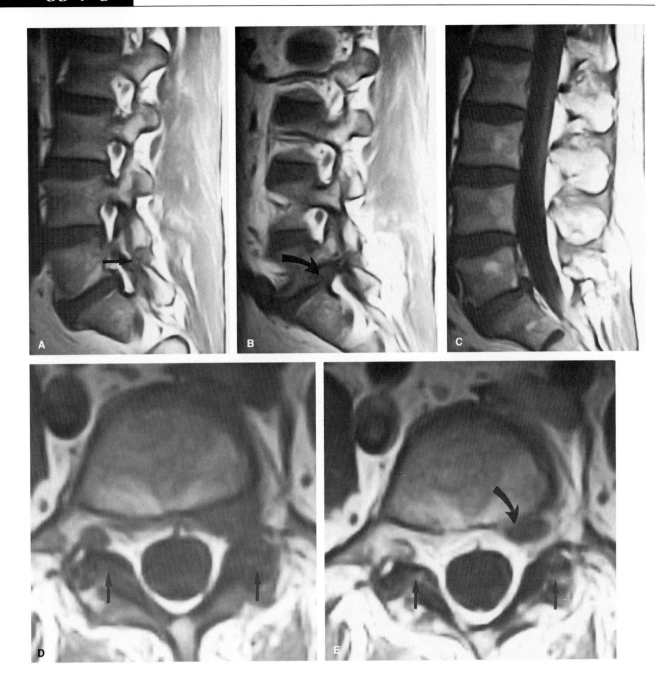

HISTORY

A 46-year-old patient with low back and left leg pain

FINDINGS

(A) A right parasagittal T1-weighted image shows a break (*arrow*) in the right pars interarticularis at the L5 level. The neural foramen is narrowed due to the anterior listhesis. (B) A left parasagittal section also demonstrates a left L5 pars interarticularis defect. A disk herniation is also present at the L5–S1 level extending into the left neural foramen (*curved arrow*). (C) The midline sagittal T1-weighted image shows grade I spondylolisthesis at the L5–S1 level. The axial (D) preinfusion and (E) postinfusion T1-weighted images show bilateral irregular pseudoarthroses (*arrows*) in the posterior ring of L5 corresponding with the pars defects. Mild enhancement of the pseudoarthroses is present, presumably due to volume averaging with the surrounding soft tissues. The disk herniation is again demonstrated (*curved arrow*). The axial

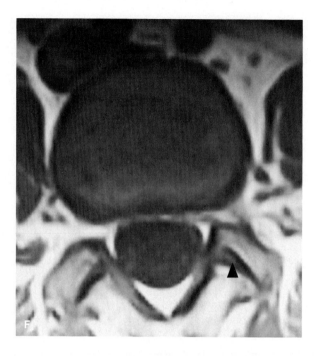

image at the level of the articular facets at L4–5 (*F*) demonstrates the appearance of the normal facet joints (*arrowhead*) above the pars defects.

DIAGNOSIS

Bilateral spondylolysis with spondylolisthesis

DISCUSSION

Spondylolysis is defined as an interruption in the pars interarticularis. The abnormality may be unilateral or bilateral. Spondylosis at the L5–S1 level is most often bilateral.[1] Bilateral interruption of the vertebral ring allows abnormal motion of the posterior elements in relation to the adjacent vertebrae. The superior and inferior facets at the involved level move independently. The superior facet remains attached to the vertebral body through the pedicle. The inferior facet continues to articulate with the superior facets of the more inferior level.

Spondylolisthesis refers to displacement or slippage of a vertebral body in relation to the adjacent body. The cause of the spondylolisthesis may be a congenital, post-traumatic, or iatrogenic disruption of the posterior elements, degenerative changes in the facet joints, an isthmic type with a defect in the pars interarticularis, or a pathologic process. This case is an example of isthmic spondylolisthesis with a defect in the pars interarticularis or spondylolysis. This most frequently results in anterior listhesis of the superior vertebral body on the body below. Anterior displacement causes narrowing of the neural foramina and may result in nerve root impinge-

ment. The neural foramen assumes a more horizontal orientation on the sagittal views.

MR Technique

Similar to CT, the site of the interruption in the pars interarticularis may be difficult to visualize on axial images. A discontinuity is usually best visualized on the parasagittal images, where it is nearly perpendicular to the imaging plane.[2]

Pitfalls in Image Interpretation

Various appearances of the pars may mimic spondylolysis on the sagittal images. These include volume averaging of the adjacent facet joint or facet spur, previous facet surgery, or sclerosis of the pars interarticularis due to benign or malignant disease.[3] Selected axial images through the level of the intervertebral disks can skip the abnormality. The defect may also be obscured on axial images due to volume averaging of the obliquely oriented abnormality.

Clinical References

1. Jinkins JR, Matthes JC, Sener RN, et al. Spondylolysis, spondylolisthesis, and associated nerve root entrapment in the lumbar spine: MR evaluation. AJR 1992;159:799–803.
2. Grenier N, Kressel HY, Schiebler ML, Grossman RI. Isthmic spondylolysis of the lumbar spine: MR imaging at 1.5 T. Radiology 1989;170:489–493.
3. Johnson DW, Farnum GN, Latchaw RE, Erba SM. MR imaging of the pars interarticularis. AJR 1989;152:327–332.

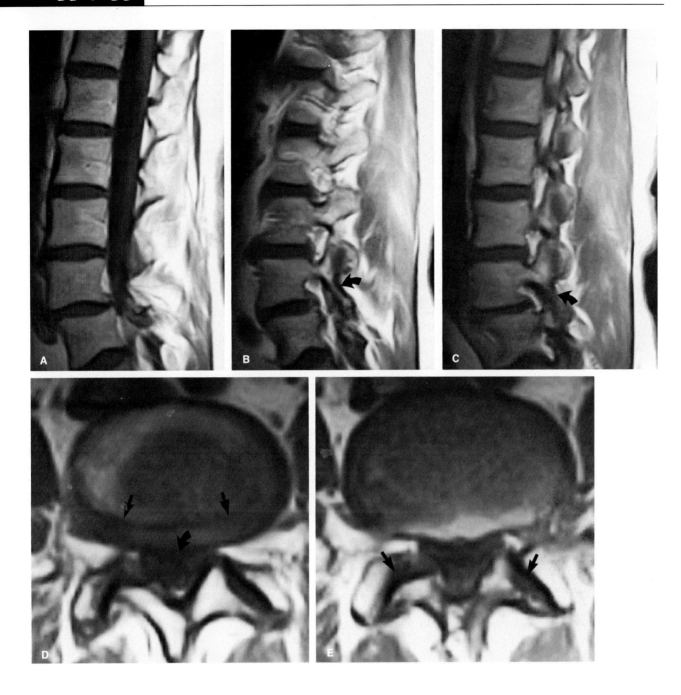

HISTORY

A 67-year-old patient with low back pain and right leg pain and weakness

FINDINGS

(A) The midline sagittal T1-weighted image demonstrates grade I anterior listhesis of L4 on L5. The (B) right and (C) left parasagittal T1-weighted images show the pars interarticularis to be intact bilaterally at L4 (*curved arrows*). This excludes spondylolysis as a cause of the spondylolisthesis. These images reveal facet degeneration with irregular, narrowed facet joints. The axial T1-weighted image through the L4–5 disk (D) again demonstrates the anterior listhesis of L4 on L5. The curvilinear low signal intensity of the posterior L4 body (*arrows*) projects 7 mm anterior to the posterior L5 body (*curved arrow*). The axial T1-weighted image through the L4–5 facets (E) reveals irregularity and narrowing of the facet joints (*arrows*). Compare these to the axial image (F) showing normal smooth facets at L3–4.

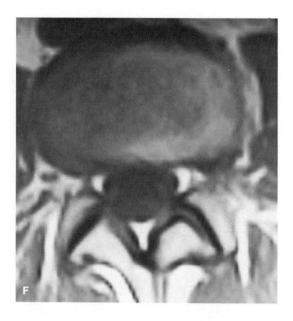

DIAGNOSIS

Spondylolisthesis secondary to degenerative facet changes

DISCUSSION

Spondylolisthesis is forward subluxation or slippage of a vertebral body in relation to the adjacent, more inferior level. The major categories of spondylolisthesis in adults are isthmic, traumatic, iatrogenic, and degenerative. Isthmic spondylolisthesis refers to subluxation due to bilateral pars interarticularis defects, which are thought to result from repeated stress.[1]

The severity of the listhesis is graded in relation to the anteroposterior dimension of the vertebral body. In the grading scale by Meyerding, grade I reflects subluxation measuring up to one fourth of the vertebral body, grade II the second quarter, grade III the third quarter, and grade IV the last quarter.[2]

Degenerative spondylolisthesis results from degeneration and narrowing of the facet joints. This occurs most commonly in the lower lumbar spine at L4–5 and L5–S1. The presence of intact pars interarticularis and other posterior elements differentiates this from other forms of spondylolisthesis. The listhesis is best evaluated on sagittal images. The parasagittal MR images through the facets demonstrate irregular low signal intensity, representing sclerosis and hypertrophic change. Axial T1- and T2-weighted images confirm the low signal intensity, narrowing, and irregularity of the facets.

With degenerative spondylolisthesis, the midline sagittal image demonstrates narrowing of the spinal canal because the posterior elements are contiguous with and therefore move anteriorly with the displaced vertebral body. With isthmic spondylolisthesis, the canal is typically not narrowed because the posterior elements move independently from the vertebral body. The adjacent posterior elements remain in alignment and the spinal canal may widen in this situation. The degenerative changes and foraminal narrowing with irritation of the nerve roots can produce symptoms in these patients.

MR Technique

Evaluation of the intact pars interarticularis is best performed on parasagittal images of the spine. The superior facet, pars interarticularis, and inferior facet are seen in continuity due to minimal obliquity in this plane.[3]

Pitfalls in Image Interpretation

Although MR is not an ideal modality for the study of bone abnormalities, contiguity of the pars can be evaluated with MR. A definitive diagnosis is not always possible, but a questionable abnormality can be further evaluated by plain films or CT.

Clinical References

1. Grenier N, Kressel HY, Schiebler ML, Grossman RI. Isthmic spondylolysis of the lumbar spine: MR imaging at 1.5 T. Radiology 1989;170:489–493.
2. Meyerding HW. Low backache and sciatic pain associated with spondylolisthesis and protruded intervertebral disc. J Bone Joint Surg 1941;23:461–470.
3. Johnson DW, Farnum GN, Latchaw RE, Erba SM. MR imaging of the pars interarticularis. AJR 1989;152:327–332.

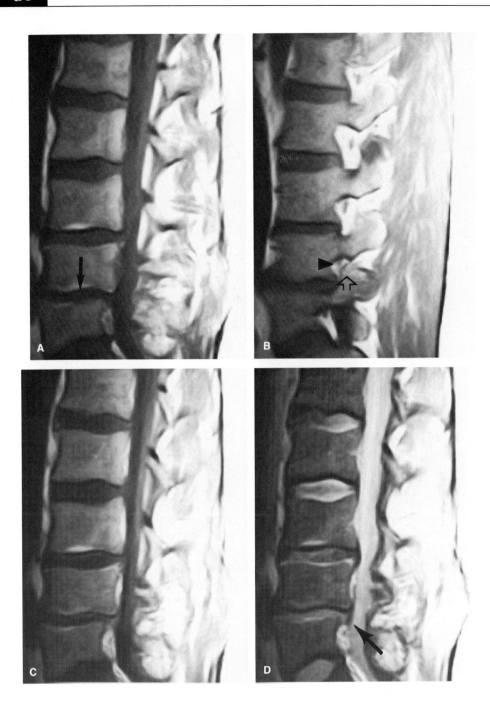

HISTORY

A 41-year-old patient with previous L4–5 disk surgery and recurrent low back and bilateral leg pain

FINDINGS

(A) The sagittal T1-weighted image near the midline shows disk space narrowing at L4–5 (*arrow*) and mild posterior displacement of the L4 vertebra on L5. A small disk bulge is present at L4–5 with thin, high-signal-intensity type II end plate changes adjacent to the L4–5 and L3–4 disks. (B) The parasagittal T1-weighted image through the right neural foramina demonstrates narrowing of the L4–5 bony foramen. The inferior aspect of the foramen is obliterated by the posteriorly displaced L4 vertebra and the associated disk bulge. The right L4 nerve root (*arrowhead*) exits under the L4 pedicle with a small amount of surrounding high-signal-intensity fat. The superior articular facet of L5 (*open arrow*) has moved in an anterior and cephalad direction, obliterating the inferior

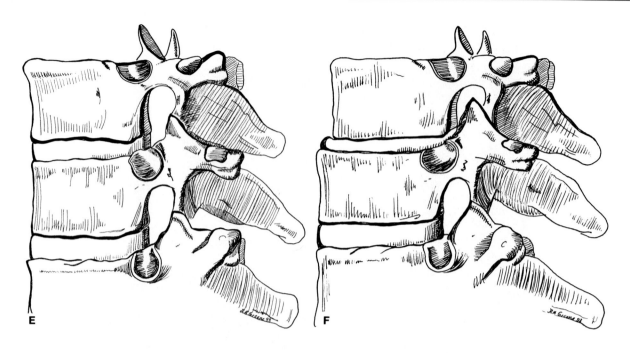

E   F

aspect and narrowing the superior aspect of the neural foramen. (*C*) The sagittal T1-weighted image following intravenous contrast administration confirms the retrolisthesis at L4–5. The malalignment is more easily detected due to enhancement of the epidural venous plexus along the posterior margin of the vertebrae. (*D*) The comparable sagittal intermediate T2-weighted image again demonstrates the malalignment at L4–5 (*arrow*). Decreased T2 signal intensity in the L3–4 and L4–5 disks is due to disk degeneration at these levels.

DIAGNOSIS

Retrolisthesis

DISCUSSION

Retrolisthesis is posterior subluxation of a vertebral body relative to the adjacent inferior vertebral body. This is usually secondary to disk degeneration with relative preservation of the facet joints. Narrowing of the disk space, combined with the effects of gravity and contraction of the paraspinous muscles, results in settling of the entire vertebra, including the facet joints. Inferior displacement of the facets causes posterior displacement of the more superior vertebral body due to the anterosuperior-to-posteroinferior slant of the facet joints. For clarity, line drawings have been included. The normal alignment of vertebral bodies in the lumbar spine is illustrated

in *E*. *F* shows disk space narrowing and retrolisthesis, with resultant foraminal narrowing.

Disk space narrowing may be caused by acute or repeated trauma, degeneration of the disk associated with aging, disk surgery, or chemolysis. Retrolisthesis following disk surgery or chemolysis with resultant foraminal narrowing and nerve root impingement is one cause of the failed back syndrome.

Retrolisthesis is most common in the lumbar and cervical spine. The L3–4 and L4–5 levels are the most commonly affected, accounting for about 85% of cases in the lumbar region.[1] Frequently, a disk bulge and spurs are also present at the affected level. This may cause mild narrowing of the spinal canal, but central canal stenosis is uncommon with retrolisthesis. Neural foraminal narrowing, however, is a common complication of retrolisthesis. Decreased height of the intervertebral disk space decreases the height of the foramen. The accompanying disk bulge narrows the anteroposterior dimension of the foramen. The anteroposterior dimension is further narrowed by posterior displacement of the more cephalad vertebral body combined with relative superior and anterior displacement of the superior articular facet of the more caudad vertebra. The foraminal narrowing can be significant and produce nerve root compression.

MR Technique

Retrolisthesis is best evaluated on midline sagittal images.

Pitfalls in Image Interpretation

Due to abnormal vertebral body alignment, axial images through the level of the interposed disk may give the impression of a disk herniation or large disk bulge. This must be verified on the sagittal images because a mild disk bulge is frequently present and, combined with the offset of the vertebrae, is accentuated on the axial image.

Clinical Reference

1. Rothman SLG, Glenn WV, Kerber CW. Multiplanar CT in the evaluation of degenerative spondylolisthesis. A review of 150 cases. Comput Radiol 1985;9:223–232.

(E and F courtesy of Robin Avison, RT)

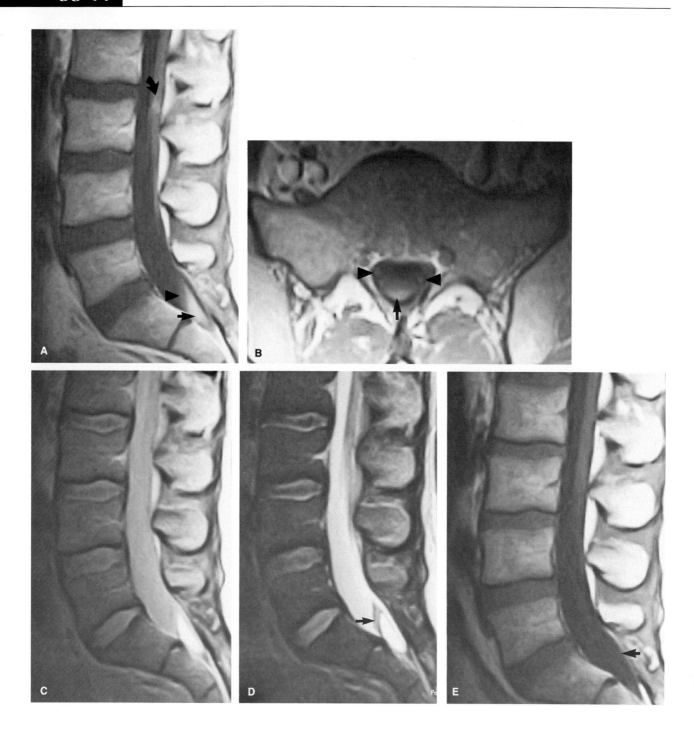

HISTORY

A patient with a cerebrospinal fluid (CSF) leak, recently treated with a blood patch

FINDINGS

(A) The sagittal T1-weighted image shows high-signal-intensity material (*arrow*) layering in the dependent portion of the thecal sac in the sacral region, representing subarachnoid blood. The more anterior portion of the blood (*arrowhead*), which is adjacent to the low-signal-intensity CSF, is of intermediate signal intensity. A focal area of high signal intensity is seen within the cauda equina at the upper L3 level (*curved arrow*). This focal high signal was slightly more apparent on the postcontrast image (*A*) than on the precontrast image (*image not shown*). (*B*) The axial T1-weighted image through S1 demonstrates high-signal-intensity (*arrow*) layering in the posterior thecal sac. A few nerve roots (*arrowheads*) are seen along the lateral margins of the thecal sac. The sagittal (*C*) intermediate and (*D*) heavily T2-weighted images again show high-signal-intensity material (*arrow*) in the distal thecal sac. The more anterior portion of the material shows progressively decreasing signal intensity with increased T2 weighting. No signal abnormality is detected in the cauda equina on the T2-weighted images. (*E*) The sagittal T1-weighted image obtained 2 months later shows complete resolution of the subarachnoid blood with CSF filling the distal thecal sac (*arrow*).

DIAGNOSIS

Subarachnoid blood secondary to a blood patch procedure

DISCUSSION

Subarachnoid blood is an uncommon finding in spine imaging. The location of the blood must be differentiated from blood within the subdural or epidural space. Subarachnoid blood follows the contour of the spinal cord and canal contents. The most common cause of subarachnoid blood in the spine is an aneurysm or arteriovenous malformation of the cord. Spinal subarachnoid blood may also originate from a cerebral source.

On MR imaging, subarachnoid blood may cause slightly increased signal intensity of the CSF. The increased signal within the thecal sac can obscure the spinal cord and nerve roots, which are usually profiled by the normal, low-signal-intensity CSF. As in this case, the blood may layer out in the dependent areas of the subarachnoid space. In vitro experiments with blood and CSF mixtures simulating subarachnoid hemorrhage revealed increased attenuation on computed tomography (CT) and decreased T1 relaxation time on MR as the concentration of blood in the mixture increased. Highly concentrated subarachnoid blood is high attenuation on CT and therefore easily differentiated from the brain. On MR, acute subarachnoid hemorrhage has signal intensity nearly isointense to the underlying brain and is less noticeable.[1] Subacute subarachnoid blood, appearing a few days to a week after the initial bleed, demonstrates high T1 signal intensity due to the presence of methemoglobin and is easily detected by MR.[2]

A blood patch is an injection of autologous blood into the epidural space, most commonly performed by an anesthesiologist. Following lumbar puncture, patients can develop a severe headache. In such patients, with a continuing CSF leak, one therapeutic option is a blood patch. The CSF leak from the puncture of the dural sac is sealed by tamponade from the mass effect of the epidural blood, or from the inflammatory response incited by the blood products, which results in fibrosis and scarring. Subarachnoid blood has been reported on MR studies following the procedure.[3]

Pitfalls in Image Interpretation

Subarachnoid blood can have high signal intensity on T1-weighted images. This should not be confused with other possible materials in the subarachnoid space, such as Pantopaque or lipomatous tissue. A negative CT or MR study does not rule out subarachnoid blood, and in patients with a high clinical suspicion for a bleed, lumbar puncture must be performed.[1]

Clinical References

1. Chakeres DW, Bryan RN. Acute subarachnoid hemorrhage: in vitro comparison of MRI and CT. AJNR 1986;7:223–228.
2. Bradley WG, Schmidt PG. Effect of methemoglobin formation on the MR appearance of subarachnoid hemorrhage. Radiology 1985;156:99–103.
3. Griffiths AG, Beards SC, Jackson A, Horsman EL. Visualization of extradural blood patch for post-lumbar puncture headache by MRI. Br J Anaesth 1993;70:223–225.

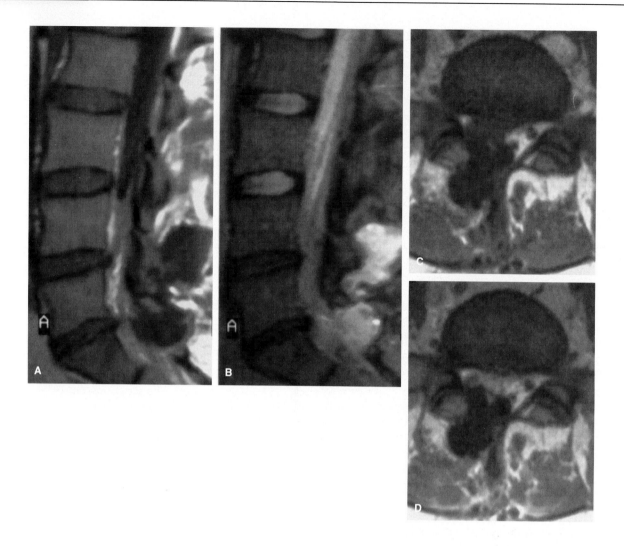

HISTORY

A 36-year-old woman with persistent back pain after a right L5 laminectomy

FINDINGS

Sagittal (*A*) T1-weighted and (*B*) heavily T2-weighted images reveal a fluid collection in the posterior soft tissues. The fluid has low signal intensity on T1-weighted images, with a progressive increase in signal intensity noted on intermediate (*image not shown*) and heavily T2-weighted images, following the signal characteristics of cerebrospinal fluid. The collection is contiguous with the thecal sac. Noncontrast (*C*) and postinfusion (*D*) axial T1-weighted images confirm the contiguity between the fluid and the subarachnoid space through a right laminectomy. Enhancing tissue within the spinal canal and surrounding the right S1 nerve root is consistent with postoperative granulation tissue.

DIAGNOSIS

Pseudomeningocele

DISCUSSION

A fluid-filled pseudomeningocele sac occurs through a tear in the dura. There may also be a tear in the arachnoid membrane. If the arachnoid layer is intact, the fluid is contained within the subarachnoid space. More commonly, there is also a tear of the arachnoid membrane. In this instance, the fluid is loculated within the posterior soft tissues. A variable-sized channel communicates with the subarachnoid space. This channel is typically visualized in at least one plane on MR. The fluid may also extend into the subcutaneous tissues and may be palpable.

Postlaminectomy meningoceles, or pseudomeningoceles, are most common in the cervical spine, usually following surgery at the occiput and upper cervical spine. Pseudomeningoceles are rare complications in the lumbar spine following diskectomy, and may produce symptoms similar to the patient's preoperative symptoms, including back pain or radicular pain.[1] Symptoms can be due to incorporation of nerve roots into the pseudomeningocele.

Pitfalls in Image Interpretation

The differential diagnosis in this instance includes a postoperative (encapsulated) fluid collection, which may be sterile or infected.

Clinical Reference

1. Lee KS, Hardy IM. Postlaminectomy lumbar pseudomeningocele: report of four cases. Neurosurgery 1992;30:111–114.

(Images courtesy of Mitchell A. Brack, MD)

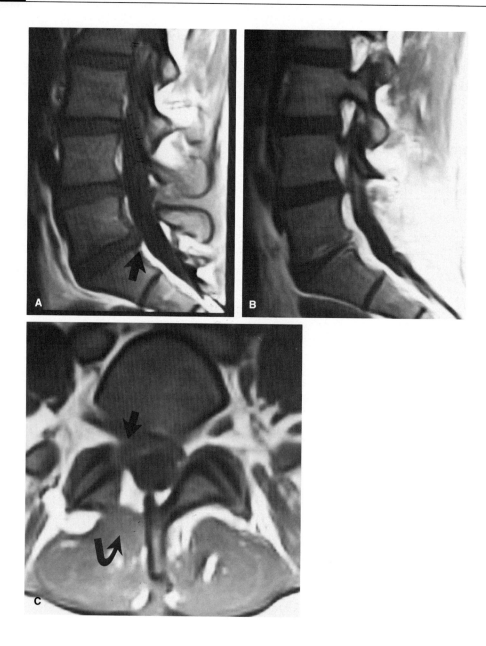

HISTORY

Continued right leg pain 2 months status post-diskectomy at L5–S1

FINDINGS

(A) The T1-weighted sagittal image to the right of midline reveals abnormal soft tissue (*arrow*) projecting posterior to the L5–S1 intervertebral disk. (B) Following contrast administration, this tissue enhances intensely. Enhancement is also apparent both superior and inferior to the the L5–S1 intervertebral disk, at the interface with the adjacent vertebral bodies. (C) A T1-weighted axial view at the inferior L5 level confirms the abnormal soft tissue (*arrow*) in the ventral epidural space. The right laminectomy defect (*curved arrow*) is also apparent. (D and E) Postinfusion T1-weighted axial views demonstrate enhancement of the extradural soft tissue; the abnormal enhancement extends around the right S1 nerve root. Enhancement within soft tissue at the laminectomy site (*arrow*), of the right S1 nerve root (*arrowheads*), and within the right paraspinal musculature (*curved arrows*) is also noted. Mild enhancement of the facet joints, right greater than left, is identified on *D*.

DIAGNOSIS

Epidural fibrosis at L5–S1 and demonstration of normal areas of postoperative contrast enhancement

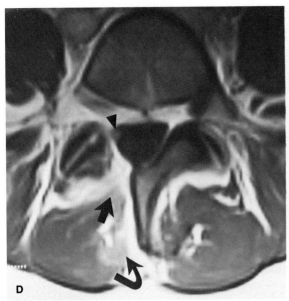
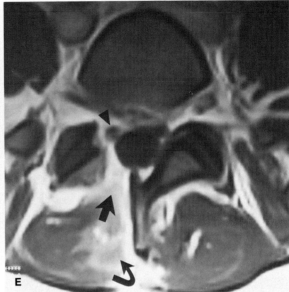

DISCUSSION

The anterior epidural mass in this case, which appears contiguous to the L5–S1 disk, would be suspicious for a recurrent disk herniation on the precontrast scans. The homogeneous enhancement of the abnormality, however, allows confident diagnosis of the lesion as epidural fibrosis.[1]

In the months following lumbar disk surgery, many types of enhancement are commonly identifiable.[2] In about one third of cases, enhancement is identified in the decompressed nerve root, often extending superiorly toward the conus. Enhancement of the facet joints and the paraspinal musculature on the side of surgery is seen in the vast majority of patients in the immediate postoperative state. Facet enhancement may be unilateral or bilateral, and may extend to levels above and below the laminectomy site. This enhancement is presumably related to surgical manipulation. In the ensuing months after surgery, enhancement of the decompressed nerve root, the facet joints, and the paraspinal muscles decreases. At the 6-month interval, nerve root enhancement should resolve and paraspinal muscle enhancement should be minimal. Facet enhancement, however, will persist in over half of patients. An additional form of enhancement seen in this case is that noted within the intervertebral disk at the operated level. This form of enhancement is not uncommon and may manifest as diffuse, mottled, or as in this case linear enhancement near the end plates at the site of surgery.[1]

Pitfalls in Image Interpretation

In the immediate postoperative period, anterior epidural mass effect at the surgical site is seen consistently, even in asymptomatic patients. This finding may be secondary to normal postoperative hematoma, which later progresses to epidural fibrosis.[2] The area of mass effect may not enhance or may enhance only peripherally, and is thus quite difficult to distinguish from a recurrent or residual disk herniation. Although the typical homogeneous enhancement of epidural fibrosis may be seen earlier, it is not consistently present until about 3 months after surgery.

Clinical References

1. Hueftle MG, Modic MT, Ross JS, et al. Lumbar spine: postoperative MR imaging with Gd-DTPA. Radiology 1988; 167:817–824.
2. Boden SD, Davis DO, Dina TS, et al. Contrast-enhanced MR imaging performed after successful lumbar disk surgery: prospective study. Radiology 1992:182:59–64.

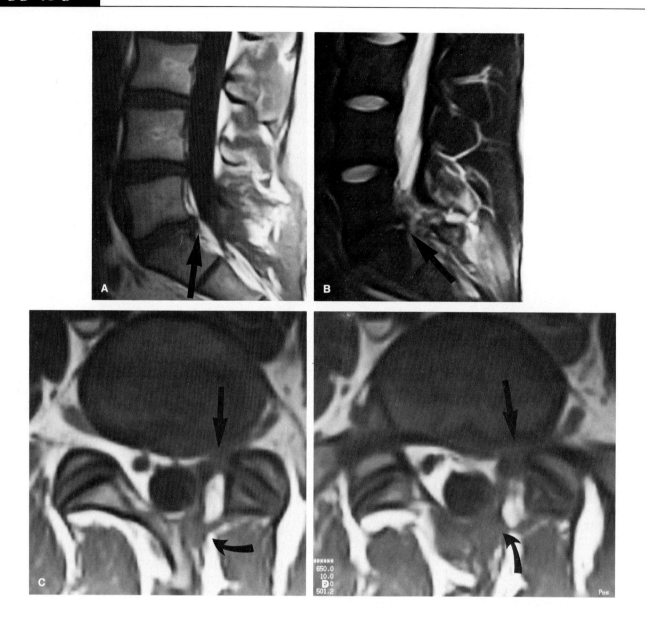

HISTORY

Persistent low back and left leg pain 2 months after diskectomy for a left paracentral disk herniation at L5–S1

FINDINGS

(A) A sagittal T1-weighted image to the left of midline
demonstrates a moderate anterior extradural defect (*arrow*) at L5–S1. This abnormality (*arrow*) is mildly hyperintense to the intervertebral disk on the T2-weighted sagittal view (*B*). T1-weighted axial images (*C and D*)
confirm the abnormal soft tissue (*arrows*) posterior to
the left side of the L5–S1 intervertebral disk and surrounding the left S1 nerve root. Additional abnormal soft
tissue (*curved arrows*) is seen in the region of the left

laminectomy. Following contrast administration (*E*), homogeneous enhancement of the abnormal soft tissue (*arrows*) is noted. Enhancing tissue envelops the left S1
nerve root (*curved arrow*).

DIAGNOSIS

Postdiskectomy fibrosis at L5–S1

DISCUSSION

Persistent pain following lumbar disk surgery is a common cause of disability in middle-aged adults. The leading causes of persistent postoperative pain include spondylolisthesis, lateral or central spinal stenosis, adhesive

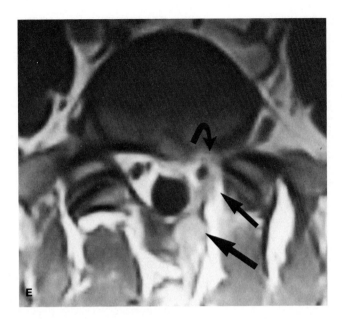

arachnoiditis, recurrent disk herniation, and epidural fibrosis.[1] The imaging characteristics of spondylolisthesis, spinal stenosis, and arachnoiditis are well known and can be demonstrated with a variety of modalities. The differentiation of recurrent disk herniation from epidural fibrosis, however, is more problematic. From both a clinical and imaging standpoint, this determination is critical. Patients may benefit from additional surgery in cases of recurrent disk herniation. Individuals with excessive intraspinal scar formation are often in considerable pain, but reoperation simply results in additional scarring.

Although CT and myelography are useful in the evaluation of bony stenosis and arachnoiditis, the superior soft tissue contrast of MR is necessary for differentiation of epidural fibrosis and scar.[2,3] The early enhancement of epidural fibrosis is the key determinant in distinguishing scar from recurrent disk herniation. Other imaging features that have been described as favoring fibrosis include the absence of mass effect, increased signal intensity on T2-weighted images, and noncontiguity to the disk space.[2] These findings, however, are often unreliable in the differentiation of disk and scar.[3]

MR Technique

When imaging the postoperative spine, axial images should always be selected through the surgical site. We routinely acquire 3-mm T1-weighted axial images before and after administration of paramagnetic contrast.

The use of thin slices reduces volume averaging artifacts. With thicker slices, partial volume effects may obscure small disk fragments, due to enhancement of surrounding granulation tissue or epidural venous plexus.

Pitfalls in Image Interpretation

In many cases of persistent pain following lumbar diskectomy, inadequate postsurgical relief is a result of failure to address lateral or central stenosis at the initial surgery.[1] One should not be satisfied with simply identifying a large disk herniation. It is critical to evaluate the size of the spinal canal and assess for possible foraminal narrowing on all preoperative studies. These abnormalities often coexist with degenerative disk disease, and the recognition of bony hypertrophic changes may drastically alter the surgical approach.

Clinical References

1. Burton CV, Kirkaldy-Willis WH, Yong-Hing K, Heithoff KB. Causes of failure of surgery on the lumbar spine. Clin Orthop 1981;157:191–199.
2. Hueftle MG, Modic MT, Ross JS, et al. Lumbar spine: postoperative MR imaging with Gd-DTPA. Radiology 1988;167:817–824.
3. Sotiropoulos S, Chafetz NI, Lang P, et al. Differentiation between postoperative scar and recurrent disk herniation: prospective comparison of MR, CT, and contrast-enhanced CT. AJNR 1989;10:639–643.

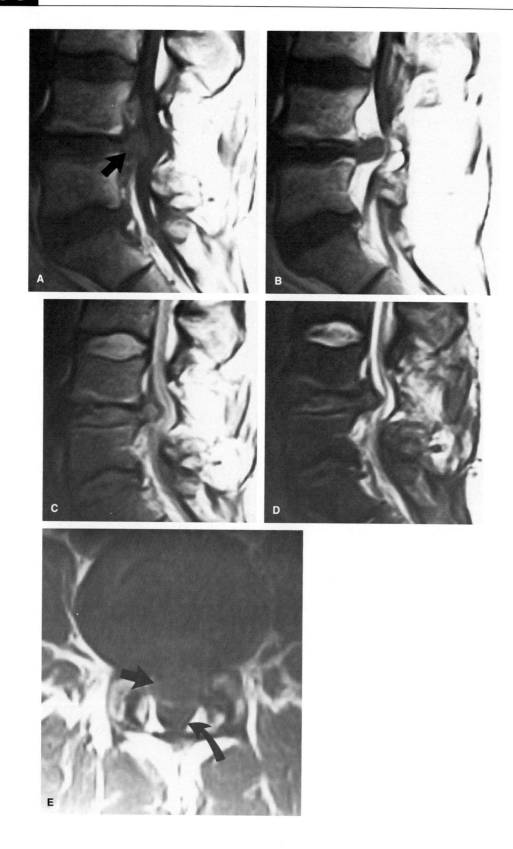

HISTORY

A 43-year-old man with bilateral leg pain and paresthesias 5 years after lumbar laminectomy

FINDINGS

(A) On the sagittal T1-weighted image, there is abnormal soft tissue posteriorly (*arrow*) at the L4–5 interspace, causing marked mass effect on the thecal sac. The posterior elements are absent at this level due to previous bilateral laminectomy. On the corresponding postcontrast image (*B*), enhancement of soft tissue above, below, and immediately posterior to the mass provides better delineation of the lesion from the thecal sac. Intermediate (*C*) and heavily (*D*) T2-weighted sagittal images confirm the contiguity of the mass with the L4–5 intervertebral disk. The central location of the lesion (*arrow*) and the resultant effacement of the thecal sac (*curved arrow*) are well demonstrated on the axial postcontrast scan (*E*).

DIAGNOSIS

Central L4–5 recurrent disk herniation

DISCUSSION

The failed back surgery syndrome (FBSS) is encountered in 25% to 40% of spinal surgery patients.[1] In this syndrome, there is continued pain and disability postoperatively. Clinical assessment of such patients is often difficult, thus increasing the importance of radiologic evaluation. MR is the modality of choice for imaging the postoperative spine.

There are many causes of persistent pain in the postoperative back. Principal among these is recurrent disk herniation, which must be differentiated from postoperative scar. A diagnosis of recurrent disk herniation is likely when a focal, smooth posterior protrusion of soft tissue contiguous with the disk is identified. The presence of mass effect also favors recurrent disk. Scar tissue often has an irregular configuration and typically is not contiguous with disk material. Early after intravenous contrast administration, limited if any enhancement of disk material should occur. Delayed enhancement (30 to 45 minutes after injection) can occur because of diffusion of contrast from nearby tissues. Conversely, scar tissue, because of its high vascularity, enhances early after administration of contrast.

The present case illustrates many of the typical findings of recurrent disk herniation. The central herniation accounts for the patient's bilateral lower extremity symptoms.

MR Technique

Because disk material enhances on delayed postcontrast images, early imaging is essential for distinguishing recurrent disk from epidural fibrosis.

Pitfalls in Image Interpretation

In the first 3 to 6 months after surgery, epidural scar tissue may possess mass effect and may enhance only peripherally.[2] Careful determination of whether the mass is contiguous with the disk and similar in signal intensity is helpful in the differentiation of disk from scar.

Clinical References

1. Djukic S, Lang P, Morris J, et al. The postoperative spine, MRI. Orthop Clin North Am 1990;21:603–624.
2. Boden SD, Davis DO, Dina TS, et al. Contrast-enhanced MR imaging performed after successful lumbar disc surgery: prospective study. Radiology 1992;182:59–64.

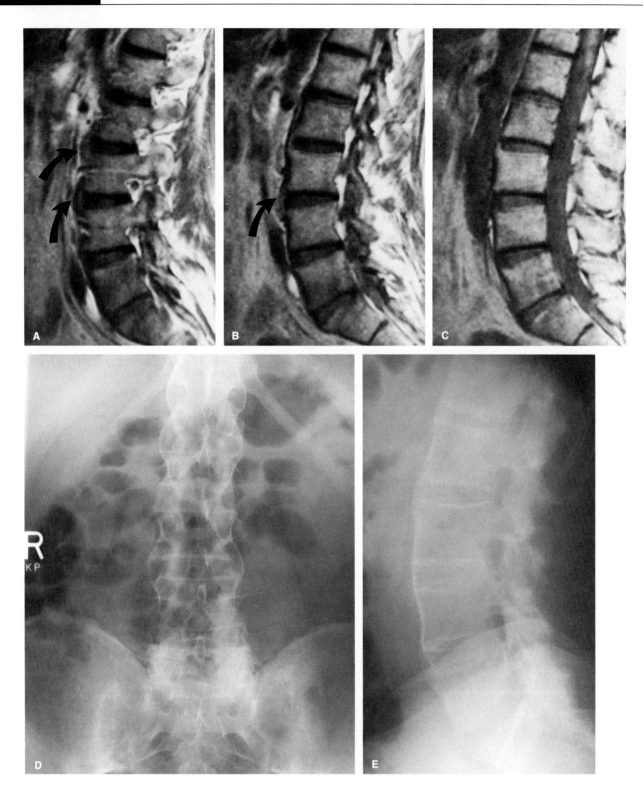

HISTORY

A 37-year-old man with an inflammatory disorder, which primarily affects the axial skeleton, and loss of spinal mobility

FINDINGS

(*A through C*) T1-weighted sagittal images of the lumbar spine are presented from far lateral to midline. The marrow signal intensity is normal. There are prominent anterior osteophytes (*curved arrows*), which appear to bridge the disk space at several levels. T2-weighted images did not reveal additional findings. AP (*D*) and lateral (*E*) plain films of the lumbar spine are also presented. The sacroiliac joints are obliterated bilaterally. Bony bridges (marginal syndesmophytes) connect adjacent vertebral bodies anteriorly and laterally.

DIAGNOSIS

Ankylosing spondylitis

DISCUSSION

Ankylosing spondylitis is an inflammatory disease of unknown etiology. The sacroiliac joint is usually involved early in the disease course. Radiographically, erosion of the cortical margins with subchondral bony sclerosis is first seen, followed by widening of the joint space due to extensive bony erosion. This may progress to fusion with obliteration of the sacroiliac joints. In the spine, inflammation occurs at the junction of the annulus fibrosus and the vertebral body. The outer annular fibers become replaced by bone, forming a syndesmophyte that eventually bridges the adjacent vertebral bodies, growing by enchondral ossification. In advanced disease, this appears radiographically as a "bamboo spine." The most serious complication of spinal disease is fracture, which can occur due to minor trauma and in the cervical spine can lead to quadriplegia. Cauda equina syndrome is an uncommon complication of long-standing disease.[1]

Clinical Reference

1. Tullous MW, Skerhut HE, Story JL, et al. Cauda equina syndrome of long-standing ankylosing spondylitis. Case report and review of the literature. J Neurosurg 1990;73:441–447.

(Images courtesy of Clifford Wolf, MD)

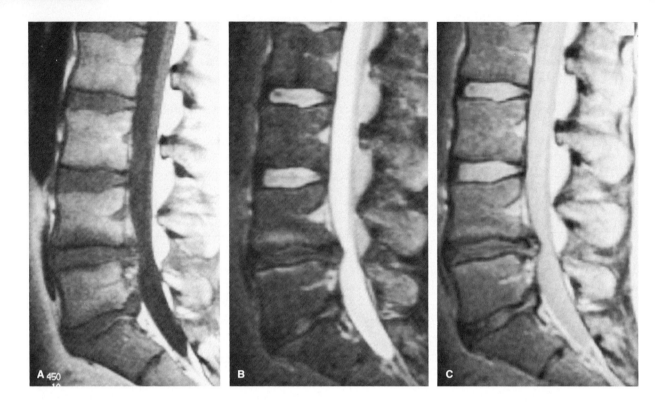

HISTORY

A 27-year-old patient with severe low back and right lower extremity pain

FINDINGS

(A) The T1-weighted midline sagittal image demonstrates large extradural defects compatible with disk herniations at both L4–5 and L5–S1. The L5–S1 disk is mildly narrowed. The signal characteristics of the lumbar intervertebral disks are normal. (B and C) Intermediate and heavily T2-weighted sagittal images confirm the disk herniations at L4–5 and L5–S1. Also apparent on these images is abnormally decreased signal intensity within the L4–5 and L5–S1 intervertebral disks. The normal high signal intensity of the disks on T2-weighted images is present at the higher lumbar levels. Mild narrowing of the L5–S1 disk is again noted. The herniated disk at L4–5 elevates the posterior longitudinal ligament. Increased signal intensity within the L4–5 end plates on the T2-weighted scans, which is of low signal intensity on the T1-weighted scans, is compatible with type I end plate degenerative changes.

DIAGNOSIS

Disk degeneration and herniation at L4–5 and L5–S1

DISCUSSION

Loss of disk height, annular tears, and decreased signal intensity on T2-weighted images are the major MR findings that indicate disk degeneration. Signal intensity changes on T2-weighted images are the most sensitive of these indicators. The significance of disk degeneration lies in its correlation with morphologic abnormalities of the disk. Disk degeneration implies a loss of integrity of the annulus fibrosus, which is necessary for the development of disk herniation.[1]

In the early days of MR, it was thought that loss of water content within the intervertebral disk was the chief determinant of variations in signal intensity on T2-weighted images. As a result, many radiologists previously described the diminished T2 signal intensity as representing disk dehydration or disk desiccation. Several recent studies, however, have revealed that loss of water content, although present, is not the key determinant of the T2 signal intensity changes,[2] and indeed may play a minor role in the signal intensity of the disk on T2-weighted scans.[3] The major factors that result in decreased signal intensity within the disk are probably a decrease in the quantity of proteoglycans within the nucleus pulposus and a decrease in the ratio of chondroitin sulfate to keratin sulfate within the disk.

MR Technique

With the exception of acute trauma, adult disk herniation in the absence of disk degeneration is very unusual. If no disk degeneration is present on T2-weighted scans, the likelihood of a disk herniation is low. Conversely, the presence of disk degeneration is useful as a marker for potential disk herniations. Axial images should be selected through areas of isolated disk degeneration to exclude focal disk abnormalities.

Clinical References

1. Yuh S, Haughton VM, Sether LA, et al. Criteria for classifying normal and degenerated lumbar intervertebral disks. Radiology 1989;170:523–526.
2. Tertii M, Paajanen H, Laato M, et al. Disk degeneration in MRI: a comparative biochemical, histologic, and radiologic study in cadaver spines. Spine 1991;16:629–634.
3. Pearce RH, Thompson JP, Bebault G, Flak B. MRI reflects the chemical changes of aging degeneration in the human intervertebral disk. J Rheumatol (Suppl) 1991;27:42–43.

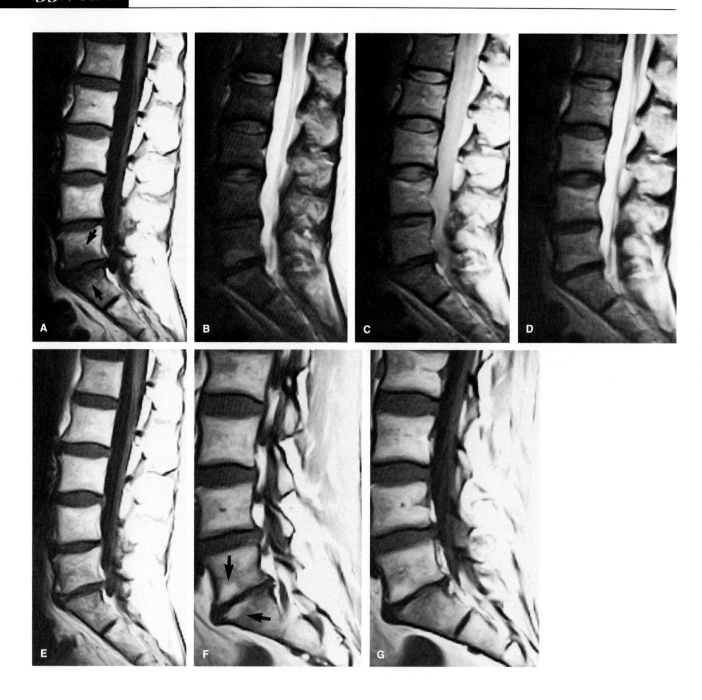

HISTORY

Patient #1: 56 years old with low back and left hip pain

Patient #2: 45 years old with low back pain

Patient #3: 76 years old with internal fixation rods and surgical fusion from L1–2 to L4–5

FINDINGS

Patient #1: The sagittal T1-weighted image through the lower lumbar spine (A) demonstrates decreased signal intensity (*arrows*) in the inferior L5 and superior S1 ver-tebral bodies. The interposed L5–S1 disk space is nar-rowed, with slight retrolisthesis of L5 on S1. (*B*) A heavily T2-weighted image through the same region reveals loss of the normal signal in the intervertebral disks, especially the L4–5 and L5–S1 levels, indicating disk degeneration. Increased T2 signal is seen in the inferior L5 and superior S1 segments corresponding with the areas of decreased T1 signal. (*C*) The proton density weighted image shows nearly homogeneous signal in the L5 and S1 bodies with loss of conspicuity of the end plate changes. (*D*) The sag-ittal fast spin echo T2-weighted image demonstrates sub-tle increased signal in the end plates. Compared to the heavily T2-weighted images, the changes are less distinct

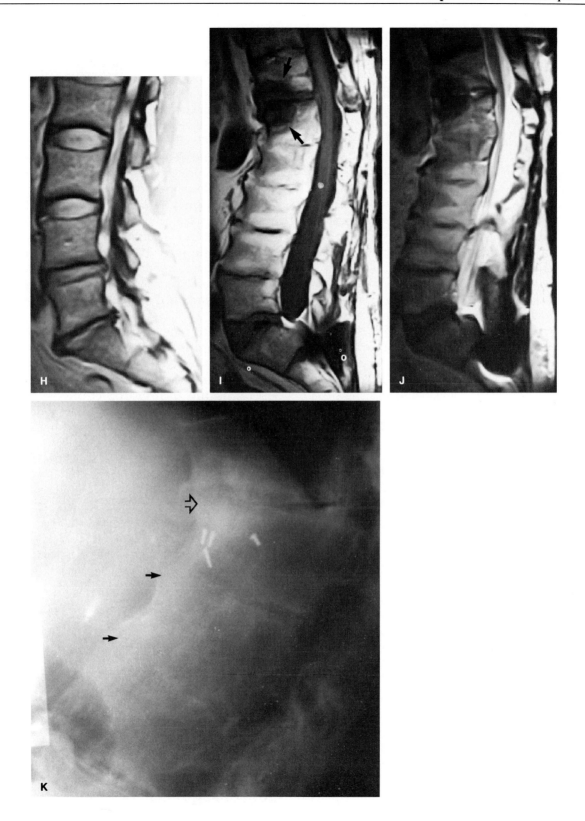

due to greater signal from fat on the fast spin echo sequences. (*E*) An image obtained after administration of intravenous contrast reveals enhancement in the affected portions of the vertebral bodies. The end plate changes become less distinct, but a subtle low-signal-intensity band demarcates the end plate enhancement from the normal marrow signal.

Patient #2: A right parasagittal T1-weighted image (*F*) demonstrates increased signal intensity in the anterior portion of the L5–S1 end plates (*arrows*). The disk space is narrowed with bulging of the disk and accompanying osteophytes. (*G*) The T1-weighted sagittal image obtained following intravenous contrast administration exhibits no enhancement of the end plates. (*H*) The proton density weighted image through this region demonstrates a slight increase in signal in the anterior end plates, compared to the adjacent marrow of L5 and S1. The signal in the end plates follows fat on all imaging sequences.

Patient #3: A midsagittal T1-weighted image of the upper lumbar spine (*I*) displays loss of height of the L1–2, L2–3, and L3–4 disk spaces. The vertebral marrow shows high T1 signal intensity secondary to fatty replacement, especially adjacent to the disk spaces. These findings are secondary to prior fusion with marked fatty marrow replacement and type II end plate changes at these levels. The T12–L1 disk is narrowed and the anterior portions of the adjacent end plates (*arrows*) display low signal intensity. (*J*) A comparable fast spin echo T2-weighted image again illustrates the changes secondary to prior fusion. The anteroinferior T12 and anterosuperior L1 vertebral bodies again demonstrate low signal intensity consistent with sclerotic, type III end plate changes. (*K*) A plain film of the upper lumbar spine confirms the end plate sclerosis at T12–L1 (*open arrow*) and fusion at L1–2 and L2–3 (*arrows*). Incidental note is made of retroperitoneal surgical clips.

DIAGNOSIS

Degenerative end plate changes

DISCUSSION

The vertebral body end plates frequently demonstrate signal changes in conjunction with degenerative disk disease. These changes by themselves are of no clinical significance; the importance is in differentiating these changes from significant pathologic processes involving the end plates.

Type I end plate changes histologically show vascular infiltration, fibrosis, and granulation tissue between thickened bony trabeculae. Increased water content results in both T1 and T2 lengthening. On MR images the end plates show decreased T1 and increased T2 signal intensity. As demonstrated in *C*, these marrow changes may become indiscernible on proton density weighted images. The signal is usually parallel to the end plates and directly adjacent to the intervertebral disk. The affected end plates commonly enhance with intravenous contrast administration.

Other important pathologic processes that could produce MR signal similar to type I end plate changes include metastatic disease and disk space infection/osteomyelitis. Metastatic disease frequently involves multiple vertebrae, and isolated involvement of a vertebral end plate is uncommon. Infection characteristically involves the disk space as well as the adjacent vertebral bodies and is not confined to the end plates alone. The demarcation between the end plates and the disk is therefore lost with infection but preserved with degenerative end plate changes. A paraspinous soft tissue mass is often present at the infected level. Both degenerative end plate changes and infection enhance following administration of intravenous contrast, so enhancement of the end plates does not differentiate these entities. However, the infected disk may enhance, and the infected paraspinous soft tissue mass typically enhances. T2-weighted images may demonstrate increased signal intensity in the infected disk.

Type II end plate changes show fatty infiltration interposed between thickened trabeculae histologically. MR reveals increased T1 and T2 signal intensity compared to normal marrow. Few significant pathologic processes would have this signal pattern confined to the end plates. Studies have shown progression of degenerative end plate changes from type I to type II, suggesting a continuum of the degenerative process.[1] Mixed type I and II changes may coexist at the same level.

Another end plate pattern, type III, consists of sclerotic changes. On MR images, the end plates are of low signal intensity on both T1 and T2 sequences. These areas correspond with sclerosis on the plain films.

End plate changes commonly involve the adjacent vertebrae to a similar degree, and the changes typically include the entire end plate. The signal changes, however, may be confined to a single end plate and may involve only a section of the end plate.

Pitfalls in Image Interpretation

The differential diagnosis for decreased signal in adjacent end plates includes disk space infection. Decreased conspicuity of the disk, evidence of end plate destruction, or a paraspinous soft tissue mass suggests the presence of infection.

Clinical Reference

1. Modic MT, Steinberg PM, Ross JS, et al. Degenerative disk disease: assessment of changes in vertebral body marrow with MR imaging. Radiology 1988;166:193–199.

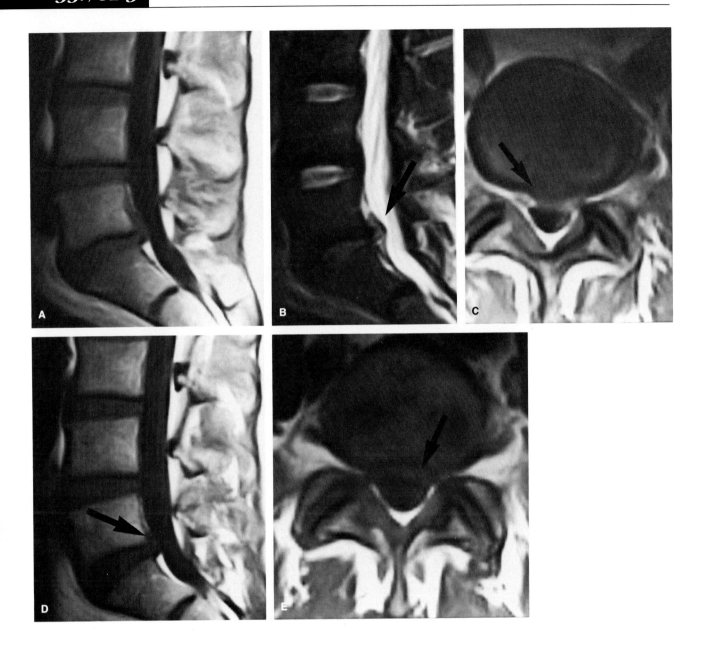

HISTORY

A 45-year-old patient with low back pain

FINDINGS

T1-weighted and (A) T2-weighted (B) sagittal images reveal an extradural lesion (*arrow*) posterior to the L5–S1 intervertebral disk, compatible with a disk herniation. Mild superior extrusion is present. (C) A postinfusion T1-weighted axial image confirms the central disk herniation (*arrow*), which causes mild mass effect on the thecal sac.

A small amount of enhancing tissue compatible with engorged epidural venous plexus or granulation tissue is present about the disk herniation. The patient was treated conservatively and presented for reevaluation 3 months later. At follow-up, T1-weighted (*D*) sagittal and (*E*) axial images reveal a persistent but slightly smaller extradural lesion (*arrow*) at L5–S1. The appearance is suspicious for residual disk herniation on these noncontrast images. (*F and G*) Corresponding postcontrast images, however, reveal homogeneous enhancement of the abnormality (*arrow*), compatible with epidural fibrosis. No evidence for residual disk herniation is seen.

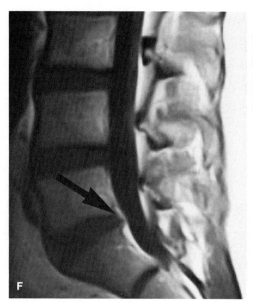
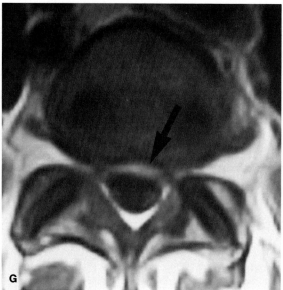

DIAGNOSIS

Resolution of central disk herniation at L5–S1

DISCUSSION

The optimal treatment for disk herniations is a subject of great controversy. Many surgeons consider the presence of an extruded disk or significant extremity weakness as an indication for surgery. Others may operate on the majority of all symptomatic herniations, with the thought that delays in treatment result in a poorer neurologic outcome. A growing body of evidence, however, indicates that conservative treatment leads to equal or superior clinical results when compared to operative therapy.[1] Indeed, a recent prospective study with MR follow-up demonstrated significant reductions in the size of disk herniations in about two thirds of patients treated conservatively.[2] Furthermore, almost half of the patients had a reduction in the size of their herniation of greater than 70%.

Although the exact mechanism of reduction of disk herniations is unknown, it is thought to be due to dehydration and shrinkage of disk material, fragmentation of herniated disk material, and regression of disk material into the original annular tear. It is also possible that granulation tissue may actually absorb or digest portions of the herniated disk.[3] The reduction in mass effect on the nerve root as the herniation decreases presumably explains the improvement in clinical symptoms that has been noted in these patients.

It is generally accepted that a disk herniation in combination with lateral stenosis necessitates surgical intervention. Coexisting lateral stenosis is believed to cause venous congestion and ischemia in the nerve root, with eventual formation of intraneural fibrosis.[1] This mechanism of injury is distinct from that seen in "pure" disk herniations, and may lead to irreversible axonal damage.

MR Technique

An example of the utility of paramagnetic contrast in the virgin back is illustrated in the current case. Without the use of contrast, a residual disk herniation would probably be diagnosed on the follow-up study. The early homogeneous enhancement of the abnormality, however, allows confident determination that the residual soft tissue is secondary to epidural fibrosis.

Clinical References

1. Saal JA, Saal JS. Nonoperative treatment of herniated lumbar intervertebral disc with radiculopathy: an outcome study. Spine 1989;14:431–437.
2. Bozzao A, Galluci M, Masciocchi C, et al. Lumbar disk herniation: MR imaging assessment of natural history in patients treated without surgery. Radiology 1992;185:135–141.
3. Ross JS, Modic MT, Masaryk TJ. Assessment of extradural degenerative disease with Gd-DTPA-enhanced MR imaging: correlation with surgical and pathologic findings. AJNR 1989;10:1243–1249.

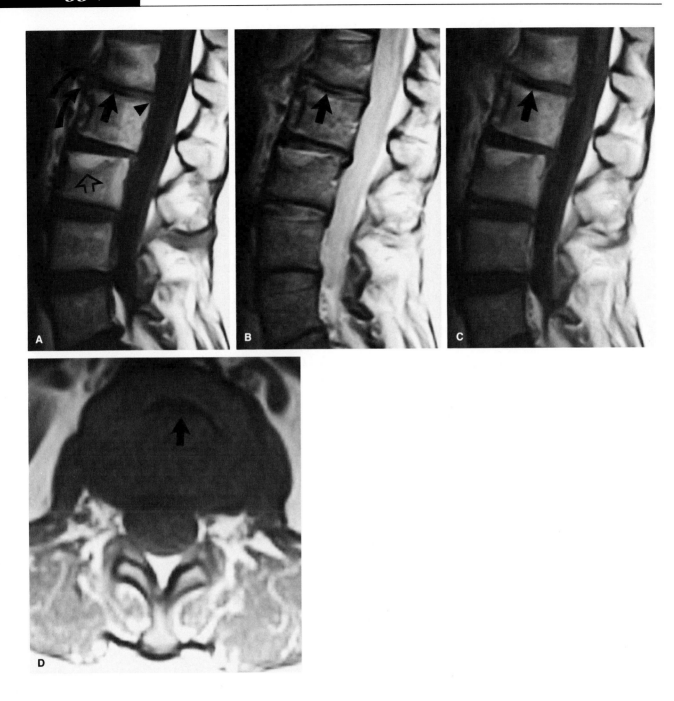

HISTORY

A 55-year-old patient with low back and right lower extremity pain

FINDINGS

(A) The T1-weighted sagittal image demonstrates a linear low-signal-intensity area (*arrow*) in the narrowed L1–2 disk. Additional degenerative changes are present at the L1–2 level, including a small posterior disk bulge (*arrowhead*) and large anterior osteophytes (*curved arrows*). Degenerative changes are also seen at the L2–3 level, including disk space narrowing, mild retrolisthesis, moderate disk bulge, osteophytic spurs, and type II changes within the superior end plate of L3 (*open arrow*). The linear low signal intensity (*arrow*) is also demonstrated on the (B) intermediate T2-weighted and (C) postcontrast T1-weighted sagittal images. The axial T1-weighted image through the L1–2 disk (D) demonstrates a curvilinear low-signal-intensity cleft (*arrow*) in the anterior disk.

The lateral plain film (*image not shown*) confirmed the presence of gas within the L1–2 disk.

DIAGNOSIS

Vacuum intervertebral disk

DISCUSSION

A vacuum disk represents a degenerated intervertebral disk with a gas collection usually within clefts in the annulus fibrosus or nucleus pulposus. The primary constituent of the gas is nitrogen. This finding is most common in the lumbar spine and appears as a low-attenuation area on plain radiographs. Reports indicate the presence of gas in up to 20% of cases, with increased incidence in older patients.[1]

MR imaging of the vacuum disk shows typical findings of signal void in the disk that is usually horizontally oriented. Because the disk is usually degenerated and therefore demonstrates low signal intensity on T2-weighted images, gas within the disk is less conspicuous on these sequences. The resultant signal void is better seen on T1-weighted images against the background of the intermediate-signal-intensity disk.

MR Technique

Small or subtle gas collections or calcifications are difficult to detect on conventional spin echo sequences. Gradient echo images are particularly sensitive in detecting air or dense calcification in the disk.

Pitfalls in Image Interpretation

Very low signal intensity in the disk space has multiple etiologies including gas, calcification, a disk tear without gas, and chemical shift artifact.[2] Gas in the disk may be due to simple disk degeneration and vacuum phenomenon, but has been reported on plain radiographs in association with disk space infection. Gas may also be seen in association with Schmorl's nodes, trauma, vertebral body collapse, neoplastic involvement of the adjacent vertebrae, and secondary forms of disk degeneration associated with crystal deposition.[1]

Clinical References

1. Resnick D, Niwayama G, Guerra J, et al. Spinal vacuum phenomena: anatomical study and review. Radiology 1981; 139:341–348.
2. Grenier N, Grossman RI, Schiebler ML, et al. Degenerative lumbar disk disease: pitfalls and usefulness of MR imaging in detection of vacuum phenomenon. Radiology 1987; 164:861–865.

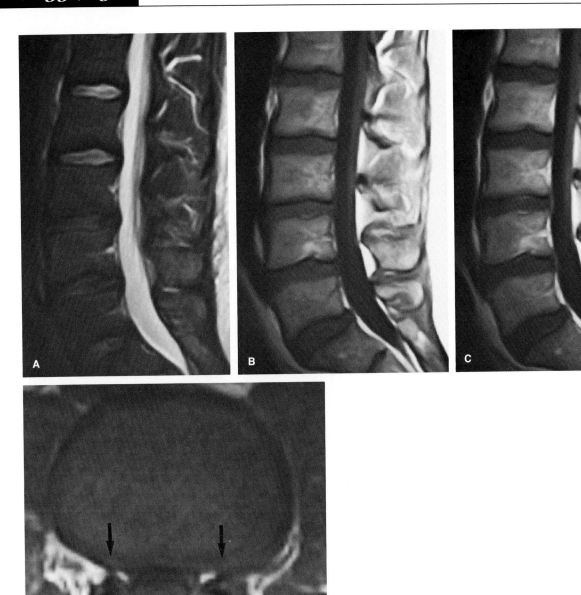

HISTORY

A 40-year-old patient with low back pain

FINDINGS

(A) The sagittal T2-weighted (TR/TE = 3000/80) image demonstrates decreased signal intensity in the L3–4, L4–5, and L5–S1 disk spaces consistent with disk degenera-

tion. The posterior disk margins extend beyond the adjacent vertebral end plates and indent the anterior thecal sac at these levels. The sagittal (B) precontrast and (C) postcontrast T1-weighted images again show mild posterior extension of disk material from L3–4 through L5–S1. The disk margin is better delineated following the administration of intravenous contrast due to enhancement of the epidural venous plexus. (D) The axial T1-weighted image through the L3–4 level reveals a generalized disk bulge with mild convexity of the posterior disk margin. The disk material narrows the lateral recesses bilaterally (*arrows*). The posterior disk margin has a smooth curvilinear contour with no focal disk protrusion.

DIAGNOSIS

Disk bulge

DISCUSSION

A disk bulge, also known as an annular bulge, occurs due to degeneration of the intervertebral disk. Initial work suggested that with a disk bulge, the annulus fibrosus was intact. An in vitro study has subsequently demonstrated the presence of annular tears in association with a disk bulge, especially with more severe bulging.[1] The presence of annular tears has also been confirmed with gadolinium enhancement.[2] The laxity and tears in the annulus fibrosus result in centrifugal extension of disk material beyond the margin of the adjacent vertebral end plates. The absence of a focal extension of disk material differentiates a disk bulge from a herniation. A disk herniation, however, may be associated with a generalized disk bulge.

On MR images, a disk bulge is most commonly associated with a degenerated intervertebral disk. The degenerated disk demonstrates decreased signal intensity on T2-weighted images. The outer annular fibers and posterior longitudinal ligament are low-signal-intensity structures on all imaging sequences. The deformity of the ventral extradural space due to a disk bulge is more easily identified on T2-weighted images because the high-signal-intensity cerebrospinal fluid profiles the disk bulge.

A disk bulge is less commonly associated with radiculopathy than disk herniation. Posterior bulging of the disk narrows the spinal canal and the inferior aspect of the neural foramina. The disk bulge is often accompanied by end plate spurs, which can also efface the ventral extradural space and foramina. These changes, combined with hypertrophic changes in the posterior osseous and soft tissues, can result in spinal stenosis and foraminal narrowing. This is particularly true when the canal is congenitally small. Lateral bulging of the intervertebral disk can cause displacement of the adjacent nerve roots.

MR Technique

The use of intravenous contrast enhancement provides greater sensitivity in the detection of tears of the annulus fibrosus compared to T2-weighted images.[2]

Pitfalls in Image Interpretation

A prominent disk bulge may appear very similar to a focal disk protrusion on sagittal images. Correlation with the axial image through the disk in question will differentiate a focal protrusion from a concentric, generalized disk bulge.

Clinical References

1. Yu S, Haughton VM, Sether LA, Wagner M. Annulus fibrosus in bulging intervertebral disks. Radiology 1988;169:761–763.
2. Ross JS, Modic MT, Masaryk TJ. Tears of the anulus fibrosus: assessment with Gd-DTPA-enhanced MR imaging. AJNR 1989;10:1251–1254.

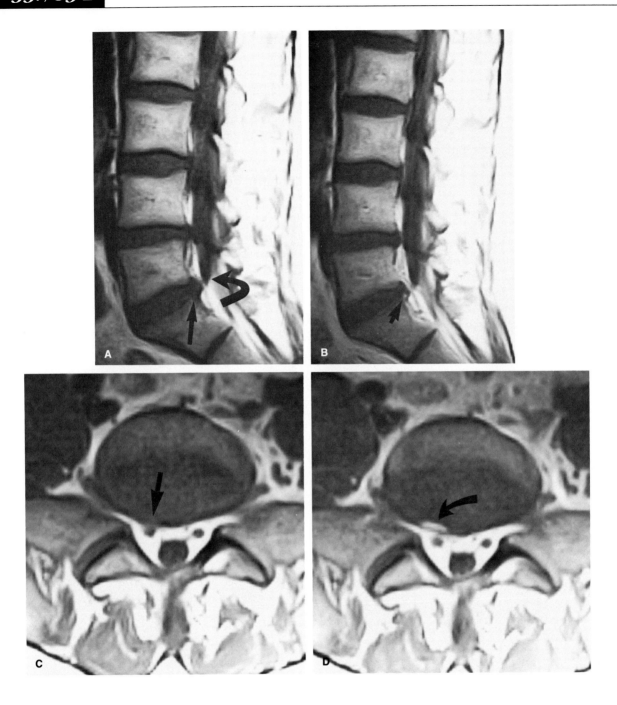

HISTORY

A 27-year-old woman with back pain

FINDINGS

(A) The sagittal T1-weighted image just to the right of midline demonstrates extension of the L5–S1 disk (*arrow*) beyond the posterior margin of the adjacent vertebral bodies. The right L5 nerve root sleeve (*curved arrow*) is filled with low-signal-intensity cerebrospinal fluid. The corresponding sagittal T1-weighted image following intravenous contrast administration (*B*) shows a small focal area of enhancement (*arrow*) along the posteroinferior margin of the disk. A focal area of high signal intensity was also apparent on the T2-weighted sagittal image (*image not shown*). The T1-weighted (*C*) precontrast and (*D*) postcontrast axial images demonstrate a mild, focal, asymmetric extension of the posterior disk margin (*arrow in C*). The disk abuts, but does not significantly displace, the right L5 nerve root sleeve. The postcontrast image shows a curvilinear area of high signal intensity (*curved arrow in D*) paralleling the posterior disk margin, representing enhancement of a concentric tear in, or separation of, the outer fibers of the annulus fibrosus.

DIAGNOSIS

Disk protrusion with a concentric tear of the annulus fibrosus

DISCUSSION

A herniated disk can be further subclassified as a protruded disk, an extruded disk, or a free fragment.[1] A disk protrusion represents a herniation of nuclear material through a tear in the annulus fibrosus, contained by the outer fibers of the annulus. A protrusion may be difficult to distinguish from a disk bulge on sagittal images, but can be differentiated on axial images. The disk bulge produces circumferential extension of the disk margin with a smooth curvilinear margin. A disk protrusion produces a focal extension of the disk margin beyond the margin of the adjacent end plates. A protrusion may occur at any location around the disk margin, but is most common along the posterior and lateral margins.

Tears of the annulus fibrosus have been subclassified as concentric, transverse, and radial.[2] Concentric tears parallel the curvature of the outer disk and represent tears in or separation of the longitudinal fibers of the annulus fibrosus. T2-weighted images frequently demonstrate high signal intensity in the torn or separated annular fibers. Images obtained following the intravenous administration of a paramagnetic contrast agent often show enhancement of the annular tear. Enhancement of annular tears probably reflects fibrovascular tissue involved in the reparative process.

MR Technique

MR has proven to be the best imaging modality for evaluation of the lumbar intervertebral disks and disk disease. High sensitivity for changes within the disk and multiplanar imaging improve the accuracy of interpretation.

Pitfalls in Image Interpretation

Correlation of findings from both the sagittal and axial planes is necessary to differentiate a generalized disk bulge from a focal disk protrusion.

Clinical References

1. Blaser SI, Modic MT. Herniation of the intervertebral disk. Top Magn Reson Imag 1988;1:25–37.
2. Yu S, Sether LA, Ho PS, et al. Tears of the anulus fibrosus: correlation between MR and pathologic findings in cadavers. AJNR 1988;9:367–371.

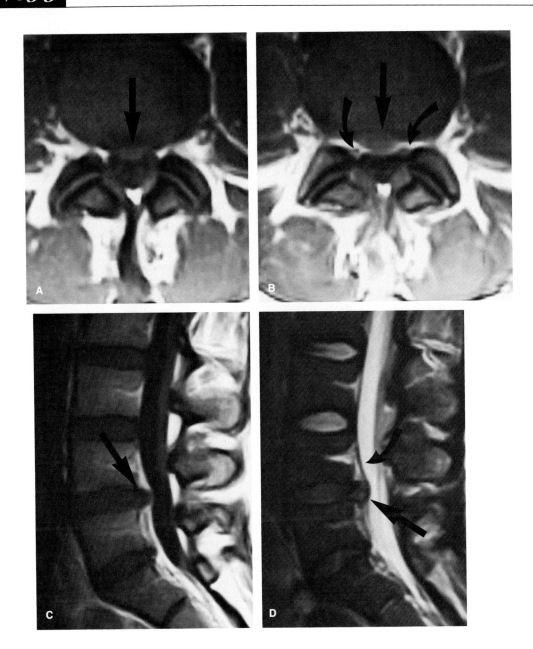

HISTORY

A 36-year-old patient with low back pain

FINDINGS

(*A*) A T1-weighted axial image at the L4–5 level demonstrates a midline anterior extradural soft tissue abnormality (*arrow*) causing moderate mass effect on the thecal sac. (*B*) Following contrast administration, the abnormality (*arrow*) is outlined by enhancing epidural venous plexus. The relationship of the abnormality to the L5 nerve roots (*curved arrows*) is well depicted. (*C*) A postinfusion T1-weighted midline sagittal image confirms the abnormality (*arrow*). The lesion is isointense to the L4–5 intervertebral disk and is contiguous to the disk.

(*D*) A T2-weighted sagittal view again displays the abnormality (*arrow*). Displacement of the posterior longitudinal ligament (*curved arrow*) is apparent. Loss of the usual high signal intensity within the intervertebral disks at L4–5 and L5–S1 is compatible with disk degeneration.

DIAGNOSIS

Central disk herniation at L4–5

DISCUSSION

Disk herniations lie at the end of a spectrum that begins with disk degeneration.[1] Almost all herniations, with the exception of posttraumatic and the rare childhood herniations, occur in degenerated disks. Bulging disks are a result of disk degeneration and laxity of the annulus, with resultant extension of the annulus beyond the vertebral body margin. Bulging disks are generally smooth and symmetric in appearance. A disk protrusion is the mildest form of disk herniation, in which nuclear material extends through a small annular defect, thereby focally extending the disk margin. Although the annulus in these cases has a small defect, it remains grossly intact. In disk extrusions, herniation of nuclear material through a ruptured annulus occurs. Extruded disks remain in contiguity with the nucleus of origin. Such herniations often result in extradural masses that are contained by the posterior longitudinal ligament. Free fragments or sequestered disks occur when the disk herniation separates from the parent disk. In most cases the free disk material penetrates the posterior longitudinal ligament.

Distinguishing between the varying degrees of disk disease is important for several reasons.[1] Clinically, bulging disks are far less likely to cause sciatica than a true herniation. Extruded or sequestered disks must be recognized because the required surgical approach is often more extensive, and percutaneous techniques such as chymopapain injection are contraindicated.

MR Technique

Sagittal images are recommended as the initial scan in lumbar disk disease. The sagittal view affords an overview of the entire lumbar region. From these views, appropriate levels for axial scan correlation can be selected.

Clinical Reference

1.   Modic MT. Degenerative disorders of the spine. In: Modic MT, Masaryk TJ, Ross JS, eds. Magnetic resonance imaging of the spine. Chicago, Year Book Medical Publishers, 1989:75–119.

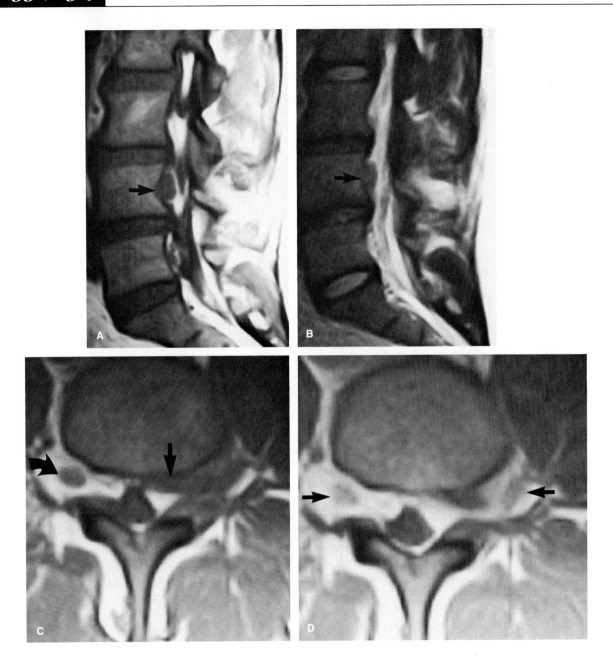

HISTORY

A 38-year-old patient with a 3-week history of severe back pain following heavy lifting

FINDINGS

(A) A T1-weighted sagittal image to the left of midline reveals an abnormal soft tissue mass (*arrow*) posterior to the mid-L4 vertebral body. (B) A fast spin echo T2-weighted sagittal image redemonstrates the soft tissue mass (*arrow*) posterior to the left L4 vertebral body. The lesion is isointense to the L3–4 and L4–5 intervertebral disks, which both appear moderately narrowed. Loss of the usual high signal intensity is seen within the L3–4 and L4–5 disks, compatible with disk degeneration. (C) A T1-weighted axial image through the mid-L4 region confirms the abnormal soft tissue (*arrow*) posterior to the left side of the vertebral body. The right L4 dorsal root ganglion is well visualized (*curved arrow*), but the left L4 ganglion is obscured by the lesion. (D) Following contrast administration, enhancing granulation tissue is seen surrounding the soft tissue mass. Normal enhancement of the dorsal root ganglia (*arrows*) is well seen, and the displacement of the left L4 ganglion is now apparent. (E) A preinfusion T1-weighted axial image at the L3–4 disk reveals a small left lateral disk herniation (*arrow*). A similar small lateral disk herniation was present at L4–5 as well (*image not shown*). (F) A postinfusion T1-weighted axial view at the L3–4 level demonstrates a prominent focus of abnormal enhancement (*arrow*) within the posterior aspect of this disk herniation.

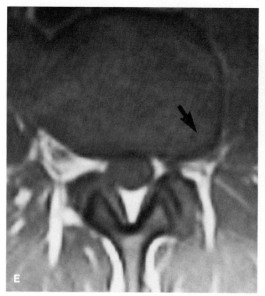 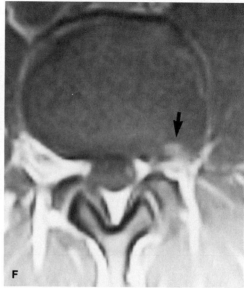

DIAGNOSIS

Left lateral disk herniation at L3–4 with large free disk fragment posterior to the L4 vertebral body

DISCUSSION

The utility of paramagnetic contrast administration in the postoperative back is well known. The early homogeneous enhancement of epidural fibrosis is the key determinant in the differentiation of recurrent disk herniation from scar tissue. The benefits of paramagnetic contrast, however, are not limited to the postoperative patient. Even in virgin disk disease, granulation tissue is known to form about a disk herniation. As a result, on noncontrast images the size of disk herniations may often be overestimated. The use of paramagnetic contrast thus allows more accurate evaluation of the size of disk herniations. Additionally, the enhancement of surrounding granulation tissue and epidural venous plexus increases the conspicuity of subtle extradural lesions.[1] Enhancement of peridiskal tissues also improves visualization of the relationship of the herniation to the thecal sac and exiting nerve roots. In lateral or foraminal disk herniations, normal enhancement of foraminal veins allows confident assessment of foraminal impingement or coexisting bony foraminal stenosis. Lateral herniations often cause mass effect on the dorsal root ganglion as well, and the normal enhancement of the ganglion provides differentiation of this structure from the nonenhancing disk herniation.

An application of paramagnetic contrast use that is particularly useful in the current case is in the detection of annular tears.[2] The presence of granulation tissue within annular tears allows visualization of these abnormalities with contrast-enhanced MR. On noncontrast MR, the source of a free fragment can often be determined by examining the size and morphology of the adjacent intervertebral disks and comparing the degree of disk degeneration at these levels. In the current example, the disks above and below the free fragment are both narrowed and degenerated, and small herniations are seen at both levels. In addition, the fragment appears to lie equidistant between the two neighboring disks. The presence of a prominent, enhancing annular tear at the margin of the L3–4 disk, however, supports the contention that the source of the free fragment is the L3–4 disk. This information is important to the surgeon, as a laminectomy in cases of free fragments is generally performed at the level of the suspected parent disk.

MR Technique

Annular tears are thought to be critical in the etiology of so-called diskogenic pain, which is believed to result from leakage of the nucleus pulposus through an annular defect in the absence of frank disk herniation. In the past, such tears have been demonstrable only with diskography. Although annular tears can occasionally be visualized with T2-weighted images, postcontrast MR appears more sensitive for the detection of these abnormalities.[2]

Pitfalls in Image Interpretation

Enhancement of the epidural venous plexus or of peridiskal fibrosis should not be confused with an annular tear. These areas of enhancement are often identified at the periphery of a disk. A diagnosis of annular tear, however, requires extension of enhancement deep to the substance of the annulus.

Clinical References

1. Ross JS, Modic MT, Masaryk TJ, et al. Assessment of extradural degenerative disease with Gd-DTPA-enhanced MR imaging: correlation with surgical and pathologic findings. AJR 1989;10:1243–1249.
2. Ross JS, Modic MT, Masaryk TJ. Tears of the anulus fibrosis: assessment with Gd-DTPA-enhanced MR imaging. AJNR 1989;10:1251–1254.

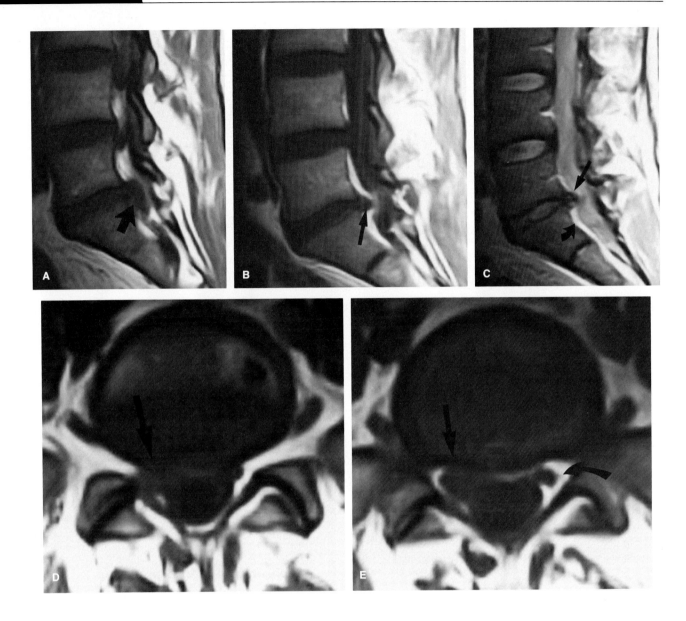

HISTORY

A 45-year-old patient with low back and right leg pain for 1 year

FINDINGS

(*A*) A T1-weighted sagittal image to the right of midline demonstrates abnormal soft tissue intensity (*arrow*) posterior to the L5–S1 intervertebral disk. Moderate inferior extension of the abnormality is present. The postinfusion T1-weighted sagittal view (*B*) reveals enhancement of much of the abnormality, although a central nonenhancing portion (*arrow*) is present. (*C*) On the intermediate T2-weighted study, the portion of the lesion directly contiguous with the L5–S1 disk (*arrow*) is isointense to the disk. The inferior component (*curved arrow*) demonstrates increased signal intensity relative to the disk. (*D and E*) T1-weighted axial images confirm the abnormal soft tissue (*arrow*) posterior to the intervertebral disk. The lesion obscures the right S1 nerve root. The left S1 nerve root (*curved arrow in E*) is well visualized. (*F and G*) Following contrast administration, the right paracentral, nonenhancing portion of the lesion (*arrow in F*) is outlined by surrounding areas of enhancement. The right S1 nerve root (*curved arrow in G*) is encircled by enhancing tissue.

DIAGNOSIS

Right paracentral disk herniation at L5–S1 with de novo scar formation

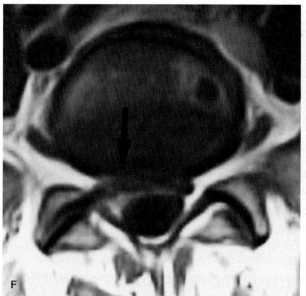
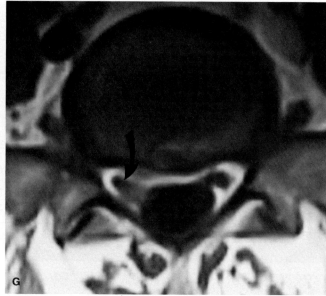

DISCUSSION

Intravenous gadolinium chelate administration can play a role in the evaluation of virgin degenerative disk disease, in addition to its established use in the postoperative back.[1] Granulation tissue forms about disk herniations even in the absence of surgery. Many feel that the formation of granulation tissue is part of the body's natural healing response to a disk herniation. Granulation tissue may actually absorb or digest disk material, with the result being a gradual decrease in the size of the disk herniation. The granulation tissue about a herniation is of course much better visualized with the use of paramagnetic contrast. Although signal characteristics on T2-weighted images, morphology, and location can aid in the differentiation of disk and scar, none of these parameters is as reliable as the characteristic early enhancement of epidural fibrosis. Recent evidence suggests that most lumbar disk herniations will significantly decrease in size with nonoperative therapy.[2] In fact, large herniations seem to be the most likely to diminish in size. This may be because large herniations develop more extensive granulation tissue, and are thus more actively resorbed. Such evidence supports the belief that lumbar disk herniation is largely a medical disease. MR provides an accurate, noninvasive means of following these patients, and the use of paramagnetic contrast allows sensitive monitoring of the transition from disk herniation to reparative granulation tissue.

MR Technique

Small disk herniations may be better detected on contrast-enhanced scans as a result of enhancement of surrounding epidural venous plexus and granulation tissue.[1] This enhancement will increase the conspicuity of subtle extradural lesions.

Pitfalls in Image Interpretation

On noncontrast MR, the presence of granulation tissue about disk herniations may result in overestimation of the size of the herniation.

Clinical References

1. Ross JS, Modic MT, Masaryk TJ, et al. Assessment of extradural degenerative disease with Gd-DTPA-enhanced MR imaging: correlation with surgical and pathologic findings. AJNR 1989;10:1243–1249.
2. Bozzao A, Gallucci M, Masciocchi C, et al. Lumbar disk herniation: MR imaging assessment of natural history in patients treated without surgery. Radiology 1992;185:135–141.

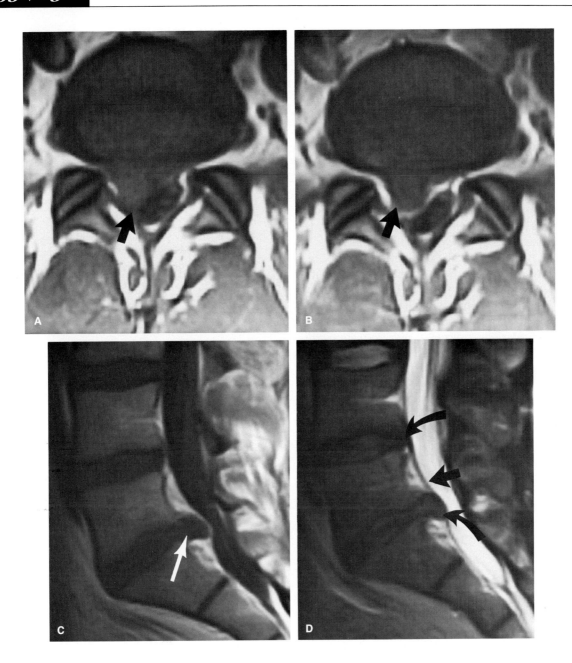

HISTORY

A 32-year-old patient with back and right leg pain

FINDINGS

(A) A T1-weighted axial image at the L5–S1 level demonstrates abnormal soft tissue intensity (*arrow*) posterior to the right side of the disk, causing moderate mass effect on the thecal sac. (B) Following contrast administration, enhancement of epidural venous plexus allows clearer definition of this extradural abnormality (*arrow*) from the adjacent thecal sac. (C) A postinfusion T1-weighted sagittal view confirms the finding and well demonstrates the continuity of the lesion with the L5–S1 intervertebral disk. The abnormality is isointense to disk material on this image and the fast spin echo T2-weighted sagittal image (D). Displacement of the posterior longitudinal ligament (*arrow*) is noted on the T2-weighted scan. Loss of the usual high signal intensity within the intervertebral disks is noted at L4–5 and L5–S1 (*curved arrows*), compatible with disk degeneration.

DIAGNOSIS

Right paracentral disk herniation at L5–S1

DISCUSSION

Lumbar disk herniation is a common cause of morbidity in middle-aged adults. Because the disk degenerates and becomes fibrotic with age, herniations in patients older than 60 years are uncommon. Symptoms attributable to lumbar disk herniation include radiculopathy, sensory loss, back pain, and weakness. The etiology of pain in lumbar disk disease is controversial.[1] Mechanical pressure from the herniated disk is important, but additional causes such as preexisting nerve root irritation, release of sensitizing substances from the herniated disk, and autoimmune causes have been proposed as contributing factors in the symptoms of disk herniation patients.

Central lumbar disk herniations may cause few clinical symptoms, because exiting lumbar nerve roots are frequently unaffected. Paracentral disk herniations, however, generally cause symptoms related to compression of nerve roots as they depart from the thecal sac. For example, an L5–S1 right paracentral disk herniation will commonly cause symptoms related to compression of the exiting right S1 nerve root.

MR Technique

L4–5 and L5–S1 are the most commonly affected levels in lumbar disk herniation, accounting for about 90% of such cases. Most of the remaining cases of disk herniation occur at L3–4. It is thus important to select axial images through the lower lumbar spine in the routine examination for lumbar disk herniation.

Pitfalls in Image Interpretation

Because lumbar nerve roots travel a considerable distance through the spinal canal before exiting, symptoms of a low lumbar disk herniation can be mimicked by abnormalities that lie higher within the lumbar spine. Attention to sagittal images of the conus and cauda equina is thus necessary in cases of suspected disk herniation.

Clinical Reference

1. Czervionke LF, Daniels DL. Degenerative disease of the spine. In: Atlas SW, ed. Magnetic resonance imaging of the brain and spine. New York, Raven Press, 1991:795–864.

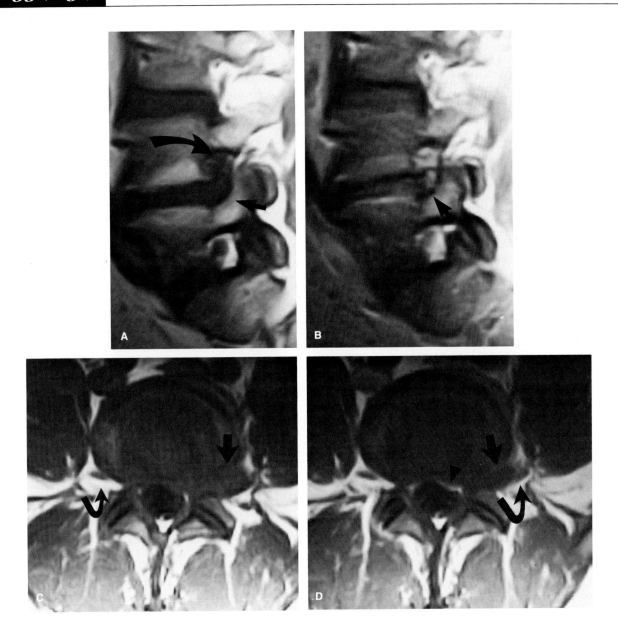

HISTORY

A 48-year-old patient with low back and left leg pain

FINDINGS

(A) A T1-weighted sagittal view to the left of midline demonstrates a soft tissue abnormality (*arrow*) extending posterior to the L4–5 intervertebral disk. The abnormality fills much of the left L4–5 neural foramen. The exiting left L4 nerve root (*curved arrow*) is identified just above the lesion. The abnormality (*arrow*) is again seen on a corresponding intermediate T2-weighted sagittal view (B). The lesion is contiguous to the intervertebral disk on both sagittal views. The signal intensity of the abnor-

mality is similar to the L4–5 intervertebral disk on the T1-weighted scan and mildly hyperintense to the disk on the T2-weighted scan. (C) An axial T1-weighted scan at the L4–5 level confirms the abnormality (*arrow*). The exiting L4 nerve root (*curved arrow*) is seen on the right, but is obscured by the lesion on the left. (D) A postinfusion T1-weighted axial view provides clearer delineation of the lesion (*arrow*) as a result of enhancement of the epidural venous plexus (*arrowhead*) and foraminal veins. The displaced left L4 nerve root (*curved arrow*) can now be distinguished from the nonenhancing mass. Mass effect on the left side of the thecal sac is also more apparent.

DIAGNOSIS

Left lateral disk herniation at L4–5

DISCUSSION

The annulus fibrosus is generally thinnest at its posterior aspect. As a result, central and paracentral disk herniations are much more common than lateral herniations. Lateral herniations behave differently than intraspinal herniations: they are often present at the L2–3 and L3–4 levels, and superior migration of disk fragments is very common.[1] Lateral disk herniations frequently result in compression of the nerve root ganglion or nerve root within the neural foramen. This results in a radiculopathy of the nerve root just above the interspace, unlike intraspinal herniations, which generally affect the nerve root below the interspace before its departure from the thecal sac. Occasionally, as in the present case, a lateral disk herniation will have a significant intraspinal component. Such herniations may result in a double radiculopathy.

Because of its multiplanar capability and superior soft tissue contrast, MR is ideally suited for imaging of lateral disk herniations.[2] A combination of imaging planes allows accurate assessment of the exact position of the disk herniation within the neural foramen, a determination that is critical in the surgeon's choice between an intraspinal or paraspinal approach. Because lateral disk herniations often occur beyond the termination of the nerve root sleeves, myelography lacks sensitivity for these abnormalities. CT is generally limited to the axial plane, and the lack of soft tissue contrast makes distinguishing disk material from an enlarged nerve root difficult.

MR Technique

The use of paramagnetic contrast agents increases accuracy in the diagnosis of lateral disk herniations. Enhancement of the epidural venous plexus and foraminal veins allows clearer depiction of the margins of a disk herniation. Without contrast, enlarged foraminal veins may mimic a disk herniation or cause overestimation of the size of a herniation.[2] A neurofibroma within the neural foramen may also simulate a lateral herniation. Unlike disk material, neurofibromas enhance homogeneously following contrast administration.

Pitfalls in Image Interpretation

In patients with scoliosis and bulging disks, disk material may project into the neural foramen on axial images and thereby simulate a lateral herniation.[1] In these cases, the disk is smooth in contour with no focal protrusions. Adjacent images often show a symmetric bulge on the contralateral side.

Clinical References

1. Osborn AG, Hood RS, Sherry RG, et al. CT/MR spectrum of far lateral and anterior lumbosacral disk herniations. AJNR 1988;9:775–778.
2. Grenier N, Greselle JF, Douws C, et al. MR imaging of foraminal and extraforaminal lumbar disk herniations. J Comput Assist Tomog 1990;14:243–249.

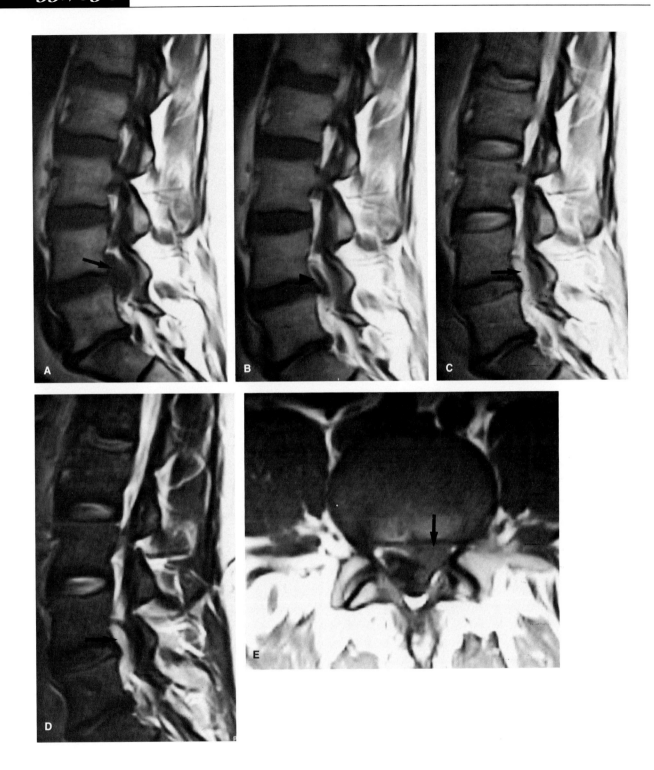

HISTORY

A 45-year-old man with low back and left leg pain

FINDINGS

The noncontrast T1-weighted sagittal image (*A*) shows an abnormal oblong area of low signal intensity (*arrow*) in the spinal canal behind the L4–5 intervertebral disk with extension posterior to the L4 and L5 vertebral bodies. The signal intensity of the mass is similar to that of the L4–5 disk. A curved low-signal-intensity line is faintly visible separating the mass from the L4–5 disk. The peripheral margin of the epidural mass enhances on the postinfusion T1-weighted sagittal image (*B*). The enhancing tissue (*arrowhead*) extends between the mass and the L4–5 disk. The (*C*) first (30 msec) and (*D*) second (80 msec) echoes of the sagittal T2-weighted pulse sequence show high signal intensity in the mass (*arrow*) compared

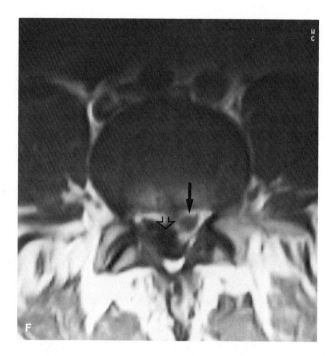

to the intensity of the L4–5 disk. The axial (*E*) preinfusion and (*F*) postinfusion T1-weighted axial images just inferior to the L4–5 level again demonstrate peripheral enhancement of the epidural mass (*arrow*). The mass deforms the thecal sac (*open arrow*) and displaces it to the right. The mass also compressed the left L5 and S1 nerve roots.

DIAGNOSIS

Large free disk fragment

DISCUSSION

Free disk fragments demonstrate low to intermediate signal intensity on T1-weighted images. T2-weighted images typically show increased signal intensity within the fragment, as demonstrated in this case, unlike most disk herniations, which have low T2 signal intensity similar to the signal in the degenerated parent disk. Free disk material is thus more easily separated from the degenerated parent disk on T2-weighted images.[1] Free fragments also frequently demonstrate some degree of enhancement following intravenous contrast administration. This can also aid in defining the separation between the free fragment and the parent disk.

A free disk fragment, also termed sequestered disk material, is a portion of disk material that has completely separated from the parent disk. The free fragment may lie anterior or posterior to the posterior longitudinal ligament, and can move superiorly and inferiorly within the epidural space. The migratory nature of the fragment may therefore produce symptoms attributable to various spinal levels. The posterior longitudinal ligament and a thin posterior midline septum direct free fragments into the paracentral regions away from the midline.[2]

MR Technique

Contrast enhancement is helpful to improve the visual conspicuity and detection of free disk fragments.

Pitfalls in Image Interpretation

The signal intensity of a free disk fragment may become bright enough on T2-weighted images that the signal approaches that of cerebrospinal fluid (CSF). The resulting decreased contrast between an intraspinal fragment and the surrounding CSF may make the fragment less perceptible.

Clinical References

1. Masaryk TJ, Ross JS, Modic MT, et al. High-resolution MR imaging of sequestered lumbar intervertebral disks. AJR 1988;150:1155–1162.
2. Schellinger D, Manz HJ, Vidic B, et al. Disk fragment migration. Radiology 1990;175:831–835.

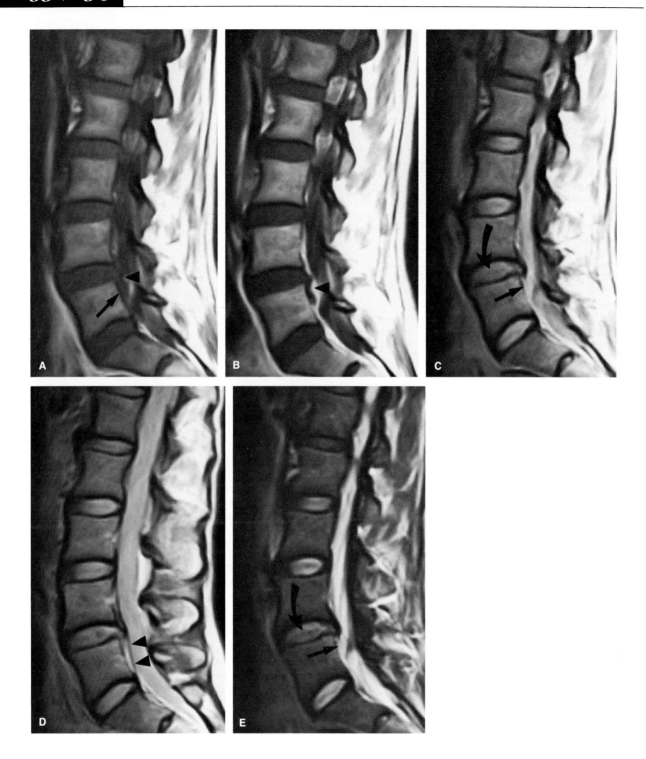

HISTORY

A 48-year-old woman who hurt her back 5 days ago, and now presents with low back and right leg pain

FINDINGS

(*A*) The precontrast T1-weighted sagittal image just to the right of midline reveals a right paracentral disk hernia-

tion with inferior extrusion (*arrow*) at the L4–5 level. The disk material extends posterior to the upper L5 vertebral body with a focal indentation in the disk material (*arrowhead*) along the posterior margin at the level of the superior L5 end plate. (*B*) The comparable image following IV administration of a gadolinium chelate demonstrates enhancement of the peripheral margin of the disk material. The posterior indentation is again seen (*arrowhead*). (*C*) The intermediate T2-weighted sagittal image shows mildly decreased signal intensity in the L4–5 disk

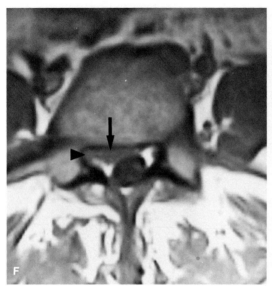

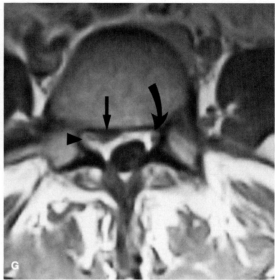

(*curved arrow*) compared to the adjacent disks, consistent with early disk degeneration. High signal intensity is seen in the sequestered fragment (*arrow*). (*D*) The midline sagittal image demonstrates elevation of the posterior longitudinal ligament (*arrowheads*) by the adjacent disk fragment. (*E*) The heavily T2-weighted image again demonstrates high signal intensity in the free fragment (*arrow*), which is higher in signal intensity than the parent L4–5 disk (*curved arrow*). The intensity of the fragment approaches that of cerebrospinal fluid within the thecal sac. Axial T1-weighted (*F*) precontrast and (*G*) postcontrast images again demonstrate the right paracentral sequestered fragment (*arrow*). The right L5 nerve root (*arrowhead*) is compressed in the right lateral recess and enhances on the postinfusion study. This abnormal enhancement is easily recognized by comparison with the contralateral normal left L5 root (*curved arrow*).

DIAGNOSIS

Large free disk fragment with a compressed, enhancing nerve root

DISCUSSION

A sequestered or free disk fragment represents material that has ruptured through a tear in the annular fibers and lost continuity with the disk of origin.[1] The fragment may be contained by the posterior longitudinal ligament or may be located posterior to it. The free fragment is most frequently located behind a vertebral body near the disk space of origin and anterior to the posterior longitudinal ligament. In this situation, sagittal and axial MR images frequently reveal the dorsally elevated posterior longitudinal ligament as curvilinear low signal intensity containing the disk material. The disk fragment may migrate superior or inferior to the interspace of origin as well as laterally, even into the neural foramen, producing radicular symptoms.[2]

Detection of a free disk fragment is particularly important to the surgeon. The surgical approach is very different when a free fragment is present, compared to a herniated or extruded disk alone. With these entities, the herniated material remains in contiguity with the parent disk. A microlaminectomy usually will not provide adequate access to remove the sequestered material. This is particularly true with migration of the free fragment. Chemolysis is contraindicated in the presence of a free fragment.

MR Technique

The possible utility of contrast enhancement for evaluation of nerve root pathology per se has yet to be fully investigated. With more widespread use of IV contrast, together with improvements in overall image quality, recognition of nerve root enhancement has become more common, with potential therapeutic implications.

Clinical References

1. Masaryk TJ, Ross JS, Modic MT, et al. High-resolution MR imaging of sequestered lumbar intervertebral disks. AJR 1988;150:1155–1162.
2. Schellinger D, Manz HJ, Vidic B, et al. Disk fragment migration. Radiology 1990;175:831–835.

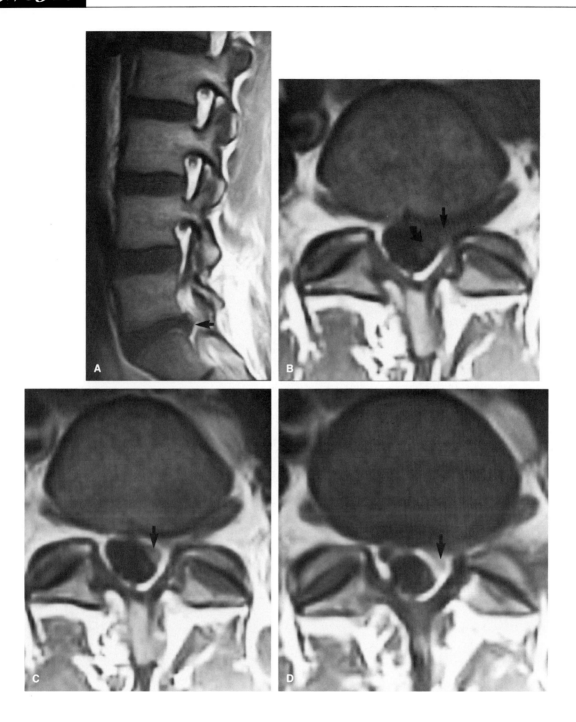

HISTORY

A 27-year-old patient with low back and left leg pain for 2 years

FINDINGS

(*A*) The postcontrast T1-weighted sagittal image to the left of midline reveals a small disk herniation (*arrow*) at the L5–S1 level. The abnormality was confirmed on the T2-weighted sagittal view (*images not shown*). (*B*) A T1-weighted axial image just above the L5–S1 disk redemonstrates the abnormal soft tissue (*arrow*) extending posterior to the vertebral margin. The left S1 nerve root (*curved arrow*) is mildly displaced and appears enlarged. (*C*) Following contrast administration, prominent enhancement of the left S1 nerve root (*arrow*) is present. The disk herniation is less apparent due to enhancement of surrounding granulation tissue and epidural venous plexus. (*D*) A postcontrast axial image at a slightly more inferior position confirms the abnormal enhancement of the displaced left S1 nerve root (*arrow*). The S1 nerve roots have exited the thecal sac bilaterally at this level.

DIAGNOSIS

Left paracentral disk herniation at L5–S1 with a displaced, enhancing left S1 nerve root

DISCUSSION

MR provides an accurate, noninvasive means of evaluating degenerative disease of the lumbar spine. However, the current ease with which patients can now be evaluated has led to an interesting clinical dilemma. Large disk herniations may be present in the absence of patient symptomatology. Furthermore, substantial morbidity from low back pain and radicular-type symptoms may occur in patients who have no obvious morphologic abnormalities of the intervertebral disks. An imaging finding that correlates well with clinical findings would, of course, thus be very useful. Recent evidence suggests that abnormal enhancement of lumbar nerve roots may have use as such a marker.[1]

The cause of abnormal nerve root enhancement is thought to be a disruption of the blood–nerve root barrier that occurs in response to any pathologic insult. Intravascular water and molecular substances may then enter the nerve, as may an intravascular contrast agent such as a gadolinium chelate. Jinkins noted enhancing nerve roots in about 5% of unoperated lumbar spine studies.[1] Seventy percent of these enhancing nerve roots were seen in association with disk herniations or focal bulges. Correlation of nerve root enhancement and clinical syndromes appeared excellent. All patients with multiple enhancing nerve roots had polyradiculopathies, and all patients with monoradiculopathies demonstrated enhancement of a single nerve root that correlated with the clinical findings. In a postoperative study by Boden and colleagues, enhancement of the nerve root that was compressed preoperatively was seen in 81% of operated levels, and enhancement diminished or disappeared by the 6-month follow-up exam in two thirds of these patients.[2] These findings indicate that enhancement of lumbar nerve roots provides insight into pathologic neural changes that may account for patient symptoms.

Pitfalls in Image Interpretation

The true clinical value of detection of an isolated enhancing nerve root on MR is unclear. While the presence of an enhancing nerve root may support the clinical significance of a compressing lesion, it has been our experience that enhancing nerve roots may be unrelated to either disk pathology or current patient symptomatology. The temporal relationship of nerve root injury and nerve root enhancement remains to be elucidated.

Clinical References

1. Jinkins JR. MR of enhancing nerve roots in the unoperated lumbosacral spine. AJNR 1993;14:193–202.
2. Boden SD, Davis DO, Dina TS, et al. Contrast-enhanced MR imaging performed after successful lumbar disk surgery: prospective surgery. Radiology 1992;182:59–64.

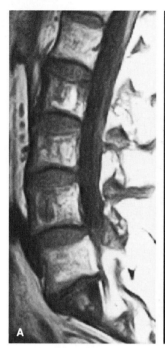
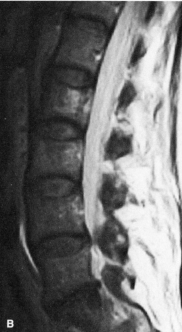
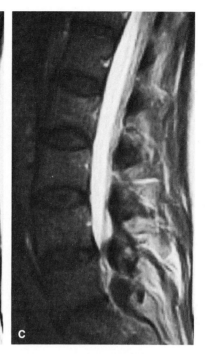

HISTORY

An elderly individual with low back pain

FINDINGS

On the sagittal T1-weighted exam (*A*), the marrow of vertebral bodies L2–4 appears inhomogeneous, with accentuated vertical-oriented trabeculae. The cortex also appears thickened, creating the appearance of a box (marrow fat) within a box (sclerotic cortex), particularly at L3 and L4. These findings are much less apparent on the first echo (TE = 45) of the T2-weighted exam (*B*), with the second echo (TE = 90) essentially normal (*C*).

Plain films of the (*D*) pelvis and (*E*) tibia in another individual with the same disease are also presented. The bony trabecular pattern is irregular and coarsened. The pelvis, femur, and tibia are enlarged. The bony cortex of the femur and tibia is thickened. The tibia is bowed anteriorly. A recent fracture of the tibia is also noted.

DIAGNOSIS

Paget disease

DISCUSSION

In Paget disease, there is both increased bone resorption and formation. Early in the disease course, bone resorption predominates, with replacement of normal marrow by vascular fibrous connective tissue. At some phase, resorbed bone is replaced by dense chaotic new bone, in which trabeculae are thickened and prominent irregular cement lines produce a mosaic pattern. The incidence of associated sarcoma is less than 1%.

Radiographic manifestations of Paget disease include cortical thickening, coarse trabeculae, and bone expansion, which are all well depicted by MR in addition to CT and plain films.[1,2] Cortical thickening is seen on MR as areas of signal void on both T1- and T2-weighted images. In some cases on MR, areas of subtle signal intensity have been noted within the thickened cortex, a finding thought to reflect bone remodeling. Bony trabeculation appears as a region of signal void on all sequences, with thickening often highlighted by adjacent marrow fat. A variable appearance of the marrow has been noted, ranging from normal to focal regions of fat to bony sclerosis, the latter with a loss of signal intensity.

By plain x-ray, the skull, lumbar spine, pelvis, and long bones are often affected. Bowing of the long bones can cause disability. Insufficiency (stress) fractures, which occur with minor or incidental trauma, are typically transverse. In the active or osteolytic phase of the disease, there is resorption of bony trabeculae, which can be seen radiographically. In the inactive or osteosclerotic phase, there is deposition of dense irregular bone. In this phase, enlargement of bone, cortical thickening, and coarsened trabeculae are prominent findings.

Many patients with Paget disease are asymptomatic. Individuals may, however, become aware of swelling or long bone deformity, with dull pain also not unusual. Pain can be caused by the primary disease process or secondary osteoarthritis. In patients with disease of the

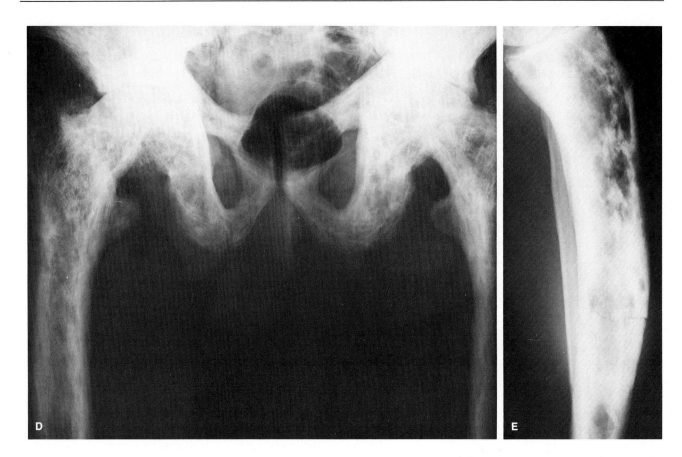

spine, spinal stenosis due to expansion of the vertebral bodies or posterior elements can cause pain and result in neurologic dysfunction. The overall incidence of Paget disease at autopsy is 3% in patients over age 40, with the incidence increasing with age. The incidence in radiologic surveys is less than 1%.

Clinical References

1. Roberts MC, Kressel HY, Fallon MD, et al. Paget disease: MR imaging findings. Radiology 1989;173:341–345.
2. Hayes CW, Jensen ME, Conway WF. Non-neoplastic lesions of vertebral bodies: findings in MRI. Radiographics 1989; 9:883–903.

(D and E *courtesy of Harold D. Rosenbaum, MD*)

Index

Page numbers followed by *f* indicate figures.

A

Achondroplasia, lumbar, 289f, 289–290
Acquisition(s), 36f, 37
Acquisition planes, multiple, 38f–39f, 38–39
AIDS, CMV polyradiculopathy in, 184, 184f
Angiolipoma, thoracic, 208f, 208–209
Angioma, cavernous, cervical, 108f, 108–109
Ankylosing spondylitis, 358f, 359
Annulus fibrosus, concentric bulge of, cervical, 246f, 246–247
Arachnoiditis, lumbar, 300f, 301
Arteriovenous malformations
  causing spontaneous hematomyelia, 98f, 98–99
  thoracic, 203f, 203–204
Artifacts
  aliasing, 32f, 32–33
  chemical shift, 29f–30f, 29–31
  flow, phase- and frequency-encoding direction related to, 44f, 44–45
  motion, phase- and frequency-encoding direction related to, 44f, 44–45
  spatial presaturation to suppress, 40f–41f, 40–41
  with spoiled GRE technique, 17f, 17–18
  truncation, 27f, 27–28, 59
Astrocytoma
  grade I, 197f–198f, 197–198
  grade II, 96f, 96–97

B

Basilar impression, cervical metastatic disease with skull base involvement causing, 94f, 94–95
Basilar invagination, 83f–84f, 83–84
Blood, subarachnoid, lumbar, secondary to blood patch procedure, 348f, 348–349
Bone marrow, fatty replacement of
  in cervical spine, due to radiation therapy, 138, 138f
  in lumbar spine, 307f, 307–308
Butterfly vertebra, at T11, 222f–223f, 222–223

C

Calcification
  disk herniation and, thoracic, 218f, 218–219
  of ligamentum flavum, lumbar spinal stenosis with, 257f, 257–258
Caudal regression, 253f, 253–254
Cerebellar tonsillar ectopia, 73, 73f
Cerebrospinal fluid, GRE and SE imaging of, 20f, 21
Cervical spinal canal
  congenital stenosis of, 66, 66f
  degenerative stenosis of, 67f, 67–68

Cervical spine, 53–170. *See also specific disorders*
  chemical shift imaging of, 24, 24f–25f
  diskectomy and fusion of, 134, 134f, 135f–136f, 135–137
  flexion-rotation injury of, 118f, 119f, 119–120
  fracture of
    dens, type II, 128f, 129
    disk herniation with, 121f, 121–122, 122f
    teardrop, at C2, 130f, 130–131
  metastatic disease of, 92f, 92–93
    with skull base involvement causing basilar impression, 94f, 94–95
  normal
    gradient echo imaging of, 60f, 60–61
    T1-weighted spin echo imaging of, 54f–56f, 54–57
      contrast media and, 64f–65f, 65
      flexion and extension views, 62f, 63
    T2-weighted spin echo imaging of, 58f, 58–59
      flexion and extension views, 62f, 63
  perched facet of, at C6–7, 130f, 130–131
  radiation therapy changes in, with fatty replacement of bone marrow, 138, 138f
  rephased gradient echo imaging of, 13, 13f–15f, 15

Cervical spine (*continued*)
spoiled gradient echo imaging of, 10,
10f–11f, 17f, 17–18
T1-weighted imaging of, 32, 32f
T1-weighted spin echo imaging of,
27f, 27–28, 34f, 35, 36f, 37, 40,
40f–41f, 44, 44f, 46f, 47
T2-weighted spin echo imaging of, 42,
42f
Cervicomedullary junction, image
interpretation and, 73
Chemical shift, of fat and water, 18
Chemical shift artifact, 29f–30f, 29–31
Chemical shift imaging, 24f–25f, 24–26
Chemical shift selective (CHESS), 25
Chiari I malformation, 74f, 74–75
with syringohydromyelia, 76, 76f
Chiari II malformation, 77f–78f, 77–79
with syringomyelia and syringobulbia,
80f–81f, 80–82
Circularly polarized (CP) coils, 51f, 51–
52
Coils
linearly and circularly polarized, 51f,
51–52
sensitivity and, 48f–49f, 48–50
Compression fracture, lumbar
osteoporotic, 340, 340f
pathologic, 338f, 338–339
Contusion, spinal, with small posterior
extradural hematoma, 123f–
124f, 123–125
Cysts
neuroenteric, thoracic, 207, 207f
perineural, lumbar, 283f, 283–284
synovial, lumbar, 261f, 261–262
Cytomegalovirus radiculopathy, in AIDS,
184, 184f

D

Dens fracture, type II, 128f, 129
Dermatomes, 56f, 57
Dermoid tumor, lumbar, with cord
tethering and lipomatous
infiltration, 321f, 321–322
Diastematomyelia
lumbar, 268f, 268–269
thoracic, 222f–223f, 222–223
Disk, vacuum, lumbar, 367f, 367–368
Disk bulge, 146f, 146–147
lumbar, 369f, 369–370
Disk degeneration, lumbar, 360f, 360–
361
Diskectomy
cervical, 134, 134f, 135f–136f, 135–
137
fibrosis following, at L5–S1, 354f–355f,
354–355
Disk fragment, free, lumbar, 383f–384f,
383–384

with compressed, enhancing nerve
root, 385f–386f, 385–386
Disk herniation
at C3–4
myelomalacia secondary to, 126f,
127
paracentral, 156f, 156–157
at C4–5, central, 148f, 148–149, 152f,
152–153
at C5–6, paracentral, 154f, 154–155
at C6–7, right foraminal, 121f, 121–
122, 122f, 158f, 158–159
cervical, paracentral, covered by
spurs, 150f, 150–151
at L4–5, 360f, 360–361
central, 356f, 357
left lateral, 381f, 381–382
at L3–4, with large free disk fragment
posterior to L4 vertebral body,
375f–376f, 375–376
at L4–L5, central, 373f, 373–374
at L5–S1, 360f, 360–361
with displaced, enhancing left S1
nerve root, 387f, 387–388
resolution of, 365f–366f, 365–366
right paracentral, 379f, 379–380
with diagnostic evaluation of de
novo scar formation, 377f–
378f, 377–378
at T8–9, left paracentral, 219f, 219–220
thoracic, calcified, 218f, 218–219
Diskitis, lumbar, postoperative, 297f–
298f, 297–299
Disk protrusion, lumbar, with concentric
tear of annulus fibrosus, 371f,
371–372
Disk space infection, lumbar, 293f, 293–
294
Dorsal dermal sinus, lumbar, 272f, 272–
273
Dysraphism, bony, by plain film, 279f,
279–280

E

ECG triggering, 42f, 42–43
Echo time (TE)
in T1-weighted spin echo technique,
2f–3f, 2–4
in T2-weighted spin echo technique, 7
End plates, lumbar, degenerative
changes of, 362f–363f, 362–
364
Ependymoma, lumbar, 325f, 325–326
Epidural abscess, 91, 91f
osteomyelitis of T6–7 with, 180f, 180–
181
Epidural fibrosis, at L5–S1, 352f–353f,
352–353
Epidural fluid collection, inflammatory,
lumbar, 295f, 295–296

Extradural hematoma, spinal contusion
with, 123f–124f, 123–125
Extramedullary hematopoiesis, with
thoracic cord compression,
210f, 210–211

F

FAST (Fourier acquired steady state). *See*
Rephased gradient echo (GRE)
technique
Fast imaging with steady precession
(FISP). *See* Rephased gradient
echo (GRE) technique
Fast low angle shot (FLASH). *See* Spoiled
gradient echo (GRE) technique
Fast spin echo (FSE) technique, 1–9,
8f–9f
Fat
chemical shift imaging of, 24f–25f,
24–26
chemical shift of, 18
focal deposits of, in lumbar vertebral
marrow, 307f, 307–308
suppression of, 25–26
STIR for, 22f, 22–23
Fibrosis
epidural, at L5–S1, 352f–353f, 352–353
postdiskectomy, at L5–S1, 354f–355f,
354–355
Field of view (FOV), 32f, 32–33
Filum terminale
fatty, 287f, 287–288
tight, 281f, 281–282
Flexion injury, lumbar, 336f, 336–337
Flow artifacts, phase- and frequency-
encoding direction related to,
44f, 44–45
Flow compensation. *See* Gradient
moment nulling
Flow-related artifacts
CSF-related, 42f, 42–43
spatial presaturation to suppress, 40f–
41f, 40–41
Foldover. *See* Image aliasing
Fourier acquired steady state (FAST). *See*
Rephased gradient echo (GRE)
technique
Free induction decay (FID) signal, in
spoiled gradient echo
technique, 11, 18
Frequency selective technique, 25
Fusion, cervical, 134, 134f, 135f–136f,
135–137

G

Ganglioneuroma, thoracic, 201f–202f,
201–202
Gibb phenomenon. *See* Truncation
artifacts

Gradient echo (GRE) technique, 20f, 21. *See also* Rephased gradient echo (GRE) technique; Spoiled gradient echo (GRE) technique pitfalls in interpretation of, 61
Gradient moment nulling, 42f, 42–43
Gradient motion refocusing/rephasing. *See* Gradient moment nulling
Gradient recalled acquisition in the steady state (GRASS). *See* Rephased gradient echo (GRE) technique

H

Hemangioblastoma, 100f, 100–101
Hemangioma, of vertebral body, lumbar, 303f, 303–304
Hematoma, extradural, spinal contusion with, 123f–124f, 123–125
Hematopoiesis, extramedullary, with thoracic cord compression, 210f, 210–211
Hemorrhage, of spinal cord, secondary to trauma, 116f, 116–117
Herniated disk. *See* Disk herniation
Histoplasmosis, lumbar, 302, 302f
Hydrogen density. *See* Spin density
Hydromyelia, tethered cord with, lumbar, 274f–275f, 274–275
Hypertrophic end plate spurs, osteophytic, cervical, 144f, 144–145

I

Image aliasing, 32f, 32–33
Image interpretation pitfalls
  in acute transverse myelitis, 168
  in arachnoiditis, 301
  in arteriovenous malformations
    cervical, 99
    thoracic, 204
  in butterfly vertebrae, 223
  in calcification, of thoracic spine, 219
  in calcification of ligamentum flavum, 259
  cervicomedullary junction and, 73
  in Chiari I malformation, 75, 76
  in Chiari II malformation, 79
  in conjoined nerve root, 286
  in contrast administration, 244
  in cord lesions in AIDS, 184
  in degenerative disk disease, cervical, 68
  in degenerative end plate changes, lumbar, 364
  in dens fractures, cervical, 129
  in diastematomyelia, 269
  in disk bulge, lumbar, 370
  in diskectomy, cervical, 134

  in disk fragments, lumbar, 384, 388
  in disk herniation
    cervical, 149, 151, 153, 155, 157, 158f, 158–159
    lumbar, 357, 376, 378, 380, 382
    thoracic, 221
  in diskitis, 299
  in disk protrusion, lumbar, 372
  in dorsal dermal sinus, 273
  in ependymoma, 326
  in epidural abscess, 181
  in epidural fibrosis, 353
  in epidural lymphoma, thoracic, 192
  in extramedullary hematopoiesis, 211
  in facet dislocations, cervical, 131
  in fatty marrow changes, cervical, 138
  in fatty tissues, 304
  in foraminal narrowing, cervical, 70
  in fusion, cervical, 137
  with gradient echo technique, 66
  in histoplasmosis, 302
  in infection, 294
  in inflammatory epidural fluid collection, 296
  in intradural lipoma, 330
  in leptomeningeal tumors
    cervical, 115
    thoracic, 213
  in lymphangioma, 324
  in marrow infiltration by myeloma, 197
  in meningioma, of posterior fossa, 170
  in meningocele, sacral, 267
  in metastatic disease, 318
    cervical, 93, 95
    lumbar, 312, 335
    thoracic, 186
  in multiple sclerosis
    cervical, 97, 166
    thoracic, 227, 229
  in myelocystocele, 280
  in myelomalacia, 127
  in nerve sheath tumors, 306
  in neurofibromas, 328
  in ossification of posterior longitudinal ligament, 161
  in osteophytic spurs, cervical, 145
  in Paget's disease, 316
  with Pantopaque, 176
  in pathologic fractures, 339
  in pediatric spine, 239, 246
  in plasmacytoma, 320
  in postdiskectomy fibrosis, 355
  in post-laminectomy patients, cervical, 133
  in pseudomeningocele, 271, 351
  in retrolisthesis, 347
  in rheumatoid arthritis, cervical, 143
  in sacralization, 250
  in sarcoidosis, cervical, 90

  in Schmorl's nodes, 252, 310
  in scoliosis, 225
  in spinal cord infarction, 217
  in spinal cord tumors, cervical, 101, 103, 111
  in spinal stenosis, 256
    cervical, 66
    lumbar, 260
  in spinal trauma, cervical, 120, 125
  in spondylolisthesis, 344
  in spondylolysis, 342
  in subarachnoid blood, 349
  in subtle bony abnormalities, 254
  in synovial cysts, 262
  in syringobulbia, 83
  in syringohydromyelia, 107
  in tethered cord, release of, 277
  in tethered cord with hydromyelia, 275
  in thoracic spine, 174
  in thoracic spine tumors, 198, 198f, 200
    neuroblastomas, 202, 206
  in vacuum intervertebral disk, 368
  in vertebral relapse of acute leukemia, 194
Imaging time, 36f, 37
Inflammatory epidural fluid collection, lumbar, 295f, 295–296
Intervertebral disk. *See* Disk *entries*
  STIR imaging of, 22, 22f
Intraspinal extrusion, in metastatic disease, thoracic, from carcinoid tumor, 187f, 187–188
Inversion recovery (IR), 23. *See also* Short tau inversion recovery (STIR) technique

K

Klippel-Feil syndrome, 71f–72f, 71–72

L

Laminectomy, multilevel, 132f, 132–133
Leptomeningeal metastases
  cervical
    from medulloblastoma, 114f, 114–115, 115f
    from pineoblastoma, 112f–113f, 112–113
  lumbar, 309f, 309–310
  lumbar spine, 331f–332f, 331–335, 334f, 335f
  thoracic, 212f, 213
Leukemia, acute lymphocytic, vertebral relapse of, thoracic, 193f, 193–194, 194f
Ligamentum flavum, thickened, lumbar spinal stenosis with, 257f, 257–258

Linearly polarized (LP) coils, 51f, 51–52
Lipoma, intradural, lumbar, 329f–330f, 329–330
Lipomatous infiltration, dermoid tumor of lumbar spine with, 321f, 321–322
Lipomyelomeningocele, 271
Longitudinal ligament, posterior, ossification of, 160f, 160–161
Longitudinal relaxation time, 4
Lumbar spine, 231–390. *See also specific disorders*
  compression fracture of
    osteoporotic, 340, 340f
    pathologic, 338f, 338–339
  fast spin echo imaging of, 8, 8f–9f
  flexion injury of, 336f, 336–337
  metastases to
    from breast cancer, 311f, 311–312
    of Ewing's sarcoma, 317f, 317–318
    leptomeningeal, 331f–332f, 331–335, 334f, 335f
    from prostate carcinoma, 315f–316f, 315–316
    vertebral and leptomeningeal, 309f, 309–310
  normal
    axial study of, 235, 235f–236f, 237
    contrast media and, 240f–243f, 241–244
    image normalization and, 238f, 238–239
    of infant, 235–246, 245f
    marrow evolution in, 247f, 247–248
    sagittal study of, 232f–233f, 232–234
  transitional vertebra with partial sacralization of L5 vertebra and, 249f, 249–250
  T1-weighted spin echo imaging of, 2f–3f, 2–3, 29f–30f, 29–30, 38, 38f–39f, 51, 51f
  T2-weighted spin echo imaging of, 5f–6f, 5–6
Lymphangioma, lumbar, 323f, 323–324
Lymphocytic leukemia, acute, vertebral relapse of, thoracic, 193f, 193–194, 194f
Lymphoma, epidural, thoracic, with spinal cord compression, 191f, 191–192, 192f

M
Magnetic susceptibility (χ), 18
Marrow evolution, in lumbar spine, 247f, 247–248
MAST (motion artifact suppression technique). *See* Gradient moment nulling
Matrix size, 27f, 27–28

Medulloblastoma, leptomeningeal metastases from, 114f, 114–115, 115f
Meningioma, 102f, 102–103
  of posterior fossa, 169f, 169–170
  thoracic, 205f, 205–206
Meningitis, lumbar, with progression to arachnoiditis, 300f, 301
Meningocele
  cervical, secondary to birth trauma, 139, 139f
  sacral, anterior, 266f–267f, 266–267
  thoracic, lateral, 177f–178f, 177–179
Meningomyelocele, lumbar, with tethered cord, 265, 265f
Metastatic disease
  cervical, 92f, 92–93
    leptomeningeal
      from medulloblastoma, 114f, 114–115, 115f
      from pineoblastoma, 112f–113f, 112–113
    with skull base involvement causing basilar impression, 94f, 94–95
  lumbar, 309f, 309–310
    from breast cancer, 311f, 311–312
    of Ewing's sarcoma, 317f, 317–318
    leptomeningeal, 309f, 309–310, 331f–332f, 331–335, 334f, 335f
    from prostate carcinoma, 315f–316f, 315–316
  sacral, with epidural tumor causing right S1 nerve root compression, 313f, 313–314
  of spinal cord, 110f, 111
  thoracic
    from breast cancer, 185f, 185–186
    with epidural extension, from lung carcinoma, 189f, 189–190, 190f
    leptomeningeal, 212f, 213
    with vertebral body destruction and intraspinal extrusion, from carcinoid tumor, 187f, 187–188
Motion, first-, second-, and higher-order, 43
Motion artifacts, phase- and frequency-encoding direction related to, 44f, 44–45
Motion artifact suppression technique (MAST). *See* Gradient moment nulling
MR technique. *See also specific techniques*
  for arachnoiditis, 301
  for arteriovenous malformations
    cervical, 99
    thoracic, 204
  for atlantoaxial subluxation, 143
  for axial imaging of lumbar spine, 237, 262
  for bony spurs, 268–269

for caudal regression, 253–254
for Chiari I malformation, 75
for Chiari II malformation, 79
for contrast administration, 244
for contrast imaging, 176
for disk bulge
  cervical, 147
  lumbar, 370
for disk fragments, 384, 386
for disk herniation
  cervical, 155, 157, 158f, 158–159
  lumbar, 357, 361, 366, 374, 376, 378, 380, 382
  thoracic, 221
for diskitis, 299
for disk protrusion, 372
for dorsal dermal sinus, 273
for ependymoma, 326
for epidural abscess
  cervical, 91
  thoracic, 181
for epidural tumors
  lumbar, 315
  thoracic, 190
  lymphoma, 192
for extradural lesions and stenoses, cervical, 149
for extramedullary hematopoiesis, 211
for fatty filum terminale, 288
for fatty marrow changes
  cervical, 138
  lumbar, 308
for fatty tissues, 304
for flexion and extension views, 63
for foraminal narrowing, cervical, 70
for fusion, cervical, 136
for gradient echo images, 219
for intervertebral disks, cervical, 131
for intradural lipoma, 330
for intramedullary lesions, cervical, 68
for leptomeningeal tumors
  cervical, 115
  thoracic, 213
for lipomyelomeningocele, 271
for marrow infiltration by myeloma, 197
for meningioma, of posterior fossa, 170
for meningocele
  sacral, 267
  thoracic, lateral, 179
for metastatic disease
  cervical, 95
  lumbar, 310, 312, 315–316, 335
  thoracic, 186
for multiple sclerosis
  cervical, 165–166
  thoracic, 227, 229
for myelocystocele, 280
for myelomalacia, 140–141

for nerve sheath tumors, 306
for neurofibromas, lumbar, 292, 328
for os odontoideum, 86
for ossification of posterior
    longitudinal ligament, 161
for osteomyelitis, 294
for osteophytic spurs, cervical, 145
for pathologic fractures, 339
for pediatric spine, 246
for polyradiculopathy, 184
for postdiskectomy fibrosis, 355
for retrolisthesis, 346
for sagittal imaging of lumbar spine,
    233–234, 264
for sarcoidosis, cervical, 90
for Schmorl's nodes, 252
for scoliosis, 225
for spinal canal and neural foramina,
    cervical, 66
for spinal cord lesions
    cervical, 101, 103, 111, 131
    thoracic, 217
for spinal dysraphism, 275
for spinal stenosis, lumbar, 256, 260
for spinal trauma, cervical, 120, 122,
    124, 129
for spondylolisthesis, 344
for spondylolysis, 342
for syringobulbia, 104–105
for syringohydromyelia, 107
for syringomyelia, 277
for thoracic spine, 174
for thoracic spine tumors, 198, 200
    neuroblastomas, 202, 206
for tuberculous spondylitis, 183
for vacuum intervertebral disk, 368
for vertebral bodies
    cervical, 131
    thoracic, fractures of, 215
for vertebral relapse of acute
    leukemia, 194
Multiplanar reformatting (MPR), 46f, 47
Multiple acquisition planes, 38f–39f, 38–
    39
Multiple myeloma, with extradural soft
    tissue mass at T6, 195f, 195–
    196
Multiple sclerosis, 97
    active
        cervical, 164f–165f, 164–166
        thoracic, 226f–227f, 226–227, 228f,
            229
    chronic
        cervical, 162f, 163
        thoracic, 226f–227f, 226–227
Myelocystocele, 280
Myeloma, multiple, with extradural soft
    tissue mass at T6, 195f, 195–
    196
Myelomalacia
    in chronic cord injury, 140f, 140–141

secondary to hard disk herniation at
    C3–4, 126f, 127

N

Nerve root, conjoined, lumbar, 285f–
    286f, 285–286
Nerve sheath tumor, malignant, lumbar,
    305f, 305–306
Neuroenteric cyst, thoracic, 207, 207f
Neurofibromas
    cervical, in type 2 neurofibromatosis,
        87f, 87–88
    lumbar, 327f–328f, 327–328
    plexiform, lumbar, 291f, 291–292

O

Os odontoideum, with stable fibrous
    union, 85f, 85–86
Ossification, of posterior longitudinal
    ligament, 160f, 160–161
Osteomyelitis
    lumbar, 293f, 293–294
    of T6–7, with epidural abscess, 180f,
        180–181
Osteophytic hypertrophic end plate
    spurs, 144f, 144–145
Osteoporosis, lumbar compression
    fracture secondary to, 340, 340f

P

Paget disease, 389f–390f, 389–390
Perineural cysts, lumbar, 283f, 283–284
Phase- and frequency-encoding
    direction, 44f, 44–45
Pineoblastoma, leptomeningeal
    metastases from, 112f–113f,
        112–113
Plasmacytoma, lumbar, 319f, 319–320
Polyradiculopathy, CMV, in AIDS, 184,
    184f
Posterior fossa, meningioma of, 169f,
    169–170
Posterior longitudinal ligament,
    ossification of, 160f, 160–161
Pseudomeningocele
    lumbar, 350f, 350–351
    postoperative, 270f, 270–271

R

Radiation therapy, cervical spine changes
    due to, with fatty replacement
    of bone marrow, 138, 138f
Rapid acquisition with relaxation
    enhancement (RARE). *See* Fast
    spin echo (FSE) technique

Repetition time (TR)
    in T1-weighted spin echo technique,
        2f–3f, 2–4
    in T2-weighted spin echo technique, 7
Rephased gradient echo (GRE)
    technique, 13f–15f, 13–16
    spoiled gradient echo technique
        compared with, 15–16
Retrolisthesis, lumbar, 345f, 345–347
RF antenna coils, sensitivity and, 49
RF pulse, in T1-weighted spin echo
    technique, 3–4
Rheumatoid arthritis, with atlantoaxial
    subluxation, 142f–143f, 142–
        143

S

Sacral agenesis, 253f, 253–254
Sacral spine, metastases to, with
    epidural tumor causing right
    S1 nerve root compression,
        313f, 313–314
Sampling bandwidth, 29f–30f, 29–31
Sarcoidosis, cervical, 89f, 89–90
Scan time, 27f, 27–28
Schmorl's nodes, 310
    of L4 body, inferior, 251f, 251–252
Schwannoma, paraspinal, thoracic, 199f,
    199–200, 200f
Scoliosis, 224f, 225
Sensitivity, coils and, 48f–49f, 48–50
Short tau inversion recovery (STIR)
    technique, 22f, 22–23
Signal-to-noise (S/N) ratio, 34f, 35, 36f,
    37
Slice thickness, 34f, 35
Spatial presaturation (SAT), 40f–41f, 40–
    41
Spatial resolution, 27f, 27–28, 32f, 32–33
Spectral saturation technique, 25
Spinal cord
    contusion of, with small posterior
        extradural hematoma, 123f–
        124f, 123–125
    hemorrhage of, secondary to trauma,
        116f, 116–117
    infarction of, thoracic, secondary to
        intradural arteriovenous fistula,
        216f, 217
    injury of, chronic, myelomalacia in,
        140f, 140–141
    metastatic disease of, 110f, 111
    tethered, lumbar
        dermoid tumor with, 321f, 321–322
        following surgical release, 276–277,
            277f
        with hydromyelia, 274f–275f, 274–
            275
        with lipoma, 276f, 276–277
        retethering and, 278, 278f

Spinal stenosis, lumbar
congenital, 255f, 255–256
at L4–5, 259f, 259–260
at L5-S1, 263f, 263–264
with thickened ligamentum flavum,
257f, 257–258
Spin density, in T1-weighted spin echo
technique, 4
Spin echo (SE) technique, 20f, 21
fast, 8f–9f, 8–9
T1-weighted, 2f–3f, 2–4, 63
T2-weighted, 5f–6f, 5–7, 59, 63
Spin-lattice relaxation time, 4
Spin-spin relaxation time, 4
Spoiled gradient echo (GRE) technique,
10f–11f, 10–12
image anomalies with, 17f, 17–18
rephased GRE compared with, 15–16
Spoiled gradient recalled acquisition in
the steady state (SP-GRASS).
See Spoiled gradient echo
(GRE) technique
Spondylitis, tuberculous, 182f–183f,
182–183
Spondylolisthesis, lumbar
secondary to degenerative facet
changes, 343f–344f, 343–344
spondylolysis with, 341f–342f, 341–
342
Spondylolysis, lumbar, bilateral, 341f–
342f, 341–342
Subarachnoid blood, lumbar, secondary
to blood patch procedure,
348f, 348–349

Surface coils, sensitivity and, 49, 50
Synovial cyst, lumbar, 261f, 261–262
Syringobulbia, 104f, 104–105
Chiari II malformation with, 80f–81f,
80–82
Syringohydromyelia
Chiari I malformation with, 76, 76f
posttraumatic, with interval shunting
and collapse, 106f, 106–107
Syringomyelia, 277
Chiari II malformation with, 80f–81f,
80–82

T

T1, 4
T2, 4
Thoracic spine, 171–229. *See also*
specific disorders
fracture-dislocation of, at T11–12,
214f–215f, 214–215
fracture of, at T12, with retropulsion
and cord compression, 214f–
215f, 214–215
normal, 172f–174f, 172–174
with pantopaque, 175f, 175–176
Three-dimensional T1-weighted
imaging, 46f, 47
Transverse myelitis, acute, 167f, 167–168
Transverse relaxation time, 4
Truncation artifact, 27f, 27–28
Truncation artifacts, 59
Tuberculous spondylitis, 182f–183f, 182–
183

T1-weighted spin echo technique, 2f–3f,
2–4, 63
T2-weighted spin echo technique, 59, 63

U

Uncovertebral joint spurring, neural
foraminal narrowing due to,
69f, 69–70

V

Vacuum intervertebral disk, lumbar,
367f, 367–368
Vertebral body destruction, in metastatic
disease, thoracic, from
carcinoid tumor, 187f, 187–188
Volume averaging, 34f, 35

W

Water
chemical shift imaging of, 24f–25f, 24–
26
chemical shift of, 18
suppression of, 25–26
Water weighting. *See* Rephased gradient
echo (GRE) technique
Whole-body RF coil, sensitivity and, 49–
50
Wraparound. *See* Image aliasing